A Pictorial History of COSTUME

From Ancient Times to the Nineteenth Century

With over 1900 Illustrated Costumes, Including 1000 in Full Color

WOLFGANG BRUHN
AND
MAX TILKE

DOVER PUBLICATIONS, INC.
Mineola, New York

Bibliographical Note

This Dover edition, first published in 2004, is a selection of plates from the work originally published by A. Zwemmer, Ltd., London, in 1955, under the title, *A Pictorial History of Costume: A Survey of Costume of All Periods and Peoples From Antiquity to Modern Times Including National Costume in Europe and Non-European Countries.* This edition contains all the plates that appear on pages 1 through 126 of the original edition.

Library of Congress Cataloging-in-Publication Data

Bruhn, Wolfgang
[Kostümwerk. English]
A pictorial history of costume from ancient times to the nineteenth century : with over 1900 illustrated costumes, including 1000 in full color / Wolfgang Bruhn and Max Tilke.
p. cm.
"This Dover edition, first published in 2004, is an abridged republication of the work originally published by A. Zwemmer, Ltd., London, in 1955, under the title A pictorial history of costume: a survey of all periods and peoples from antiquity to modern times including national costume in Europe and non-European countries"—T.p. verso.
Includes index.
ISBN 0-486-43542-3 (pbk.)
1. Clothing and dress—History—Pictorial works. I. Tilke, Max, 1869-1942. II. Title.

GT511.B763 2004
391'.0022'2—dc22

2003070051

Manufactured in the United States of America
Dover Publications, Inc., 31 East 2nd Street, Mineola, N.Y. 11501

INDEX OF PLATES

1. Ancient Egypt. Old Kingdom till about 2200 B.C. Middle Kingdom, about 2100 B.C., New Kingdom about 1530 B.C.
2. Ancient Egypt. Times of Rameses I. to Rameses III. 1350–1200 B.C.
3. Ancient Egypt. New Kingdom (about 1530 B.C.).
4. Ancient Egypt. New Kingdom (Late Period).
5. Assyria and Neighbouring peoples (12th–7th centuries B.C.).
6. Babylonia and Assyria.
7. Western Asia in Antiquity, Sumerians, Hittites and West-Asiatics.
8. Western Asia in Antiquity, Phoenicians, Hittites, Syrians (Canaanites).
9. Mycenae, Crete, Cyprus (Aegean and Phoenician cultures, 2000 to 500 B.C.).
10. Persia in Antiquity and the Early Middle Ages.
11. Scythians and inhabitants of Asia Minor. (Early Greek culture).
12. Greece. Early Period (6th and 5th centuries B.C.).
13. Greece. Great Period of Greek Art (5th and 4th centuries B.C.).
14. Greece. Armour, banquets, games and music.
15. Late Greek town costume of the Hellenic Period on painted terra-cottas of the 4th century B.C. (mostly from Tanagra and Boeotia).
16. Etruscans. About 750 B.C.
17. Rome. Men's costume.
18. Rome. Ordinary people. Priestesses, women.
19. Greece and Rome. Hair styles and head-dresses.
20. Footwear in ancient times.
21. Teutons. Prehistoric and Early Historic Periods.
22. Teutons. Roman Period, partly earlier.
23. Persia. Sassanian Period in the Early Middle Ages (227–636 A.D.)
24. Gauls, Vikings and Normans.
25. Rome. Equipment of soldiers and gladiators at the time of the Empire.
26. Early Christian Period. 300–600 A.D.
27. Byzantine Empire 4th–11th centuries.
28. Monastic Orders and Orders of Knights.
29. Ecclesistical garments and Orders of Knights.
30. Germany from the times of the Merovingians to those of the Hohenstaufen Emperors 500–1200.
31. Europe. Early Middle Ages (300–1000) and Byzantine Empire (9th–11th centuries).
32. Germany. Time of the "minnesingers" and crusades, 12th–13th centuries.
33. France in the Middle Ages. 900–1400.
34. Normans and Anglo-Saxons. 11th–14th centuries.
35. Middle Ages. Armoured knights (800–1300). Crusaders (1100 to 1300).
36. Europe. Knights. 14th and 15th centuries (Burgundy, France, England, Italy, Poland).
37. England in the Middle Ages. 10th–15th centuries.
38. Armoured knights. France and Germany. 15th century.
39. Italian monuments representing knights. 13th–15th centuries.
40. Germany. Garments of people of rank as represented by 13th century sculpture.
41. German and Burgundian knights. (1300–1380).
42. Knights' armour and weapons (1500–1575).
43. Europe. Middle Ages. Helmets and swords.
44. France. 14th century.
45. Burgundian fashion on Flemish book illustrations (miniatures) of the 15th century.
46. Burgundy. Head-dress and hair styles. 15th century.
47. Late Middle Ages. Footwear. Pointed shoes and wooden sandals.
48. Italy. Early Renaissance. 1485–90. Mural paintings by Domenico Ghirlandajo.
49. German tournament apparel.
50. France. First half of 15th century.
51. France. (Charles VIII 1483–98, Louis XII 1498–1515).
52. Burgundian fashion. 1425–90.
53. Italian Early Renaissance. 14th century.
54. Italian Early Renaissance (about 1425–1480).
55. Northern Italy. Early Renaissance (1440–90) under the influence of Burgundian fashion.
56. Italian Early Renaissance (1350–1500).
57. Italy. Early Renaissance. Hair styles.
58. Germany in the Late Middle Ages. Burghers and craftsmen's costume (1475–1500).
59. Spain in the Middle Ages (late 13th–15th centuries).
60. Germany about 1500.
61. Italy. Renaissance 1520–30. According to contemporary paintings.
62. Germany at the time of the Reformation. Head-dress. (1500–50).
63. England at the time of the Reformation (Henry VIII, 1509–47).
64. Spanish fashion, 1550–80, according to contemporary paintings.
65. Germany at the time of the Reformation. Citizens' costume. 1510–50.
66. Italy. Renaissance. Head-dress and hair styles. (1500–50).
67. Italy. Early Renaissance. 1460–90.
68. Italian. Renaissance about 1500.
69. Germany under Burgundian influence (15th century).
70. Germany. Mercenaries. 1500–40. Slahed garments.
71. Germany. Mercenaries (1520–60). The "trunk-hose".
72. Germany at the time of the Reformation (1500–30).
73. Germany. Spanish fashion. 1550–1600.
74. Spain and Portugal. 1500–40. Spanish Moors, 15th century.
75. France at the time of the Renaissance. 1500–75 (Francis I and Henry II).
76. France. Spanish fashion. 1560–90 (Charles IX).
77. France. Spanish fashion. 1575–90 (Henry III).
78. Italy. Spanish fashion. 1590–1610.
79. France. Late Spanish fashion. 1600–40. (Henry IV and Maria de Medici).
80. Spain in the 16th and 17th centuries. (Spanish fashion from 1540–1660).
81. Russia. 16th–17th centuries.
82. Poland, Hungary and Ukraine 16th and 17th centuries.
83. Germany. Time of the Reformation and Spanish fashion. Paintings by Lucas Cranach (Father and Son, 1514–64).
84. German citizens' costume, about 1560–80.
85. Military costume. Europe. End of the 16th century.
86. Germany. Head-dress (Spanish fashion) 1550–1600.
87. Germany, the Netherlands, France. Costume at the time of the Thirty-Years War (about 1630–35).

88. England. Spanish fashion (at the time of Queen Elizabeth) as represented on contemporary pictures.
89. Spanish court costume (about 1630–60) according to paintings by Diego Velasquez.
90. Turkey. 16th and 17th centuries.
91. Turkey. 17th century. Costume at the Sultan's court, represented on miniatures.
92. Europe. Military costume 1600–1650.
93. France at the time of Louis XIV. 1660–1700.
94. France. Régence and Rococo, 1700–40. Theatre and dance.
95. Germany. 1625–75. Citizens' costume, partly under French influence.
96. The Netherlands, 17th century. Contemporary pictures.
97. The Netherlands, 1650–80, partly under French influence.
98. The Netherlands. Ruffs and collars, hair and beard styles in the 17th century.
99. England about 1640 according to etchings by Wenzel Hollar.
100. France. Court dress at Versailles after engravings dating from about 1700.
101. France at the time of Louis XIV. 1695–1700.
102. France. Time of the Régence about 1715–20.
103. The Italian Comedy in Paris, about 1730.
104. Holland and England. Rococo about 1740–50.
105. France and Germany. Rococo about 1730–60.
106. Italy. Rococo. Venice about 1750.
107. France. Rococo. Paris street life about 1740.
108. Street life in Vienna and Venice. 1770–90.
109. France. Late Rococo. 1776.
110. England. 1770–1800. Rococo and Late Georgian.
111. France. Late Rococo. Women's hair styles, 1775–95.
112. Germany and Austria. China figures' costume. 1750–75.
113. France. Rococo. 1730–75.
114. France. Late Rococo 1775–85.
115. France. Late Rococo (1780–89).
116. Paris fashion. 1790–95. Revolution and "Directory".
117. French Revolution, "Directory" and Consulate. (1790–1803).
118. Uniforms. Germany and France (1680–1790).
119. England and France. 1800–30. French Empire (Late Georgian) and "Biedermeier" styles.
120. Germany. 1815–35. "Biedermeier" fashion.
121. Europe. Uniforms. 1795–1815. Revolution till French Restoration.
122. Prussia. Uniforms. 1730–70.
123. Germany and France. Late Rococo about 1788.
124. France. Paris fashions. 1830–35. ("Biedermeier" and "Romantic" fashion).
125. France and Germany. Fashion of 1850–60. The crinoline.
126. France and Germany. Fashion of 1870–75. The "tournure" (cul de Paris).

DETAILS OF THE PLATES

DETAILS OF THE PLATES

ANTIQUITY

ANCIENT EGYPT. *Old Kingdom till about 2000 B.C., Middle Kingdom about 2100, New Kingdom about 1530 B.C.* 1

Top Group

1. King of the 5th Dynasty wearing a loin-cloth of pleated gold material, with a lion's tail fixed at the back. (Privilege of the king, probably of the early times when the chiefs of the African primitive race ornamented themselves with such trophies). In front of the loin-cloth a stiff triangular piece of linen, and over it the regal ornaments. The head is covered with the striped head-cloth with the sacred uraeus (cf. 10 side view). Further royal insignia: The artificial medium-sized beard and the two types of sceptre, the crook and the whip (probably originally a symbol of agriculture and stock-rearing).
2. Egyptian of rank. His high rank is shown by the ceremonial loin-cloth (partly made of golden material like the king's) and by the stick and club (commander's baton). He wears a short curled wig.
3. Egyptian woman, grinding grain with an ancient hand-mill. The tunic indicates a better class woman; the slave women usually wear hardly any clothes. The hair is tied up by bands.
4. Woman of rank dressed in a tunic; the original braces for keeping up the garment are widened here and cover the breasts, thus forming a V-neck. The material is light and diaphanous. In addition a linen mantle, coloured collar embroidered with glass beads. Wrist and ankle bracelets. Over the parted hair a wig with a decorated metal fillet or diadem.
5. Woman returning from the market in a checked tunic with wide white braces. Ornamental collar, bracelets, large black kerchief (obviously not a wig).

Centre Group

6. Official or man of rank with a stick. Simple loin-cloth in the style of the Old Kingdom. The shaven head is not covered by a cap or wig, which is necessary in the hot sun.
7. Official (Middle Kingdom) with a lengthened loin-cloth, neck decoration, wig and short beard as a sign of rank. The beard, not favoured by the Egyptians, is shaved off. But on ceremonial occasions in order to enhance the dignity of the wearer, an artificial beard is fixed by means of ribbons to the ears. The longest beard was worn by the king.
8. Egyptian of the 5th Dynasty with the linen triangle in front of the loin-cloth (cf. 1). Collar with pendant. Wig.
9. Woman of the Middle Kingdom. Patterned tunic (similar to 5). Wig, fan.

10–16. New Kingdom from 1600 B.C.

10. King of the New Kingdom acting as sacrificial priest.

Bottom Group

11. Man of rank in a shirt-like garment with two loin-cloths, collar and wig with a feather stuck into it and carrying a stick with an animal's head (originally a king's sceptre, later on carried by high officials and ordinary people).
12. Man with shirt-like garment, but only one loin-cloth visible; collar; band tied round the wig.
13. Mourner from a funeral procession.
14. Woman wearing a mantle. The greater variety in garments corresponds to that of the men. In the New Kingdom, fashion requires a tight fitting garment, exposing one shoulder, and a wide mantle, carried across the front and draped over one shoulder. Both are often quite diaphanous allowing the shape of the body to be seen.
15. Man of rank in a shirt-like garment with two sleeves and a very small loin-cloth on top. Neck ornamentation and wig.
16. Lower official or king's servant. Neck decoration, bracelets and loin-cloth with a heart-shaped piece of material in front. On the head a perfume container which slowly drips.

ANCIENT EGYPT. *Times of Rameses I. – Rameses III. 1350–1200 B.C.* 2

Top Group

1. High Official with the white ostrich feather fan, a high decoration of honour, which gradually became the emblem of rank, for instance for *King's Favourite* and other titles of honour. Princes and the highest officials or army commanders were given the feather fan. Collar (round collar), wig and bast sandals. The loin-cloth is wrapped over the long tunic.
2. Scribe; a vocation found frequently in ancient Egypt. The reed pen is stuck into the wig behind the ear. He carries the paint box with red and black under his arm, and the papyrus scroll in his hand. The boxes on the floor with protecting bags are for the rolled-up papyri.
3. Temple attendant carrying a vessel with sacrificial liquid.
4. High Priest from Heliopolis with a leopard's skin (decorated with silver stars). Priests' garments were not sewn. The hair is shorn. He wears a wig which is seldom worn by priests.
5. Sacrificial priest with incense burner. Loin-cloth, leopard skin, white band on upper part of body. Straw sandals.

Centre Group

6 and 10. Royal princes in war apparel, distinguished by a long plaited lock on the side of their heads. This lock, originally only worn by children, was later, in a conventionalized form, a prerogative of princes. The armour consists of leather covered with metal pieces. No. 10 has leather strips wound spirally round the body. He has also a feather fan.

7. Companion of the Prince, with his master's bow and shield, covered with skin.

8. The King with the characteristic regal girdle decoration hanging down in front (cf. Plate I, 1). The Pharaoh wears the peculiar royal helmet (chepereshh) with the uraeus; the sacred vulture who protects the king in war is embroidered on the armoured jacket as though enfolding him with its wings.

9. The King's bow-bearer dressed in a tight protective quilted garment covered with small bronze plates. On his head a quilted cap.

Bottom Group

11 and 12. Nubian archers.

13–15. Soldiers with ordinary kerchief and heart-shaped leather front piece over the loin-cloth or (14 and 15) a quilted outer tunic carrying sickle-shaped knives, clubs or battle-axe. Shields with eye-holes.

3 ANCIENT EGYPT. *New Kingdom about 1350 B.C.*

Top Group

1. The King. The hood with the uraeus falls down on both sides in two pleated strips and is gathered on his back like a plait. He wears an artificial beard as a sign of a king, a diaphanous garment over the loin-cloth (invisible), girdle decoration and sandals made of papyrus (cf. Plate I, 1).
2. The King's footman or runner wearing an outer garment interwoven with gold. He carries quiver and bow, stick or club by means of which the runners made way for the royal procession.
3. Queen of the 19th Dynasty (14th cent. B.C.) in her hand the scourge, one of the royal insignia. On her wig the sacred vulture head-dress, usually worn by queens. She is dressed in two diaphanous garments (the new fashion for noble ladies): the light tunic and the light mantle fastened on the chest. The old tunic has been discarded. Not until the end of the 20th Dynasty is a short undergarment of thicker material worn again under tunic and mantle.
4. King with a blue wig, diadem with the sacred uraeus, artificial beard, collar, girdle decorations and two sceptres or insignia: scourge and crook.
5. Princess. Around the wig an ornamental band; collar, tunic, mantle, bare footed. (According to a wooden statuette in the Louvre, Paris).

Centre Group

6. King performing the sacrificial ritual and offering a golden ointment box. The king, like all officiating priests, is scantily clad, bare-footed and does not wear anything besides the two crowns, the neck decoration, the wide royal loin-cloth and girdle decoration.
7. Blind priest playing the harp. The head is shaven, without a wig. Flowing mantle.
8. The god Mônt of Hermonthis, with a hawk's head and feather decoration, also with solar disk and sacred uraeus. He carries the handle-cross, the so-called Nile-key which was the symbol of life and the attribute of many gods. (Hermonthis is the modern Erment near Thebes). The god Horus (light and sun-god) with the hawk's head is often similarly represented, the hawk was his sacred emblem.
9. The Queen as *wife of a god*. The Egyptian gods had a harem of living noble ladies; especially the god Ammon (the chief deity at Thebes with a human or a ram's head). Usually the queen (the Pharaoh's wife) is the earthly wife of Ammon, the *wife of a god*. Her attributes are plumes, solar disk, diadem, neck ornaments, the handle-cross and lotus sceptre. According to the old rite she wears the tight fitting tunic widening from below the knees and leaving the breasts exposed, a garment worn by the women of older times. Even Cleopatra, the friend of Anthony and Caesar, was represented as *wife of a god* in this costume. The light-bronze colour of the women is depicted as yellow, the colour of the men's skin is red.
10. The god Osiris in human form. He is the god of a younger popular legend symbolizing the master of the earth who gave the Egyptians laws and taught them agriculture. Killed later on by Seth or Typhon, the god of darkness, he reigned as king of the dead in the nether world, while Horus, the son of Osiris and Isis became the god of light and lord of the living. Osiris as a king wears a gold crown similar to the one worn by Upper-Egyptian kings with feathers on its sides, a white royal beard, he carries the two regal sceptres: scourge and crook and wears a coloured mantle. The skin is represented as green in accordance with the myth.

Bottom Group

11. Woman playing the harp dressed in a long tunic with slits for the arms; flower garlands on head and neck.
12. Woman playing the tambourine, collar, embroidered chastity belt, light mantle tied by a knot on the breast.
13. Slave girls with earthenware jug and leather bag, collar and chastity belt which (like the one of No. 12) holds up the narrow leather strip between the legs.
14. Slave girl with a light cloth extending from the hips to the knees, carrying so-called lotus flowers (Nelumbinum). Hair band and garland of flowers.
15. Hired female mourner from a funeral procession.

4 ANCIENT EGYPT. *New Kingdom (Late Period)*

1. Rameses II. (1324–1258 B.C.) on his war-chariot. The king as an archer; the reins attached to the girdle; two uraeus serpents, the symbol of royal dignity, are floating over his war-helmet (chepereshh). Quivers, long daggers or straight narrow swords, are attached to his girdle and chariot. (Relief according to Lepsius).

2. King Harmahib (1374–1350 B.C.) carried by soldiers on a litter. By the side of the king walks the *fan-bearer* whose office is only honorary. The real lower *fan-bearers* walk in front and behind the soldiers. In front of the procession: captives. The king holds the crook, which is a royal insignium like the scourge and the sickle-shaped sword. (Relief according to Lepsius).
3. Priests carrying in procession the sacred barge of Ammon Re. The barge which was kept in the holy of holies of the temple is adorned with the head of the animal sacred to the god. It has side rudders and a cabin is provided with fans and manned with bronze figurines. (Relief, according to Lepsius.)
4. A quilted armoured shirt with embroidery. Illustration at the tomb of Rameses III. (Rampsinit, about 1180) the last efficient king of the declining New Kingdom.

5 and 7. Banners and standards.

6. Soldier with a large shield from the Middle Kingdom. The New Kingdom adopted a different shape of shields (Cf. Pl.2)

Bottom Group

8. Isis priestess dressed in Graeco-Roman style. (Marble statuette, Rome, Capitoline Museum).
9. Isis priestess in Egyptian style with a mantle tied in a knot over the right shoulder while the left lappet falls loosely over the arm (Bronze figure, formerly Berlin Altes Museum).
10. Woman's costume. Mantle as No. 9. (Basalt figure, Munich, Antiquarium).

11 and 12. Saïte Priests with a mantle with jagged edges (Saïte Period, 7th and 6th centuries B.C.)

13. Egyptian clad in a mantle.
14. Ptolemy Euergétes (247–221 B.C.) with crown and mantle, sceptre and handle-cross.

ASSYRIA AND NEIGHBOURING PEOPLES *(12th–7th centuries B.C.)* 5

The Kingdom of Assur on the upper Tigris about 1500; from 885 (Asurnazirpal) great power, in 729 united with Babylonia; 606 end of Assyria.

Top Group

1. High dignitary in a long fringed tunic with short sleeves. Tasselled sash, fillet, neck ornaments. Bracelets on the upper arms and wrists. A sword worn by the aristocracy even in peace time. The sheath mounted with metal.
2. Assyrian king as officiating priest with a high cap and short tunic, the ceremonial garment of the priests. Priest's sticks with knobs or fan- or brush-shaped ends. His royal rank is marked by the mantle thrown over one shoulder and the tassels attached to the girdle.
3. Simple official with boots and hose (from a later period).
4. King with a cap decorated with gold braid, ends of which hang down the back. Fringed garment and mantle thrown over one shoulder. Purple-violet colour. Bracelets on the upper arm and wrists. Ear-rings (as 1–3). In his right hand, the long royal official staff. (Asurnazirpal, 884–860 B.C., according to a relief in the British Museum, London).

5 and 6. Canopy and fan-bearers of the king, beardless with broad sashes.

7. Bow-bearers of the king with a fringed skirt (as 5 and 6).

Centre Group

8. Warrior with metal helmet, double sword-belt with a metal buckle as a protection where the bands are crossed. Sword, long spear, round shield, hose and boots.
9. Lightly armed archer, with sword and simple cap.
10. Heavily armed warrior with coat of mail made of small metal pieces.
11. Ordinary woman with fringed skirt and mantle thrown over one shoulder.
12. Man in a short tunic and sash.
13. Captive with felt cap (member of a non-Assyrian tribe).

Bottom Group

14. Tribute-bearer from Northwest Mesopotamia.
15. Citizen from Nineveh (Capital of Assyria).
16. Prince from *Muzri* (modern Kurdistan).
17. Tribute-bearers from Palestine in the reign of King Jehu.

18 and 19. The Assyrian sacrificial mantle, front and back view. (18 King Asurnazirpal; 19 King Salmanassar III. 860–826 B.C.) According to originals and Layard: *Discoveries in the Ruins of Nineveh and Babylon*, with use of O. Jones, *Grammar of Ornament*, for the colouring.

BABYLONIA AND ASSYRIA 6

(Babylonia, the country between the Euphrates and Tigris was divided into Southern Sumer and Northern Akkad; south of the Euphrates was Chaldea)

Top Group

1. Old Babylonian priest-king (Gudea about 2250 B.C.) in a wide woven mantle, led by a god wearing the traditional skin mantle and horned cap.
2. King Khammurabi (about 2000 B.C.) wearing a Sumerian mantle and lamb skin cap. Relief.
3. Idol of the Babylonian-Assyrian weather god Adad with metal disks hanging down from the girdle.
4. King Merodach-Baladan of Babylonia (722–710 B.C.) dressed in a white tunic, held together by a girdle. At the back the tunic is pleated and the edge is fringed. Pointed cap elongated into a kind of tube.
5. Noble Babylonian lady in a long-sleeved tunic and fringed cape. Metal rings round the neck. Reconstructed by Max Tilke after an ivory figure in the Louvre, Paris.
6. Shows the head of a similar figure with cap and fillet tying up the hair at the nape of the neck.

Centre Group

7. King Asurbanipal (668–626 B.C., called *Sardanapalus* by the Greeks) on a couch in the garden of his harem. His head is encircled by a diadem with long bands falling down on his back and by a string of pearls. Richly decorated garment. Bracelets and ear-rings.

8. The queen on a high chair in a richly decorated tunic with tight ornamented sleeves; the long fringed mantle over it. Soft shoes. Star-shaped ear-rings, neck band, bracelets and a diadem in the shape of battlements. Feather fan on the small table.

9–12. Servant girls in long-sleeved tunics partly covered by a mantle. All garments with fringed borders. Sandals tied together with bands, probably worn over shoes made out of material. Turban-like head gear (fillets). Neck ornamentations and ear-rings. They wave the fan against flies and hold a plate with fruit and also a fringed cloth (possibly a napkin, Fig. 12). Incense burners on the floor.

Bottom Group

13. Armoured archer, shooting with his left hand.
14. Warrior with helmet, broad girdle over a short-sleeved tunic; lance, sword, round shield. The sword is usually fixed in a horizontal position to the sword-belt. The helmet has the small horse-hair curved metal decoration (which was further developed on the Greek helmet).
15. Horseman with pointed helmet in a short tunic, the upper part covered by a short ornamental garment (upper coat of mail). Fringed girdle, armoured hose, knee bands, laced boots, weapons: lance, sword, bow and arrows in the quiver. The horse's cover resembles an animal's skin. Ornamental straps are wound round the neck over the clipped mane. On the head part of the bridle an ornamental hair-tuft. Snaffle (similar to the bridles of today in Western Asia and Turkestan). The background shows how they shot from behind large shields fixed into the ground. According to original monuments in different museums and Layard, Discoveries. Cf. also C. Bezold: *Ninive und Babylon.*

7 WESTERN ASIA IN ANTIQUITY *Sumerians, Hittites, and West-Asiatics*

(The non-semitic Sumerians about 3000 B.C. in Southern Babylonia; Hittites from the 2nd millennium rulers over Asia Minor as far as Syria; their empire was destroyed about 715 B.C., with the conquest of Carchemish.)

1. Seated figure with tablet on his knees, wearing a Sumerian mantle (From Tello).
2. Head of a similar figure with astrakhan cap.
3. Head of a commander with helmet and skin mantle; from the stele of Egyptian King Echnaton (Amenophis IV.) 14th century B.C., Paris, Louvre.
4. Woman in a shaggy lambskin mantle (arranged in flounces). Alabaster statuette from Ur in Chaldea (old cultural centre of the Sumerians).
5. Warrior from the ranks with axe, the bronze head fixed to a wooden shaft. Time of the Egyptian King Echnaton (cf. 3).
6. The oldest chariot represented in art. A leopard's skin is thrown over the seat. Drawn by four mules. The driver, unlike all other Sumerians, protects part of his head with a wig and wears a beard against evil spirits.
7. Hittite weather-god. Leather shoes with turned-up points as still worn in the Orient. Basalt relief, 2nd millennium B.C.
8. Hittite warrior. Leather shoes as No. 7. Basalt relief from Sendshirli. 2nd millennium B.C.
9. Hittite chief with pointed cap and ear-rings.
10. Cilician god. He wears a horned cap, and in his hands grapes and ears of corn. Leather shoes as in No. 7.
11. Priest praying to a god or Cilician prince. (Cf. the Assyrian sacrificial mantle, Plate 5 which is draped round the body in the same way). One should notice the clean-shaven upper lip of figures 10 and 11. 10 and 11 form a rock-relief in Northern Syria.
12. Arabian warrior in a short tunic, with bow, arrow and quiver. From an Assyrian representation.
13. Hittite warrior with sickle-shaped sword.
14. Hittite prince in a wide mantle, the borders richly decorated.
15. Deity with peculiar trailing garment (perhaps a mantle held in place round the hips by a girdle. Found at Jerabis.
16. Hittite woman from a procession, wearing a crown in the form of battlements.
17. Hittite woman, in a large wrap which also covers the head, sitting in front of a folding table and holding a metal mirror. Pointed turned-up leather shoes.
18. Hittite figure in a long mantle. From Boghaskoi, the former Chatti (capital of the Hittites about 1800 B.C.).
19. Head of the Armenian king Tigranes I. with an indented crown with animal frieze over the fillet.
20. Head of a Parthian King. Helmet over fillet.
21. Warrior of a sea-faring nation attacking Palestine.
22. Philistine warrior wearing cap with chin-strap and feather-like crest.

8 WESTERN ASIA IN ANTIQUITY *Phoenicians, Hittites, Syrians (Canaanites)*

The most powerful neighbouring people of the Egyptians in the north were the Hittites (Kheta, Chatti, cf. Plate 7; Kefti: Crete; Retenu: Palestine); this plate also includes West-Asiatic tribes, nomad Bedouins or those in settlements as well as sea-faring nations.

Top Group

1. Man from Kefti with fillet, multi-coloured loin-cloth with tassels, bobs and socks woven in many colours to protect the ankles. Skin-sandals.
2. Hittite or Kheta. Fillet, long, simple garment (as still common in the Orient today), short shoulder cape. Clean-shaven.
3. Man of a desert tribe east of Palestine. Decorated skin mantle fastened on one shoulder. Tattooing on the legs.
4. Man of the Purasate, a hostile sea-faring people from the time of Rameses III. – Feather head dress which does not denote a chief but is worn by every one. The Purasate or Pulasate can probably be identified with the Philistines of the Bible. (Not Semites but probably coming from Aegean countries).
5. Syrian of rank from the interior of the country.

Centre Group

6. Bedouin (nomad hunter and breeder). Loin-cloth woven in gay colours and leather sandals. Bow and arrows, wooden hunting stick for throwing made of hard wood and bent in a special way (cf. the Australian Aborigine's boomerang).

7. Bedouin woman in a mantle woven in many colours; actually a cloth fastened on one shoulder. Fillet, shoes made of one piece of leather. The leather bottle was used for keeping fat, ointment or rouge.
8. Syrian or Canaanite. (According to an Egyptian representation dating from the end of the 18th Dynasty. Perhaps a rich merchant). Yellow tunic with tight sleeves and trousers, covered by a richly embroidered outer garment draped so that the blue and red stripes alternate. Short beard.
9. Man from a South Palestinian tribe.
10. Man belonging to a primitive South Palestinian tribe. The body painted and tattooed in the fashion of primitive people. Fair or dyed hair.
11. Man from *Retenu* (Palestine or Syria) with tassels and coloured borders.
1–11. Partly according to Egyptian representations in *Manners and Customs of the Ancient Egyptians* by Wilkinson, London 1878.

Bottom Group

12–17. Hebrews.
12. Hebrew in a short sleeved long fringed woollen tunic, an oblong piece of material worn over it and decorated with tassels at the lower corners (according to Mosaic law). He wears a pointed cap of bands wound round the head.
13. Street vendor wearing an outer wrap with fringes.
14. Priest with the vessel for the sacrificial blood (cf. 15).
15. High Priest. The priestly costume consisted of breeches or a loin-cloth (second book of Moses 28, 42), a white linen tunic with long sleeves, a long girdle wound several times round the body; the head-dress consisted of a band wound round a large tube (or open cap). During the ritual he was bare footed. In addition, the High Priest wore a sleeveless mantle reaching down to the knees and over that the *ephod* or shoulder garment made of two seperate back and front parts and fastened on the shoulders by means of onyx brooches and round the waist by a girdle made out of gold and coloured threads. Four rows of three jewels were fixed to the breastplate of the *ephod* as emblems of the twelve tribes of Judah. Besides the fillet a golden plate was worn by the High Priest with the inscription: Holy to Jehovah Yahweh).
16. Hebrew with prayer mantle and prayer strap, the longer tassels of the mantle manifesting his great piety and obedience to the law.
17. Ordinary man in a fringed tunic with sash and high boots (According to reliefs on the black Obelisk of Salmanassar in the British Museum, 9th Century B.C.). 1 and 2 according to the same reliefs.

MYCENAE, CRETE, CYPRUS *(Aegean and Phoenician Cultures 2000–500 B.C.)* 9

1–11. Mycenae.
1. Fragment with representation of warriors and woman. National Museum, Athens.
2. Warriors with large leather shields. From a Mycenaen sword blade.
3–7. Ornamental objects made of gold plate, frequently used as decoration on garments.
8–11. Female figures from gold and copper signet rings, Mycenae.
12–18. Crete.
12. Bronze statuette of a woman wearing flounced skirt.
13–16. Snake goddess with bodice and frills. Flounced skirt.
17. Statuette similar to No. 12.
18. Women carrying pails of water, a harpist behind. Painting on a sarcophagus from Crete. The Crete male figures (bull-fighters, equilibrists, etc.) are mostly represented as naked, pale or reddish as, for instance, the harpist, but they wear a sort of coat of mail round the hips or a loin-cloth corresponding exactly to the women's, who, however, wear in addition the flounced skirt and the bodice which leaves the breasts exposed.
19–23. Cyprus.
19 and 20. Cyprian warrior, terra-cotta statuette.
21. Cyprian prince with double loin-cloth and ornamental collar, cyprian hat (Egyptian style).
22. Man's head (Cyprus).
23. Woman's head with ear-rings, diadem covered by a veil. (Terra-cotta in Creek style).
24. Man's head with a Cyprian straw hat or cap as still worn today.
25. Cypriot wearing a sort of himation (cf. Greece) with ornamental border. (Early Greek period). According to Bossert, *Altkreta*. Berlin, 1937, also F. Winter, *Kretisch-mykenische Kunst*, 1913.

PERSIA IN ANTIQUITY AND THE EARLY MIDDLE AGES 10

Top Group

1–15. Ancient Persia 6th–5th centuries B.C.
1. King Darius in a long trailing Median outer garment, the superfluous length of which is pulled up at the left side and allowed to fall down in rich folds. Wide sleeves. Stick as carried by the Assyrian kings (cf. Plate 5) and a bunch of flowers in his hand. Long beard which was a royal privilege all other men wearing a short round beard. Regal cap richly decorated and serrated at the edge which is worn by the body guard in similar form. All ancient Persian caps are worn so as to show part of the hair over the forehead.
2 and 3. Fan and canopy-bearers according to ancient Assyrian court custom.
4. Companion of the king with fillet and carrying spear and bow.
5 and 6. Bodyguard. The bodyguard consisted of a whole army mostly dressed in Median garments. Arms: spear, bow, oval shield with semi-circle cut out at the sides. Ordinary warriors carried round shields.

Centre Group

7–9. Warriors in ancient Persian knee-length tunics with girdle and long trousers. Leather cap and shoes fastened on the instep with bands. Short broad sword (or dagger) hanging from the belt. Figure 7 carries the peculiar Persian case for the short bow and arrows.

10. Distinguished Persian in a long Median outer garment with wide sleeves and pleated cap. Beard and medium long curls. Laced leather shoes.
11. Persian in travelling costume with mantle open in front.
12. Court servant in a long outer garment with fan for flies and combined cape and hood consisting of a large piece of cloth wrapped round the neck and head.

1–12. Mostly from representations found in the ruins of Pasargadae and Persepolis, the palaces built by Cyrus (died 529 B.C.), Darius (died 485 B.C.) and Xerxes (died 465 B.C.). Another source is the Mosaic at Naples, an imitation of a much older picture.

13 and 14. Men's heads from Xerxes' reign (485–465 B. C.).
15. Woman's head from the same period, with a veiled mouth as is still customary with Armenian women.

16–25. Persian at the time Khoshu II. (591–628 A.D.).
16. Servant girl in a long tunic.
17–19. The ruler with servants and pages.
20–25. Persian Ambassador according to cave paintings from Ajanta (formerly Berlin, Museum für Völkerkunde).

11 SCYTHIANS AND INHABITANTS OF ASIA MINOR *(Early Greek Culture)*

The Scythians (Saks) often mentioned by Herodotus were a mounted stock breeding people north of the lower Danube and in modern southern Russia, who invaded Asia Minor in the 7th century.

Presumably they are a European tribe of the Iranians and related to the Persians, thus being Indo-Europeans.

Top Group

1–6. Scythians according to representations in tombs. Leningrad, Ermitage.
1. Archer in a leather tunic with long embroidered leather trousers, decorated with small metal plates, called Scythian leather trousers, and soft medium-high leather boots. Band round the long hair.
2. Warrior with a conical cap tied under the chin. Trousers like No. 1.

3–6. Archers with large pocket-like quivers. Cap like 2, trousers like 1. Also two warriors in similar costume.

Centre Group

7–11. Phrygians, i. e. a people related to the Armenians, thus they were Indo-Europeans living in Asia Minor. Agricultural people of a certain cultural standard, they lived partly in towns and cultivated handicrafts, (especially carpet weaving and embroidery).

7. Phrygian shepherd. (A representation of the mythological Attis or Atys, the Phrygian Adonis, who was usually represented as a youthful shepherd and was the favourite of the goddess Cybele.
8. A similar figure from a West Asiatic relief of hellenistic times.
9. Girl in a Phrygian patterned costume as seen on Greek vase paintings, wearing the so-called Phrygian cap.
10. The Trojan Paris in a Phrygian costume with long hose and hood-like head-dress (Phrygian cap).
11. Amazon from a Greek vase painting. It shows her wearing the Phrygian cap, hose and high laced boots. She carries a battle-axe, a small shield (and also often a bow).

Bottom Group

12–21. Costume and arms of Asia Minor.

12. Medea wearing a gaily coloured Phrygian costume, her home being in Colchis in Asia Minor. According to a vase painting of the later classical Greek period.
13. One of the body guard of the Persian king in Phrygian costume. According to the Greek vase, called Darius vase; Naples Museum.

14–21. Arms from Asia Minor according to Greek vase paintings.

12 GREECE. *Early Period (6th and 5th centuries B.C.)*

Top Group (According to black vase paintings)

1, 2, 4, 6. Women and girls in the archaic stiff Doric chiton *(tunic)* which reached down to the feet and was decorated with bands of ornaments and patterns. A girdle was worn round the waist. Chest and shoulders are covered by a short jacket or kerchief which, however, is often produced and arranged by way of pulling the superfluous length of the chiton up through the girdle and allowing it to fall down over the upper part of the body. It was usually fastened with safety-pins and brooches on the shoulders.
This upper part of the garment, when dresses became softer and fuller (linen instead of wool), gradually develops in a way to fall down in a baggy fold which is the beginning of the later forms of garments. In addition the himation, a loosely wrapped cloak, is worn and is sometimes drawn over the head by women.

3. Man in a dignified long chiton with flower patterns and a himation. The borders of both garments are ornamented. Beard and long hair.
5. Youth only wearing a short mantle called chlaina (without chiton).

Centre Group (according to later vase painting. 6th–5th centuries.)

7–9. Women and girls dressed in garments made of thinner material (linen or crêpe, byssus or cotton) and arranged in fine narrow pleats, many bulges and folds, falling down on the upper or lower part of the body. The pleats were produced by stitches on the upper seam or by pressing and ironing. The garment, originally sewn and meant to be pulled over the head like a tunic, is later wrapped and draped round the body (cf. bottom group). A himation is worn over head and shoulders.

10–11. Youth wearing a short linen chiton fastened on the shoulders and held together by a girdle.

11. With the short mantle *(chlaina)* and the petasos worn on journeys (or a travelling hat).
12. Man wearing a long chiton with many folds and a draped mantle *(himation)* having little lead weights at the ends.

Bottom Group

13 and 14. Women assisting at a burial and death ritual.
15. Woman putting on the Doric woollen chiton (cf. upper group) with part of it falling down from the shoulders.
16. Girl (before dressing) wrapping a band or girdle round her breast.
17. Girl in a short-sleeved linen chiton draping the mantle, Chlamis and fastening it with brooches or safety-pins on the shoulder.

GREECE. *Great Period of Greek Art. (5th and 4th centuries B.C.)* 13

Top Group

1–4. Examples showing different ways of draping the outer garment *(himation)* without the chiton.
1. According to a tomb stele from Orchomenos.
2. According to a statue.
3. Roman marble copy after a Greek bronze statue of Demosthenes, about 280 B.C.
4. After a statue of Sophocles about 340 B.C.

Centre Group

5. Short chiton, pulled over the left shoulder, in order to leave the right arm free. Craftsmen's costume. The left shoulder and arm are covered by a small wrapper. (Statue of Hephaestus, god of fire and the smiths.
6. Apollo Citharoedus and conductor of the Muses in a long woman's peplos. Roman marble copy after a Greek original of the 5th century B.C.
7. Pallas Athene in a woman's peplos with an outer wrapper, the Aegis, the mythological goat skin with the Gorgon's head (so-called Athena Lemnia. Bronze statue by Pheidias).
8. Delphic charioteer in a long chiton with a girdle (Bronze statue in Delphi, about 470 B.C.).

Bottom Group

9. Amazon by Polycletus in a short chiton with girdle (Bronze statue from Delphi about 470 B.C.).
10 and 11. Attic tomb relief: woman and servant.
12. Resting pugilist wearing a chlamis similar to the Abyssinian mantle *shama*.

GREECE. *Armour, Banquets, Games and Music* 14

1. Chariot which replaced the cavalry in Homer's description according to a later representation. Coat of mail with metal shoulder plates. Helmet with cheek-guards which can be turned up.
The sword is strapped very high to the belt.
2. Tomb stele of Aristion (end of 6th century). A star on the shoulder plates; a lion's head on the breast plate. The coat of mail is decorated all round with three ornamental metal bands. The short chiton can be seen on the upper arm and the thighs.
3. Achilles bandaging the wounded Patroclus who is sitting on his shield with his helmet taken off so that the felt hair cap can be seen. Coat of mail with movable shoulder plates and studded leather or linen elongations hanging down from the coat of mail for protection of the lower part of the body. Under the coat of mail the short chiton. The cheek-guards on Achilles' helmet are turned up. The armour is that of the time of the Persian Wars.
4. Heavily armed soldier.
5. Heavily armed soldier with greaves connected by springs. Oval shield cut out at the sides.
6. Warrior with spear. Large crest on his helmet, turned up cheek-guards, decorated greaves. The coat of mail protecting the ships consists of several layers.
7. Helmet with fixed cheek-guards and two crests placed across the helmet.
8. Helmet of the late archaic epoch before the great period of art.
9. Banquet *(Symposion)*. The members wearing garlands on their heads, the one on the right with a cup *(skyphos)* the one on the left holds out the goblet to the young slave with a jug. The ornamental border of this painted vase shows cooling vessels, jug, goblet and shoes.
10. Banquet, the man lying, the girl sitting.
11. Member of a banquet wearing a garland and holding goblet and drinking horn.
12. Cup *(Kantharos)* with large rounded handles used for official ceremonies.
13. Bowl without handle *(phiale)* which was filled from a jug.
14. Tumbler *(rhyton)* in the shape of a bull's head, through the nostrils of which the wine flowed into the mouth.
15. Bowl with handle and stem.
16. Jug with handle.
17. Greek woman carrying honey in the comb with the left hand and a kantharos in her right hand.
18. Female tumbler in a loin-cloth moving on her hands between pointed swords.
19. Male figure from the retenue of Dionysus (Bacchus).
20. Wandering minstrel with flute and lyre.
21. Man blowing the flute and wearing a fillet to which the flute can be attached. He wears the peculiar ceremonial garment: the long chiton with a sleeveless jacket. So-called *aulet* (derived from *aulos*: flute with mouth-piece, usually applied to a twin flute).
22. Pipes *(syrinx)* the simple natural instrument of Greek shepherds, each pipe of different length.
23. Woman playing the *psalterion*. (This was the old lyre with strings.)
24. Lyre *(psalterion)* with a roundish sounding-box.
25. Woman with a string-instrument (in the shape of a *kithara*, which was being plucked by the *plektron*.
26. Woman tuning her lyre.
27. Harp *(trigonon*, called thus from its three-cornered shape). The sounding-board faces the harpist.

15 LATE GREEK TOWN COSTUME

of the Hellenistic period on painted Terra-cottas of the 4th Century B.C. (mostly from Tanagra, Boeotia)

1. Female dancer in a flounced skirt.
2. Boy wearing a *petasos* (wide, soft sun-hat).
3. Boy wearing chiton and chlamis, as well as *petasos*.
4. Girl in a full-pleated chiton and mantle *(himation)* and well dressed hair (front view).
5. Girl wearing a mantle and pointed sun-hat (so-called Thessalian hat), white and red border.
6. cf. 4 (side view).
7. Girl (Artemis with her hunting dog) wearing a costume suitable for sport and similar to that of the Amazons: Chiton and pink chlamis. The doe skin of the hunter (nebris) over it is fastened by means of a blue girdle. High hunting-boots fastened by bands cross-laced. From Tanagra, 4th century B.C.
8. Two girls putting their arms round each other and wearing the so-called sleeveless Doric chitons and over it a short mantle *(himation)*, the right one being blue, the left red. The girl on the left has her hair combed up carefully, the one on the right has thick plaits laid round the head. From Corinth.
9. Young woman with Eros, wearing chiton and himation.

1–6. According to original statuettes from the Munich Collection of Antiques.

7 and 8. According to A. Furtwängler, Sabouroff collection, vol. 2 (Berlin 1883–87).

9. From a photo in the Loeb collection, Munich.

16 ETRUSCANS. *About 750 B.C.*

1, 5, 11 and 18. Woman in a long close-fitting dress. (1, back view, 5, front view).

2. Woman's shoes made of one piece with holes for laces.

3 and 12. Woman with a conical head-dress and with a spiral garment decorated with flowers and the ends of which are pulled over the shoulders from the back and allowed to fall down over the chest.

12. back view.

4 and 7. Golden ear-rings.

6 and 9. Man before arranging his garment and after having draped it round the body (9: is a free drawing in order to illustrate the way the garment is worn).

8 and 16. Ear plates with gold pendants.

10. Head of a female statuette with hood and neck bands.

13. Bronze votive statuette, for protection and healing.

14 and 15. Heads from Etruscan mural paintings from the tomb-grottoes near Corneto.

17. Terra-cotta sarcophagus (from Caere, now Cervetri) a leather wine bottle is placed near the couple on the couch.

19–24. Home-coming warriors, Samnites, enemies of Rome, who, in the 5th century B.C. pushed part of the Etruscans out of Southern Italy (Mural painting from a tomb in Ruvo di Puglia, now in the Museum at Naples).

25–35. The two lower rows: Etruscan banquet: a memorial feast for the dead. The participants lie next to the table, and in addition there are the usual servants, flautists, jugglers and dancers, both male and female (Mural painting from an Etruscan tomb, now in the Vatican Museum, Rome).

17 ROME. *Men's Costume*

1. Toga draped over the tunica in the old simple way. According to a so-called statua togata, statue representing an Etruscan in peace time attire.
2. Priest (Pontifex) performing a sacrifice. His toga drawn over his head.
3. Dealer of sacrificial animals or sacrificial attendant (victimarius).
4. Inhabitant of Gabii in Latium wearing his toga in a special way: the end of the toga is drawn tightly round the waist thus forming a girdle (cinctus Gabinus). Left: coin showing Julius Caesar's head with a laurel garland. Right: coin of Aurelian with the emperor's crown as worn at the time.
5. Julius Caesar addressing his soldiers. The *paludamentum*, the general's mantle only worn in war-time over the armour, covers the coat of mail with its bronze decorations. It was longer than the simple war mantle, the *sagum* and was fastened on the right shoulder with a brooch (according to a statue in Naples).
6. Julius Caesar wearing the *toga pura* or *virilis*, the simple white toga as worn by men from their seventeenth year (according to a statue in the Alte Museum, Berlin).
7. Dignitary in the stance of an orator in the *toga praetexta* which had a purple border to indicate high office.
8. Emperor wearing the long military mantle *(paludamentum)*.
9. Lictor, i. e. attendant or honorary guard who were attached to the high officials in different numbers. In his hand the fasces (bundle of rods).
10. Emperor wearing the long trailing purple toga, originally worn by the censors. (Since the Emperor Domitian it became the customary imperial garment.)
11. Emperor with the purple mantle embroidered with gold threads over the toga fastened by a girdle.
12. Emperor performing a sacrifice wearing tunica and paenula (mantle) thrown back over both shoulders (cf. Plate 19, fig. 5).
13. Youth wearing paenula.
14. Cape with hood *(cucullus)*.
15. Sun-hat with a narrow point similar to the woman's hat on the statuette from Tanagra (Pompeiian representation) cf. plate 15: Hellenistic costume.

ROME. *Ordinary People, Priestesses, Women* 18

Top Group

1. Auriga (charioteer in the arena in a coloured tunica, carrying victor's palm.
2. Man in the long sleeveless, full *tunica talaris* (ankle length).
3. Peasant wearing a tunic made of sheepskin with high boots and broad-brimmed hat.
4. Fisherman wearing the *exomis* (a short tunic exposing the right breast).
5. Representation of the *paenula* (cloak with hood), back view. Pattern of the north African burnous (cf. Plate 187–88, Algeria and Tunis as well as text: African peoples).

Centre Group

6. Slave wearing a tunica with a girdle and sandals with straps wound round the ankle and calf.
7. Sacrificial attendant (Camillus) wearing a tunica with a girdle. Long hair adorned with a garland.
8. Woman wearing a mantle thrown back over one shoulder and showing a short tunica with a girdle. The under-garment is a long tight-sleeved *tunica interior* or also called *subucula*.
9. *Tunica recta* made of one piece of material and reaching down to the feet. Long veil and a crown on her head.
10. The wife of Drusus.
11. Women wearing the tunica with a girdle *(tunica muliebris)* the customary garment for women.
12. Veiled vestals with mantle drawn over the head, over long tunica.
13. A middle-aged vestal (priestess of Vesta).
14. The empress Agrippina the Elder (wife of Germanicus and the mother of Caligula, who died 33 A. D.), wearing pleated tunica with half-long sleeves and a mantle thrown over. Wig with plaits hanging down at the sides.

Bottom Group

15–19. Roman women in different stances wearing the *palla*, a sort of himation or mantle draped in various ways.

GREECE AND ROME. *Hair styles and head-dresses* 19

1. Greece

The man belonging to early Greek culture wears locks and plaits skilfully arranged in various ways often intertwined with the fillet or hair band (1–7). Only from the 5th century is men's hair shorn or cropped and arranged in a simpler way (Fig. 8). Women in early times have their hair dressed in a very elaborate way with locks and plaits (11–14), obviously produced by curling-irons or by means of false locks. Probably these elaborate and painfully created styles were not worn every day, as some representations – also from the 9th century – show much simpler styles. Bands and kerchiefs were amply applied (Figs. 15–19).
Men's head-dress was the plain cap and the soft more elongated woollen cap with the edge turned up. The well-known Phrygian cap is only a special form of this kind, which by the way is still worn today by Italian or Portuguese fishermen in red or black colours. The stiffer hat with a turned-up brim has probably developed from the soft cap. The pointed hat with a narrow brim (*pilos*, fig. 10) and the one with the wide brim called *petasos*, the Greek travelling hat, represent the main types of hats. The *petasos* could be hung over the back by its bands (fig. 8).

2. Rome

Already at the time of Ovid (in the reign of the emperor Augustus), the hair styles of Roman women must have been extremely varied, as ladies of rank kept several slave girls for the purpose of dressing their hair. Those who were not in a position to do so had to resort to simpler styles or kerchiefs. Women with simpler styles wore a parting and gathered their hair in a knot similar to the Greek fashion. But it was the women of rank and the elderly women who prefered the more elaborate styles. Fig. 28 has a parting and her hair is laid round the head in a complicated way, interlaced with a ribbon and ending on the head (*nodus*). Besides ribbons they wore hair-nets, fillets and diadems or simple metal bands. Fig. 26 (Bust in the Capitoline Museum, Rome) wears her hair set in waves according to Greek fashion. Figs. 27, 23 and its back view 25 show the way plaits were fastened on the head. There were numerous variations in which little round curls were arranged in tight rolls on the heads of noble Roman women, of which figs. 20, 22, 23 are examples; fig. 20 has, in addition, two long locks hanging down at the sides. Elaborate and majestic (resembling battlements) is the empress Messalina's hairstyle (fig. 21) according to a bust in the Capitoline Museum, Rome.

FOOTWEAR in ANCIENT TIMES 20

At first the shoe served only as a protection with the Greeks; people went bare-foot at home; it was only in the streets that shoes were worn. The Romans as a rule travelled and marched more frequently than the Greeks, also entered colder countries more often and therefore gave more attention to footwear.
The Greek woman, mostly confined to the house, is seldom represented with shoes. She prefers soles fastened with straps, or sandals. Later on, as shown by the Tanagra statuettes, dating from the 4th century B.C., more elegant shoes were worn by women, for instance red ones with yellow edged soles. There were no special types of shoes. There were many forms varying from the simple sandals to the high laced boots partly with rich decorations and slits as can be seen on Greek representations.

The simplest form is the *karbatine* (fig. 16) worn by both Greeks and Romans which consisted of a piece of cow's hide turned up around the foot and fastened by straps. It is in fact the old strapped shoe as also worn by the Teutons and up to the 16th century by German peasants and even today by Rumanians, Slovaks, and other peoples. The main part of all footwear remains the sole (fig. 5), the solid support of the foot as a protection against the cold, dampness and rough ground; then the straps for fastening were added, later the toe-caps and finally the upper part of the shoes, which according to need or taste have slits or are decorated (figs. 9, 10, 12). Figs. 9, 10, 12–16, also 1–3 show Greek styles. These represent the kind called *krepis* or *krepide*. In fig. 17 the foot under the strap is bandaged with linen bands. Figs. 13–15 and 19 resemble more our shoe and boot, but are not of a more recent Greek origin. Fig. 22 is a type between the two, as the toes are exposed again. The simplest Roman footwear were the *soleae* (fig. 5). Figs 7 and 8 show the Roman *calceus*. The colour of fig. 4 is red as a sign of distinction for the high officials of the Republic (*mulleus*). The *calceus* when worn by the soldiers is called *caliga* (figs. 11 and 23) and is represented here as a heavy hobnailed sandal. Fig. 6 has been drawn after an original from a museum in the Rhine Province. Fig. 21 is again the Greek *krepide*, worn by a Roman, fig. 20 is a Roman example from the time of the Imperium. Figs. 24, 26 and 27, 29, 32, 34 are Coptic footwear (slippers, sandals of all types); fig. 28 represents a Coptic straw sandal, 26 is a Coptic laced shoe. Fig. 25 is a late Roman slipper from the time of the Emperor Justinian, 30 is a Roman boot (similar to fig. 20, fig. 31 is a Roman spur).

The Coptic shoes are represented according to *Antike und frühmittelalterliche Fußbekleidung aus Achmim-Panopolis* by Frauberger. Düsseldorf, 1896.

21 TEUTONS. *Prehistoric and Early Historic Periods*

1–5. Teutons in Jutland and Schleswig-Holstein. Bronze Age about 2000 B.C.
1. From the finds at Borum Eshöi (Jutland).
2. Girls garments from the finds at Egtved. Linen tunic and outer garment reaching below the hips, a cord gathering this short tunic at the waist.
3. Man's costume from the finds at Trinohi. Oval shaped woollen mantle. A short tunic-like garment is wrapped round the body, the ends of which are knotted at the back.

4 and 5. Women's and men's costume according to the reconstructions in the Copenhagen Museum. No description can be given of the linen undergarment which was probably worn (like fig. 2 where the linen tunic has been added) as all the linen has perished in the wooden coffins. The outer garments were mostly made of brown shorn wool.

6–10. Teutons in Northern Germany.

6. Frisian youth after the find by Max Etzel. Sleeveless short tunic, short breeches. Laced shoes.
7. Man of the Marcomanni tribe in a short tunic with sleeves gathered at the waist by a girdle and wearing mantle fastened on the right shoulder and long hose. Under his coat he carries a sack on his left shoulder.
8. Girl dressed in a long sleeveless tunic with a girdle and a broad richly decorated sash-like band passed over one shoulder. According to a find near Hamburg.
9. Teuton with short tunic and breeches similar to 6. In addition hose (or high gaiters). Find at Oberaltendorf.
10. Man dressed in a long sleeved tunic, putties, mantle fastened on the right shoulder and collar hood. Find at Bermethsfeld near Hanover.

11–15. Eastern Teutons of the Roman period.

11. Cymbric warrior (according to a find at Gundestrup, near Cassel).
12. East Germanic warrior (according to finds reconstructed in Silesia).
13. Fettered warrior belonging to the tribe of the Bastarnae (now settled in Rumania) wearing very long pleated hose as still worn in Rumania.
14. Captive of the Daci tribe (province of Dacia) in the retinue of a prince. (Figs. 13 and 14 according to the Tropaeum-victory memorial monument – at Adamkliss (Dobrudja).
15. Man belonging to the tribe of the Bastarnae (cf. fig. 13). He wears, like fig. 13, a tunica with girdle and over it the narrow paenula (cf. Roman costume) and the Roman hair style.

22 TEUTONS. *Roman Period, partly older*

1. Figure of the *Germania*. The legs covered like those of warriors. The lozenge-shaped pattern has also been found on materials on the bodies found in the moors. Relief from the stone rampart of the *practorium* in the legions' camp at Mayence. Time of the emperor Vespasian (died 79 A. D.).
2. A man of the Suevi tribe, half naked, (with breeches), overthrown by a Roman horseman. Tombstone of a Roman horseman.
3. Kneeling, imploring Germanic youth covered with hose which have fallen down in front from the girdle; hair gathered in a tuft at the back of the head, mantle and shoes. (Roman bronze figure. Paris. Bibliothèque Nationale.)

4 and 5. House urns.

6. Daci wearing long hose tied at the ankles, tunic with girdle, mantle, oval shields. From Trajan's column erected 113 A.D.
7. Man with a sling. Man of the tribe of the Marcomanni. Relief from the column of Marcus Aurelius, Rome (after 173 A.D.). Similar to fig. 6.
8. Warrior with sword, with the upper part of the body exposed and wearing shaggy woollen trousers. Statuette on an ivory box from Frankish-Merovingian Gaul (about 6th–7th century).
9. Teuton wearing mantle or cape-like sleeveless garment made of wool or fur and with a hole for the neck. Roman triumphal relief in the Vatican Museum, Rome.
10. Germanic woman (so-called Thusnelda) dressed in a Graeco-Roman garment with the left breast exposed as described by Tacitus in the *Germania*. Roman marble statue, now in Florence, Loggia dei Lanzi.
11. Woollen tunic of a Germanic body discovered in the moors, from Thorsbjerg (Jutland). The sleeves are sewn on and show lozenge pattern.
12. Woollen trousers found in the same moors. The foot part of one leg is sewn on.

13–15. Bronze helmets and bronze cap found in Germany but of uncertain origin.

16. Shoe found in the moors. It is in one piece, and is fur-lined. It is the shape of the ancient laced shoe worn by German peasants until the late 16th century.

17 and 18. Shoes found in Swabia, flattened out.

19. High woollen cap, found in the moors, Jutland. Copenhagen Museum.
20. Frankish axe.
21. Short sword, dagger.

22. Axe with shaft, natural shape. According to a find near Reichenhall.
23. Head of one axe with loop and socket.
24. Axe; old emblem of dignity and office. Instead of a blade, a hammer is often attached. Find from Schleswig.
25. Blade of an axe from near Osnabrück. 1–25 according to photographs in *Deutsche Geschichte* by Heyck. Vol. I.
26 and 27. East Teuton with tuft of hair gathered on one side of the head (seen from the two angles).
28 and 29. Men belonging to the tribe of the Bastarnae from the *Tropaeum Trajani* at Adamkliss (Rumania). Cf. plate 22.
30 and 31. Teuton's heads according to Rhenish finds.
32 and 33. Marcomanni from the Column of Marcus Aurelius. (Max Tilke says of the woman's costume that Indian women of Arizona still wear a similar primitive garment). 26–33 according to *Tracht der Germanen* by J. Girke (Leipzig 1922).

PERSIA. *Sassanian Period in the Early Middle Ages (227–636 A.D.).* 23

1. Head of a deity.
2. King Narsahe (Narses) 293–302 A.D.
3. Companion of the king.
4. Official, according to a seal in the British Museum.
5. King on horseback wearing a garment and very wide trousers.
6, 7 and 10. Parthians dressed in tunics and long, close fitting trousers (5) or wide trousers (10), according to Sassanian reliefs.
5–7 and 10. according to *Kostümkunde* by Weiss.
8. King or prince hunting. (From a silver vessel in the Paris Collection of Coins).
9. King Ardeshir.
11. The god Ahura-Mazda, Ormuzd (right) gives King Ardeshir the ring of sovereignty. Rock relief near Naksch-i-Rustam.
12 and 13. Statue of King Sapor from a grotto near Shapur. According to Texier.
14–17. Parthians wearing different helmets and fillets.
18–24. Parthian according to Iranian rock reliefs. The relief representations according to *Iranische Felsreliefs* by Sarre-Herzfeld, 1910.
25. Long-sleeved original garment of a Parthian, wool dyed green. Discovered by Max Tilke in the former Berlin Museum für Völkerkunde (about 600 A.D.).
26. Sassanian horseman.
27. King with halo over the crown placed on a head with long curls.

GAULS, VIKINGS AND NORSEMEN 24

Top Group

1–10. Gauls.
1 and 2. Gallic warrior (1) with leather cuirass over the short tunic.
3. Gallic woman wearing a long blouse without a girdle.

Centre Group

4 and 5. Gallic peasants with hooded collars *(cucullus)*.
6–8. Warriors, the middle one with a bronze trumpet similar to an alpine horn, (6) wearing a *sagum*.
9. Chief with insignia.
10. Warrior. Reconstructed from preserved pieces of weapons and ornaments by French experts (perhaps not quite correctly). The special Gallic breeches *(bracca, braca* = Celtic word, in German *Bruch*) reach only down to the knees.

Bottom Group

11–14. Vikings.
11. Viking wearing skin trousers.
12. Viking (Norseman) with bronze helmet wearing a gaily bordered tunic. (11 and 12) according to bronze plates from Öland.
13 and 14. Scandinavian Norsemen from the 7th to 10th centuries wearing iron or bronze helmets of different shapes. (14) wearing bronze helmet with movable front piece, a coat of mail and carrying a wooden shield mounted with bronze. Copenhagen Museum.
15. Norseman (warrior) with jagged leather coat (from Britain, 9th century A.D.). (11–14) partly according to A. von Jenny: *Germanische Frühkunst*, 1937.

ROME. *Equipment of Army and Gladiators.* 25

Top Group

1. Soldier of the Roman legions with leather cuirass, leather breeches, studded girdle, rectangular shield *(scutum)*, sword attached to the sword-belt *(balteus)*, javelin *(pilum)* and metal helmet *(cussis)* with a crest *(crista)*.
2. Soldier of the Roman legions (similar to those represented on Trajan's Column). The leather cuirass mounted with iron bands *(lorica segmentata)*.
3. Ensign (standard-bearer) (signifer, vexillarius) vexillum-bearer, wearing lion's or bear's skin, coat of mail, leather cuirass with sword, dagger and round shield *(clipeus)* made of mounted leather and with a handle on the inner side.
4. Standard-bearer with the insignia of the legion (4200–6000 men: 10 cohorts, each consisting of 3 maniples). With scale armour *(locica squamata)*. Sword and dagger. In camp the eagle was stuck into the ground.

Centre Group

5. Captain (centurio) of a century or half a maniple with scale-armour, over it decorations of merit (silver phalerne), decorated greaves *(ocreae)*, doubled wrap or mantle and vine-wood stick, the mark of a centurion. Next to 5: helmet with crest placed cross-ways (cf. 1), sword in its scabbard.
6. High officer (Trajan's Column) mantle made of fine purple woollen material. Crest like a caterpillar, round metal shield (in early Greek style).

7. Horseman with leather cuirass and oval leather shield with six corners and elaborately mounted; horseman's spear and long sword *(spatha)*, used by horsemen from 100 A.D. onwards.
8. Soldier of a Germanic auxiliary tribe (auxiliaris) with loin-cloth, girdle, the outer garment *(paenula)* is fastened up and has a hood. He carries an oval shield, sword, dagger and two javelins (According to a tombstone in Mayence). 1, 3–5, 7 according to Lindenschmit: *Tracht und Bewaffnung des römischen Heeres*, 1882, – 2 and 6 after photographs of Trajan's Column.

Bottom Group

9. Horn-blower with the cornu, a large, round metal horn, dressed in the tunica with wide border in the middle.
10. Net-fighter (retiarius) who tried to throw his net over his opponent, for instance the heavily armed gladiator with sword *(gladius)* and tried to pierce him with long trident. He is only slightly protected by his bandaged left cuirass sleeve which is widened on top into a metal shoulder plate. Otherwise only girdle with loin-cloth, greaves with bands wound round them.
11. Gladiator (myrmillo), armed in the Gallic way with vizor helmet, shield, belt, leg protection and sword.
12. Fencer in Thracian armour *(thrax)* with the same protective armour as the myrmillo (11), but two greaves and the short Thracian dagger *(sica)*.
13. Fencing-master (lanista) at the gladiatorial games, with official's rod and wide tunic decorated with two stripes; he is raising his hand to stop the game. Half-open sandals.

26 EARLY CHRISTIAN PERIOD. *300–600 A.D.*

Christianization of the Roman Empire in the 4th century did not change costume decisively. The early Middle Ages developed the traditional forms and added some features different from those of the Antique. The classic folds had partly to give way to the preference for ornament and gay colours. From the Romans came the name *clavus* (stripe) for the striped ornament on garments which originally were reserved for Romans of rank. This clavus ran down from the shoulders to the seam of the garment. There was also the round clavus. All these stripes were either sewn or embroidered on, or woven or inserted into the material. Christian initials were also used as inserted decorations, i. e. the Greek X and P, which mean Ch and R (Christ's initials) or the anchor cross, i. e. X and P to which were added *A* and *Ω* (alpha and omega), beginning and end, furthermore the cross † with X and P and the old T-cross (Anthony's cross) in addition with *A* and *Ω* (A and O).

Top Group

1. Lady wearing a dalmatica as an outer garment first worn in the East Roman Empire. This became the official costume of deacons. Wide head band the ends of which fall over the shoulders (Catacomb painting, 4th century).
2. Evangelist in the costume of the 5th century (Mosaic at Ravenna).
3. Elderly Christian woman wearing a mantle in the shape of the casula, the costume of officiating priests. Kerchief.
4. Lady of rank wearing striped dalmatica.
5. Youth wearing a tunica (shirt-like garment) with round stripes. Sandals with straps.

Centre Group

6. Shepherd with girdled tunica, bands wound round the legs and protective collar.
7. Apostle according to the conception of the Early Middle Ages wearing a dignified large toga-like mantle.
8. Elderly woman (really a picture of the Virgin) with fringed mantle.
9. Young woman wearing tunica and dalmatica as well as head and praying with uplifted arms.
10. *The good shepherd* with the ancient reed-pipe or Pan flute (like 6). (1–10) according to catacomb paintings and mosaics of Early Christian times. Cf. R. Forrer, *Reallexikon der prähistorischen frühchristlichen Altertümer* (1907).

Bottom Group

11. Richly decorated sleeved tunica partly covered by the so-called hoodless *pluviale*, both woven of fine wool.

12 and 13. Late forms of the antique toga. The upper part is narrowly pleated. Time of the Emperor Justinian (527–565).

14. Warrior in a leather cuirass with mantle tied up on one shoulder. Phrygian cap and round shield. Mosaic in San Marco, Venice.
15. Woman wearing very wide woman's tunica with slits for the arms.

27 BYZANTINE EMPIRE. *4th–11th Centuries.*

Through the destruction of the Ostrogothic kingdom in 552 A.D. Italy was re-conquered by the Byzantine Empire. Ravenna became the residence of the Byzantine governors and is today a major source of our knowledge of Byzantine culture and costume. This is characterized by great magnificence; much silk, gold, jewelry and gaily coloured and patterned materials.

Top Group

1. The Emperor Arcadius (since 395 A.D. Emperor of the Eastern Empire, i. e. Byzantine Empire). The imperial orb was originally the imperial Roman emblem of the earth and world dominion. Later the Christian cross was added as an attribute of the western Emperors.
2. Consul from the first half of the 5th century. Consuls, although of no importance any more since the institution of emperors, were still nominated by the Senate. The years were named after them (until 541). From then on the emperor became *Consul Perpetuus*.
3. Galla Placidia, sister of the emperors Arcadius (Eastern Empire) and Honorius (Western Empire), wife of Athaulf, king of the Visigoths, lived at Ravenna after his death. (Ivory carving in the cathedral of Monza).
4. The Emperor Valentinian III. (435–455 A.D.) of the Western Empire, son of Galla Placidia.

Centre Group

5–11. Figures important for their costume from the choir of the Church of San Vitale, Ravenna. Mosaics after 552 A.D. The Emperor Justinian (9) and the Empress Theodora (11) with offerings accompanied by their retinue. 5. Companion of the Empress. 6. Lady in waiting to the Empress. 7. Distinguished courtier. 8. Weapon-bearer of the Emperor. His magnificent shield studded with jewels and decorated with the initials of Christ: X and P (Ch and R).

9. The Emperor Justinian. 10. Bishop Maximinian in the Emperor's retinue.

11. The Empress Theodora.

12. Byzantine warrior (7th–8th centuries). According to an ivory carving in the cathedral, Aix-la-Chapelle.

Bottom Group

13. The Emperor Nicephorus III. (died 1081) wearing a rich outer garment exposing the lower part of the tight sleeves of the tunic. Triangular neck and shoulder collar, from the 10th century on, part of the ruler's official costume. Beard (in fashion in the Byzantine Empire from the 7th to the 14th centuries). Crown with ornamental chains.

14. Dignitary from the same period (11th century) wearing a mantle in the shape of the Greek chlamis. Red socks, sandals with white straps.

15. The Emperor Romanus II. (died 963).

16 and 17. The Emperor Nicephorus III. (cf. 13) and his consort in official costume; the emperor wears the *pallium* wrapped round shoulders and hips, originally a clerical garment. It is made of coloured brocade (in contradistinction to the clerical pallium, which was white and decorated with crosses). The empress, too, wears the insignia of a ruler: pallium, sceptre, crown.

MIDDLE AGES. MONASTIC ORDERS AND ORDERS OF KNIGHTS. 28

Top Group

1–5. Orders of Knights.

1. Templars. The Order of the Knights Templar was founded at Jerusalem in 1119 by French crusaders. Their headquarters were south from the Mosque of Omar on the Temple site from whence they derived their name. Red cross on white linen mantle.

2. Armoured Templar: coat of mail covered by a girdled tunic with sword, belt and sword.

3. Knight of the Teutonic Order. Representation of 1243. It was in 1189/90, during the third crusade, that crusaders from Bremen and Lübeck laid the foundation of a hospital near Acre, whose brethren were raised to the rank of an Order of Knights by German princes in 1196. The order consisted of knight-brethren and priest-brethren. In 1211 the order received as a gift the district of Burgenland in Transylvania and later on the Kulmerland and parts of East and West-Prussia. White mantle with black cross.

4. Knight of the Order of the Hospitallers of St. John of Jerusalem (16th century). Originally founded about 1048 in Jerusalem for the purpose of nursing sick pilgrims (Hospital and hostel near the Church of the Holy Sepulchre). After the first Crusade the hospitallers were raised to the rank of an Order of Knights, the oldest of such orders, in 1113 was reorganized and received special rules. The order consisted of three classes of brethren: knights, priests, serving brethren. Their first headquarters were in Ptolemais, from 1291 in Cyprus, 1309 in the island of Rhodes (hence called Knights of Rhodes), 1530–1798 in Malta (Knights of Malta), 1826 in Ferrara, 1834 in Rome. Oldest costume of the Order: black mantle with a white linen eight-cornered cross.

5. Lady of honour of the Order of St. John of Jerusalem. Costume of a later period (18th century).

6–16. Monastic Orders.

Centre Group

6. Dominican. The preaching order of the Dominicans was founded in 1215 by the Castilian Dominic. Costume: white garment, white *scapulary*, large cloth made of two pieces, covering back and chest and a hole for the head. Black hooded mantle.

7. Franciscan. The order was founded by the layman Francis of Assisi in 1208. The Franciscans' garb is the brown cotton cowl with a rope in place of a girdle and sandals on bare feet.

8. Augustinian monk. It was not until 1244, after having been founded years, that the Augustinians had their rule formally confirmed. Indoor garment: white woollen cowl and *scapulary*. Outdoor garb: wide black cowl with long wide sleeves and hood. Through Luther, who had been an Augustinian monk, this garment was adopted by the Reformers and Protestant preachers.

9. Benedictine monk. The order of the Benedictines was founded by St. Benedict of Nursia in 528 as the first residential monastic order at the monastery of Monte Cassino near Naples. His statutes became the foundations of the whole monastic life. They vowed obedience, chastity and poverty. The abbot was the head of the monks whose time was divided into periods of prayer and labour (*ora et labora*). Later on science and art as well as teaching children were some of the tasks of these monks. Their garb, although differing according to districts, consisted in the main of a black cowl, mantle and *scapulary*.

10. Carthusian monk. The order of Carthusian monks was founded in 1084 by St. Bruno of Cologne at Chartreuse near Grenoble. The rule of the order demanded an ascetic life and silence outside the Holy Service, forgoing meat dishes and living in solitary cells. Costume: white cloth cowl with leather girdle, white *scapulary* both parts connected by a broad strip of material at the back and front, black mantle. The order exists in France, Italy and Switzerland.

11. Capuchin monk. The order of Capuchins is one of the many branches of the Franciscan order (cf. 7) also called Minorites, founded in 1527 in Italy. They are named after the pointed brown capouch attached to the cowl. The mantle reaches down to below the arms. In place of a girdle they wear a knotted rope. The cowl was rather tight, just wide enough to allow it to be slipped over. Sandals, socks only in emergency. The costume is brown. They wear a beard and carry a rosary.

Bottom Group

12. Carmelite monk on outdoor costume. The order was founded on Mount Carmel in the Holy Land in 1156 by the South Italian crusador Bertold and confirmed by the Pope in 1226. Among the younger branches of the order the Observants, or barefooted Carmelites follow a more severe rule. The picture shows a shoeless Carmelite monk in a brown woollen cowl and *scapulary*. Outer garment: a tight white hooded mantle. Rosary.
13. Carthusian monk in outdoor garb: soutane (cloth tunic), white *scapulary*. black hooded mantle which is gathered at the shoulders. Black shoes.
14. Carthusian monk wearing indoor garb: white cowl, white scapulary with hood (cf. 10).
15. Carthusian nun during the ceremony of investiture when taking the veil. Ornaments for this special occasion: Over the white woollen garment the scapulary held together by bands. Full white mantle, white neck-cloth. Brown veil. Blue stole with golden crosses. Blue maniple hanging over left arm. In her left hand she carries a burning candle and wears a five pointed crown on her head. Doyé in *Die alten Trachten der männlichen und weiblichen Orden.* (Leipzig, 1929), says that "*this garb, if historically true, was worn against the rule.*" The indoor outfit consisted of white skirt, white scapulary and neck-cloth, white veil which was also lined with white material. Black shoes, white cloth mantle.
16. Nun of the order of the Visitation, so-called Salesian nun. The order was founded in 1610. Black pleated dress of coarse wool with long, fairly wide sleeves which are turned back exposing tight sleeves underneath. Silver cross attached to a black woollen ribbon hanging down over her breast. White neck-cloth *(barbette)* tied round the neck. Black fillet, black veil. The Salesian order, like numerous others, followed the Augustinian rule.

29 ECCLESIASTICAL COSTUME AND ORDERS OF KNIGHTS. *1400–1800.*

Top Group

1. Roman Deacon (1450) wearing a long white dalmatica *(subucula)*.
2. Flemish Deacon (1460) wearing a short outer dalmatica over the long *subucula*.
3. Priest about 1470 wearing vestments for the mass with chasuble (round bell-shaped mantle, cut out at the sides) and stole only the fringed ends of which are visible over the dalmatica.
4. Bishop wearing double chasuble over the dalmatica and alba and a mitre, a bishop's crozier and maniple (originally a linen sudarium). According to Matthias Grünewald's painting in Munich, about 1525.
5. Pope in ceremonial costume, that is as a bishop of the Lateran church, Rome. His mass vestments consist of a shoulder wrap *(humerale)*, an alba (white gown), a cingulum girdle, not visible in this picture), a tunicella (fringed dalmatica reaching down below the knees) and outer and more richly decorated dalmatica, a stole (a narrow band), a chasuble, embroidered gloves and mitre (the papal tiara consisting of three crowns). Crozier with double cross. According to a Low-Rhenish painting about 1480.

Centre Group

6. Bishop of the 17th century wearing ceremonial robes with richly decorated chasuble. Bands *(fanones)* are hanging down from the mitre. Dutch (After a painting by Rubens).
7. Pope Pius VI. (1775–99) pronouncing the benediction in Vienna and wearing the white chasuble over the stole, tunicella and alba, as well as the mitre.
8. Bishop wearing canon's vestments: violet soutane and over it a surplice. Over the shoulders a short cape *(manteletta)*. Violet beret *(biretta)*.
9. Pope when appearing in public (not at holy service), wearing white silk soutane, surplice, red velvet cape *(mozetta)* richly trimmed with ermine, red gold-embroidered stole. Red velvet hat. In addition to the white papal garments he wears the scarlet of a cardinal in his position as Cardinal-bishop of Rome.
10. Priest of the Order of the Knights of Our Lady of Mount Carmel and St. Lazarus in Jerusalem. Costume as 8.

6–10. After Schwan, *Abbildungen der geistlichen Orden*, 1791.

Bottom Group

11. Lady of Honour or *Lady of Devotion* of the Order of St. John in the 18th century, wearing black garment with black mantle, tight-fitting linen cap over the shorn head and over this a black stiff veil like a cap with lappets. (The veil is the symbol of betrothal to Christ. The linen headdress is a reminder of Christ's shroud). White cross on breast and left side of the mantle.
12. Knight of the Spanish Order of St. James of the Sword, founded in 1170 by King Ferdinand of Leon and Galicia, 14th century. White garment with girdle. Mantle fastened by a cord. Gauntlets. Beret with St. Andrew's scallop shell. Red cross on white mantle.
13. Knight of the Order of the Golden Fleece (18th century), founded in 1429 by Philip the Good, duke of Burgundy at Bruges (in remembrance of the ancient Greek legend according to which the Argonauts sailed off to Colchis to carry home the Golden Fleece (ram's skin). Bright red robe and wine-red wide mantle lined with white material and richly embroidered. Golden chain of the Order with the golden fleece *(toison d'or)* pendent on it. White shoes with red heels.
14. Knight of the Order of St. Stephen, Hungary, founded in 1764 by Maria Theresia, the robe resembling the costume of the Hungarian magnates.
15. Teutonic Knight of the 18th century (the Teutonic Order was founded in 1189). The costume reflects the rococo fashion but the colour of the material is black without pattern or embroidery. The special costume of the Order is represented by the white mantle (with lapels) ornamented with a black cross, the simple scarf and the high boots (cf. Doyé, *Die alten Trachten der Orden.* 1929).

GERMANY *from the Merovingians to the Hohenstaufen emperors, 500–1200.* 30

Top Group

1–3. Frankish noblemen of the Merovingian and Carolingian times. Long-sleeved tunic decorated with silk braids or embroidered patterns. Girdle. Mantle fastened on the right shoulder by a brooch. Long hose bound with bands at the knees and the lower part of the leg bandaged according to old Germanic fashion leaving the toes exposed. Otherwise soft leather boots.

4. Frankish warrior with round shield with the buckle fixed on the crossed iron frame. Carolingian iron helmet with crest. Breeches. Bands wound round the legs and sandals. About 850.

5. Warrior with helmet and the rest of the head protected by armour. Coat of mail with skirt studded with metal plates. About 900–950.

Centre Group

6. Frankish woman in a long-sleeved tunic the borders gaily decorated. Mantle fastened on the breast by a brooch. Soft pointed leather shoes in the Roman fashion.

7. Frankish noble lady wearing two garments, the one underneath with long tight sleeves, which are visible. Embroidered long mantle pulled over the head.

8. Charles the Bold (youngest son of the Emperor Louis the Pious (le Pieux) first King of France (Western Frankish kingdom 840–877).

9. A Princess. 8 and 9 according to a miniature. (Bible of Charles the Bold).

10. Carolingian king according to a relief on a book cover.

11. The German king Henry II. (1022–1024) according to a miniature.

12. Frankish man of the 10th century (cf. 1–3) wearing boots.

13. Frankish woman wearing linen kerchief over her head.

Bottom Group

14. The Emperor Rudolph of Swabia (chosen in opposition to Henry IV. of Germany, died 1080) in coronation robes. According to a tombstone at Merseburg.

15–17. Women's costume of the later 11th century. Girdled garments which are slipped over long-sleeved tunics. 15 and 17 wear a long fur-lined mantle, fastened over the breast with a cord. 16 wears an unusual undergarment which is open in front and exposes the long tight-fitting hose.

18. Sword-bearer of the time of the crusades with parti-coloured garment; two pieces differing in colour sewn together down the middle.

19. Noble youth in a long tunic with high collar and gathered by a girdle.

EUROPE. *Early Middle Ages (300–1000) and Byzantine Empire, 9th–11th Centuries.* 31

Top Group

1 and 2. Men of the earliest Middle Ages (according to ivory carvings) in Florence, 4th century.

3. Warrior in the late Roman costume (ivory carving from the episcopal throne of St. Maximilianus at Ravenna).

4. South European man of rank (according to an ivory carving).

5. Warrior (according to the mosaics of San Marco, Venice).

Centre Group

6. Man of rank of the 10th century (ivory slab in the museum at Milan. The Emperor Otto I. and his family kneeling).

7. Woman of rank of the early Middle Ages with the draped veil-like mantle. (Mosaic in San Marco).

8. The Emperor Honorius, 5th century (ivory slab at Aosta).

9. Figure (servant girl from the mosaics of the church of Santa Maria Maggiore, Rome. Triumphal arch, 5th century).

10. Warrior (according to an ivory carving formerly in the Kaiser Friedrich Museum, Berlin).

Bottom Group

11. Greek (Byzantine) patriarch of the 9th century. The ecclesiastical stole is seen hanging down. It was a wide band put round the neck, made of gold thread. The shoulders are covered by a cape (instead of the palladium), woven through with gold threads. Along the right leg hangs the so-called *hypogonation*: the bag with tassel of the higher clergy.

12. Bishop (Pontifex) of the Greek church with the *pallium*. With the Romans the pallium was originally a mantle which in clerical costume was reduced to a wide band (similar to the stole). In the Roman Catholic Church it was bestowed by the Pope on the archbishops, rarely on bishops, as a special sign of distinction. The bishops of the Greek church generally wear it. The ecclesiastical pallium is always white with red crosses.

13. Representation of a priest of high rank wearing a pallium (but with black crosses for a religious festival). From the mosaics of the Church of San Marco, Venice.

14. Byzantine monk with a tunic arranged in folds and mantle. High leather boots over the patterned hose.

15. Greek-Byzantine empress from the time of the first crusade about 1096.

GERMANY. *Time of the Minnesingers and Crusades. 12th–13th Centuries.* 32

1. Woman of rank in a long close fitting garment with tight sleeves above the elbow, and falling down wide and open below it. 12th century.

2. The Emperor Frederick I. (Barbarossa) as a crusader (according to a miniature from Northern Italy, end of 12th century).

3. Woman of rank wearing a short-sleeved tunic-like garment over the long under garment with long ermine trimmed sleeves. Shoulder mantle. Kerchief. Late 12th century.

5. Peasant in a girdled tunic with pleated skirt. Long hose. Hood.

5. Jew with a long girdled tunic and mantle trimmed with yellow stripes. Pointed yellow hat (Jew's hat).

6. Vagrant minstrel with fiddle wearing a furred tunic.

7–19. Costumes from the so-called *Manesse-Liederhandschrift* (a manuscript of songs) in the University library of Heidelberg.

7. Princely minnesinger.
8. Man of rank.
9. and 10. Woman and girl belonging to the court.
11. Man in travelling attire.
12. The Jewish minnesinger Süsskind with the pointed *Jew's hat* as prescribed by the Lateran Council of 1215.
13–17. Ordinary minnesingers, dancing and playing instruments.
18 and 19. Minstrels.

33 FRANCE IN THE MIDDLE AGES. *900–1400.*

1–6. French Costume in the 11th century (partly according to frescos in the vaulting of the Abbey Church of St. Savin at Poitou). The peculiar pointed conical caps partly with the point bent down, (similar to the ancient *Phrygian* cap) are striking. Similar in shape is the helmet with bands (3 and 6): Knights in the coat of mail over the tunic.

Centre Group

7. Knight wearing scale armour over coat of mail and a flat iron hat.
8 and 9. Squires in girdled tunics with caps also covering the ears and tied under the chin.
10. Knight with battle-axe wearing a material garment over the coat of mail.
11. Elderly man with sleeveless tunic falling in folds down to the knees and a hood attached to it.
12. Falcon-bearer with a head-dress tied under the chin (similar to 8 and 9) and wearing long hooded cloak and gauntlets.
13 and 14. Youth and woman in hooded cloaks (13 shows the hood hanging down over the back; 14 has drawn it over the head.
15. Girl in long-sleeved garment, the upper part close-fitting. 7–15 Miniature paintings from the 12th–13th centuries.

34 NORMANS AND ANGLO-SAXONS. *11th to 14th Centuries.*

Top Group

1–9. According to representations on the embroidered tapestry at Bayeux (Normandy) after 1066 (Battle of Hastings).
1. Fully armed Norman horseman. The coat of mail consists of material with rings sewn on. The legs are protected in the same way. Over the hood of mail is the basinet reinforced by bands with nose guard. Wooden shield, lance.
2. Light-armed Norman. The hair at the back of his head shorn in the Norman fashion.
3. Dismounted horseman from the army of the Anglo-Saxon King Harold. Armour like No. 1. Legs bandaged with leather bands. Buckle shield.
4. Anglo-Saxon warrior with club and large wooden shield.

Centre Group

5. Norman warrior with battle axe (not used by the Anglo-Saxons). Scaled hawberk, mantle fastened by a brooch, calves bandaged.
6. Light-armed Norman in a short girdled tunic.
7. Anglo-Saxon archer. The small conical cap covers half long hair.
8. Norman with a large wooden shield.
9. Light-armed Anglo-Saxon with a moustache and long hose.

Bottom Group

10–12. Norman peasants (12th century).
13 and 14. Peasant women (13th–14th centuries); 14: hood with nape protection.
15. Man of rank in fur-lined travelling dress. Hood with collar and fur cap (14th century).

35 ARMOURED KNIGHTS *(800–1300)* CRUSADERS *(1100–1300).*

Top Group

Protective armour: helmet, coat of mail, shield.
Offensive weapons: lance, sword, dagger, battle-axe and mace.

1. Knight with iron helmet over leather cap, scaled coat of mail (iron plates fixed on leather doublet) over pleated leather skirt; round buckler, lance, long sword, calves bandaged, shoulder mantle *(sagum)* from the Carolingian period about 800.
2. Knight wearing helmet with iron bands and nose guard *(nasale)* chain mail (with hose all in one piece). Elongated, large three-cornered shield with rounded corners. Short sword.
3. Knight with iron helmet and short chain hawberk. Round shield and battle-axe.
4. Knight covered by barrel helmet (flat-topped helmet; *heaume*). Over the ringed coat of mail *(byrnie)* the girdled and sleeveless surcoat falling down to the knees and called *cote armure*. Small pointed shield.
5. Knight wearing on his head a basinet with nose-guard *(nasale* cf. 2). Surcoat over coat of mail. Large shield. Horn.

Centre Group

6–12. Crusaders.
6. Crusader, wearing helmet, strengthened by a band, from the time of the German Emperor Henry VI.
7. Crusader from the time of Barbarossa. Barrel helmet. The horse's trappings ornamented with coat of arms.

Bottom Group

8. Knight wearing chain mail. 12th century.
9. Saracen warrior with two lances and large round shield. Short girdled and quilted tunic over loin-skirt. In front of him the small Saracen fist-shield. On his head a turban.
10. Knight covered by an iron hat. 13th century, time of the crusades.
11. High helmet resembling bishop's mitre.
12. Knight wearing ringed mail *(byrnie)* with hood under the surcoat. In his right hand the barrel helmet. 13th century.

EUROPE, KNIGHTS. *14th and 15th Centuries.* 36

Burgundy, France, England, Italy, Poland

Top Group

1. Burgundian armour about 1450. Plate mail over chain mail. Barrel-like cap made of jagged pieces of cloth. From the girdle hang the then fashionable bells.
2. Burgundian armour about 1425.
3. English armour. 15th century. Plate mail which replaced the older chain mail in England about 1450. Battle-axe for beating and pushing, still in use with lance and sword. The long handle indicates the further development towards a *partisan* or halberd about this time.
4. English armour. 14th century (Edward, the Black Prince, died 1376). Chain mail with hood of mail, rerebrace of plate to defend the arms and greaves to protect the legs, close fitting surcoat. It is decorated with the owner's coat of arms.
5. French armoured horseman, archer. He wears *brigantine*, i. e. plate armour. About 1450. At this time the cross-bow replaces the bow in battle.

Centre Group

6. Young Burgundian knight, 14th century, with upright wings or *ailettes* fixed as shoulder or neck pieces to the ringed or chain mail.
7. Knight with bells hanging from the girdle, about 1350.
8. Polish archer. 14th century. From his girdle hangs the hook to stretch the bow.
9. Polish nobleman. 15th century.
10. Horseman alighted, about 1375.

Bottom Group

11–16. Italian battle dress in the 14th century.
11. Armoured soldier protected by numerous plates.
12. Condottiere (Italian general) in mangnificent ceremonial outfit, with field marshal's baton, chain mail covered by plates, surcoat, beret. Decorated horse trappings.
13 and 14. Foot soldiers, mercenaries.
15. Italian knight.
16. Mercenary wearing ringed mail under the *brigantine*. Naked legs. Calves and feet bandaged over pieces of material, narrow shield. Partly after paintings in the Campo-santo at Pisa (about 1350–60).

ENGLAND IN THE MIDDLE AGES. *10th–15th Centuries.* 37

Top Group

1. Anglo-Saxon, 10th century in a long-sleeved tunic gathered by a girdle with a short cape-like mantle fastened by a clasp or brooch on the right shoulder. Hose (in fact stockings sewn together) bandaged with straps or bands. Shoes made of soft material or leather.
2. Irish monk, 10th century.
3. Warrior of the 11th century (time of the Norsemen's invasions) in a thick armoured coat with small iron plates sewn on and a hood attached to it. Underneath tunic reaching down to the calves. Helmet with chinstrap and nose-protection. High soft leather boots.

4 and 5. Women of the 12th century in long-sleeved garments with small girdles and mantles fastened by a cord, a costume which was also common in Germany at the time of the Hohenstaufen. The hair was gathered in the nape by a net. A *chapel* (crown-like cap with cheek and chin band).

6. Girl of the 13th century in a short-sleeved outer garment (cf. the *Suckenie* of the German costume of that period) over the long under garment with tight sleeves. Hooded collar for protection.

Centre Group

7–13. English costume of the 14th century, on the whole corresponding to the prevailing Burgundian-French fashion of the continent.

Bottom Group

14–20. English costume of the 15th century, also following the fashion on the continent. According to examples in Strutt: *Dress and Habits of the People of England*, 1862.

ARMOURED KNIGHTS. FRANCE AND GERMANY. *15th Century.* 38

Top Group

1–5. French.
1. French knight about 1405 in the earlier plate armour. Basinet with movable vizor, underneath the hood of mail with large camail. The plating of the armour which is laced at the back consists of small studded plates on which the skirt of tonlets is fastened as a protection of the loins.
2. French foot soldier under Charles VII. at the time of Joan of Arc about 1430 during the Hundred Years' War.
3. Archer from the same period.
4. French knight of the same period in plated armour. Helmet in the shape of a *salet* with vizor, shield with three buckles, battle axe.
5. Ceremonial armour from the time of King Louis XI. (1461 to 1483).

Centre Group

6–15. German
6. Armour in the princely armoury at Sigmaringen, supposed to have belonged to Count Eitel Friedrich I. of Hohenzollern (died 1439).
7. St. George from the altar by Hans Multscher (died 1463) in Sterzing, Tyrol.
8. St. George (after the wood carving of about 1420, formerly at Kaiser Friedrich Museum, Berlin).
9. St. Gereon (according to a painting in the Museum at Cologne).
10. Knight Konrad of Schauenburg (according to the tomb by Tilman Riemenschneider at Würzburg).

Bottom Group

11. Johann von Eschbach (according to the tomb at Lorch on the Rhine).
12. St. Victor (according to a wood carving in the museum at Wiesbaden).
13. Plate armour about 1450.

14 and 15. Fluted harnesses about 1500. So-called Maximilian armour.

39 ITALIAN MONUMENTS REPRESENTING KNIGHTS. *13th to 15th Centuries.*

1. Statue of a horseman representing Mastino II. (died 1289), by Perino Milanese. 13th century, Verona, tomb of the Scaliger near the church of Santa Maria Antica, Verona.
2. Statue of a horseman, representing Can grande da Verona by Giovanni da Campione. 1329.
3. Tomb of Guglielmo Berardi near the church of Santissima Anunziata at Florence. 14th century.
4. Relief of a horseman (St. George with the dragon) with two bearers of coats of arms. The armour in the antique tradition. Door lintel (sopraporta) on the palace at Vico Mele, Genoa. Lombard school. 15th century.

1–3. Show battle horses with large wide partly decorated trappings. The armoured knights wear 1. the high barrel helmet, 2. the basinet with a barrel helmet hanging down on the back, 3. the iron helmet over the hood of mail and 4. the *salet* with neck plate and vizor.

40 GERMANY. *Garments of People of Rank as represented by 13th Century Sculpture.*

1. Margrave Hermann von Meissen (died 1032) and his consort Reglindis. Statues in the west choir of the cathedral at Naumburg about 1250–70. Both wear the girdled long tunic with close fitting sleeves. The slit to widen the hole for slipping over the head is fastened on the breast by a brooch. Hermann also wears as an outer garment a sleeveless mantle *(Schaperun)* with six ornamental buttons and without girdle. The wide semi-circular mantle is kept in place by means of a band over the chest with flat brooches on both sides. The woman's hair is veiled by a kerchief passed round the chin. Over it she wears the *chapel* in the shape of a cap held in place by a crown-like fillet.
2. Margrave Ekkehard II. von Meissen (died 1046) and his consort Uta. Statues in the west choir of the cathedral at Naumburg. Costume like 1. The man in a long girdled tunic with mantle. The soft cap on his head does not entirely cover his curly hair. The woman's mantle has a high collar. Over the barbe (cf. 1) the cap-like *chapel* but a higher crown-shaped fillet.
3. *Foolish Virgin* and prince of the world as seducer. Statues on the south portal of the west façade of Strasbourg cathedral in Alsace (about 1280–1300). Both their garments consist of the long-sleeved long tunic gathered by a girdle (not visible) which is covered by a wide sleeveless outer garment, the so-called *schaperun*, that of the man having short wide sleeves hanging down from the shoulders as well as ornamental buttons on the chest. The outer garment has slits at the sides which are fastened by buttons. Both wear the fillet-like *chapel* on their heads. The one of the man decorated like a crown.
4. *Synagogue* (Old Testament) with broken rod and veiled eyes. Statue at the side of the *princes* portal on the northern aisle of the Bamberg cathedral. About 1250. Long trailing garment of finest diaphanous material gathered by a girdle. A brooch at the base of the neck.
5. The Emperor Heinrich II. and his consort Kunigunde, the founders of the cathedral at Bamberg. Statues on the left jambs of the south-east portal (Adam's gate) of the cathedral at Bamberg. About 1240. The woman wears a long outer garment *(schaperun)* with girdle over the long girdled tunic, the man wears a mantle draped over one shoulder.
6. *Ekklesia* (the Church, the New Testament). Girdled garment with brooch like 4, covered by a shoulder mantle held by a band across the chest.

41 ARMOURED KNIGHTS. GERMANY AND BURGUNDY. *14th Century.*

Top Group

1–8. German.

1. Over the chain mail short leather doublet reaching down only as far as the loins; breast plate, helmet and helmet-protection. Legs cased in plate; knee cops.

2 and 3. Chain mail covered by leather doublet with chain sewn in.

4. Knight in indoor costume. Doublet, short close fitting cape over chest and back.

Centre Group

5. Knight wearing ermine coat and iron *knee cops* which are attached separately. They later on developed into greaves.
6. Leather doublet down to the loins, leather hose, knee cops.
7. Leather doublet worn over complete chain mail.
8. Doublet with pleated skirt both decorated with embroidered or woven coat of arms.

Bottom Group

9–12. Burgundian.

9 and 9a. Burgundian knight (about 1380) covered by a steel basinet with movable vizor. This form of helmet was called *Hundsgugel* in Germany. Small shield cut out at the side.

10. Knight from Neufchatel, without vizor, about 1370, wearing basinet with camail edge.
11. Standard-bearer about 1300 with the insignia of a crusader who has taken the vows (cross and pilgrim's staff). Flat topped helmet *(heaume)* with the vizor screwed on.
12. Knight's armour about 1370. Lance, large shield for horsemen who had alighted and tried to protect themselves with several of such shields against archers, etc.

KNIGHTS ARMOUR AND WEAPONS. *1500–1575.* 42

Plate armour consisted of the following pieces: helmet with gorget, shoulder plates with pieces connecting them with breast and back plate casing for the arms, elbow cops, gauntlets, coat of mail with steel bands, loin covering, knee cops, greaves, iron shoes (following the fashion of the wide shoes after 1500). This armour of overlapping and movable plates and greaves was even more perfected under Maximilian I. by fluted plates which increased the power of resistance against attack. These coats of mail were called Maximilian armour or Milan armour.

1. German armour made of polished iron with movable iron bands. The metal is either polished or tarnished by oxidizing or applying acids or by painting it black.
2. German steel armour about 1515 with high shoulder plates (French: *passe-gardes*). The right shoulder plate is much smaller and appears as a sort of free-standing disk in order to leave room for fixing the jousting lance. The steel tonlets are rigid, not overlapping and movable.
3. Italian armour. The polished iron decorated by patterns produced by etching.
4. Italian round shield, made of six pieces, similar to the ones in use in Germany about 1500. In France called *rondache*.
5. Heavy helmet with vizor of polished iron (cf. plate 43).
6. Helmet with ear-like appliances standing out (called horse's face, i. e. *Roßstirn* in German). Iron, studded with brass nails and a thorn.
7. Burgundian helmet of polished iron with crest, with protruding nose and nape guards and cheek plates.
8. Iron cap with cheek guards.
9. Pointed iron cap, (called *Birnenhelm*=pear-shaped helmet in German).

10 and 11. Sword hilts with the so-called ass's hoof, ornamental bands surrounding hilt and blade.

Bottom Group

Tilting over the lists with coronet on the end of the lances (cf. plate 43). On the right: Frederick, Count Palatine; on the left: Duke Wilhelm IV. of Bavaria. According to the *Turnierbuch* (Tournament book) of the Bavarian Dukedom 1510–18. Original miniatures. Munich, Bayrische Staatsbibliothek.

EUROPE. MIDDLE AGES. *Helmets and Swords.* 43

1. Pointed helmet with nose guard *(nasal)*.
2. French copper helmet of the 12th century.

3 and 4. Flat topped helmet *(heaume)* with movable vizor, 1280.

5. Painted flat topped helmet *(heaume)*, 1240.
6. Italian flat topped helmet *(heaume)*. About 1250.
7. Head protection from a picture of the 9th century.

8 and 9. German swords 1100–1400.

10. Bassinet with vizor, a close fitting round cap. 1310.
11. Pointed helmet with side wings. French and English. About 1270. Not used after 1325.
12. German basinet. 1370.
13. Pointed basinet with vizor.

14–16. and 21. Northern swords. From the Copenhagen National Museum. 1000–1450.

17. Basinet with nose guard *(nasal)*. 1350.
18. German helmet worn for tilting. 1370.
19. Spanish basinet.
20. English basinet. 1380–90.
22. French sword. About 1375.
23. French basinet with vizor. 1350–90.
24. Spanish sword. 1480.
25. *Salet* with the Wittelsbach crest. 1449.
26. Danish sword. 1400.

27 and 29. Early spear heads of Norsemen.

28. French helmet. 1430.
30. Tournament helmet for fighting with swords and maces. About 1450.
31. French *salade* or salet. 1420.
32. Iron hat. 1460
33. Iron hat, Danish. About 1475.

34 and 36. Salets resembling more modern helmets.

35 a and b. Salets with *mentonnière*, chin protection. 1480.

37. Striped helmet *(armet)* with simple vizor. 1506.
38. Striped helmet *(armet)* with chin guard *(mentonnière)* and vizor.

Bottom Group

39. German knights tilting, from the end of the 12th century. (Reign of the Emperor Heinrich VI.). Helmets with nose guards *(nasals)*; Italian nasale; cf. fig. 1. Small shields, lances with pennons. Right: large horse-cover. From the manuscript of a south-Italian Norman.
40. Spanish knight in the tourney yard. According to a representation in the Alhambra near Granada.
41. Knight, jousting. Beginning of the 14th century. The spear of the opponent (whose picture has not been preserved) is not pointed but shows the little coronal usual at tournaments (sometimes a pointless metal end was fixed). Crested flat-topped helmet *(heaume)*. Surcoat and large horse cover (French: housse). From the Codex Balduini Trevirensis about 1330.
42. Helmet with crest (in the shape of a dragon) of King James I. of Aragon (died 1276). Imitating Oriental forms. Madrid. Armeria Real.

As to the development of helmets: The conical form of the 11th century develops into a large flat-topped (barrel-shaped) helmet *(heaume)* in the 12th century. This flat-topped helmet wrought in one piece is worn over the basinet which, from the 13th century replaced the hood of mail. From about 1300 onwards the basinet is worn without the heaume, developing into a more conical shape in the 14th century and later on becoming more pointed, and is completed by a nose-guard *(nasal)* and vizor. – The iron hat (32–33) is an old independent shape of helmet disdained by knights but worn by the ordinary soldiers, vassals, archers and cross-bow men. When later adopted by knights two slits were pierced into the front brim, through which the horseman with his head bent could look. This is the origin of the salet (French: salade = bowl. 35 a and 35 b) of the late 15th century which adopts the long horizontal slit for the eyes from the iron hat but has a less projecting brim. It also adds the *mentonnière* (35 b and 25) as a characteristic novelty. This mentonnière, a movable chin protection, is the forerunner of the vizor, also the neck guard of the salet, which originally is a rigid protecting part of the helmet (see figs. 31 and 35 a) becomes a movable joint made of several plates (36) – Tournament helmets vary according to purpose whether for tilting or jousting and often have the vizor made of steel bands or trellissed rods (30). (They were specially favoured in heraldry). – In the time of Maximilian I. the so-called knight's helmet appears. It originated from the basinet, but the camail of the basinet gave way to the rigid steel plates, the gorget (as a protection of the neck) while the vizor consisted of two movable overlapping parts: the chin-guard and the vizor proper, which turn on the same pivot.

44 FRANCE. *14th Century.*

Top Group

1. Youth in a semi-long girdled doublet, hooded shoulder cape, hose and pointed shoes.
2. Girl wearing a long outer garment gathered by a girdle just below the breasts with wide low neck and sleeves hanging down to the knees. Her hair braided at the sides. (1 and 2 according to ivory tablets).
3. Princess wearing a long trailing garment with long sleeves and outer garment gathered at the waist in rich folds.
4. Prince wearing a close-fitting short doublet fastened in front by buttons and a low belt. The long open sleeves expose the long and patterned sleeves of the under garment. Hooded cape and parti-coloured hose (so-called *mi-parti*).
5. Courtier wearing jagged coat with jagged hooded cape (cf. German *Gugel*, plate 53, 9 and 10).
6. Girl wearing parti-coloured outer garment slashed open at the sides, with long hanging sleeves.
7. Figure similar to 5; back view, the hood *(gugel)* pulled over the head.

Centre Group

8. Knight wearing a girdled short close-fitting tunic with hood and a tight fitting hat with the narrow brim turned up.
9. Similar to 3, the garment shows a close fitting bodice.
10. Dandy in a short tight-fitting coat buttoned down the front, a belt round the hips, a collar with hood ending in a long liripipe.
11. Woman of rank wearing a long garment with long sleeves hanging down to the ground and having slits for the arms. As an outer garment she wears the so-called surcoat, a sleeveless low-necked jacket which looks like a shoulder cape on this figure.
12. Prince at the court of Charles V. of France (died 1380) with a cloak-like outer garment with long padded sleeves (so-called *tabard*). On his head a cap with a liripipe worn round the neck. The high, upright collar is attached to the short tunic under the coat.

Bottom Group

13. Women of rank in a long-sleeved gown with a girdle right under the breasts. Head-dress: the new-fashioned conical hat (steeple cap) with a long flowing veil.
14. Judge wearing a long fur trimmed tunic *(tabard*, cf. 12) slashed open at the sides, slit sleeves padded at the shoulders. Narrow-brimmed hat.
15. Youth wearing the new-fashioned short and close-fitting jacket with wide sleeves exposing the tight sleeves of the under garment.
16. Prince wearing the knee-length bell-shaped outer cloak *(heuque* or *huque*; in German: *Hoike* or *Heuke)*. Slit sleeves over the short tunic with standing collar. Hat with liripipe.
17. Distinguished citizen in a long wide outer cloak *(tabard)*.
18. Young courtier in a short, girdled outer jacket with half open hanging sleeves over the short under jacket which has standing collar and tight sleeves. Turban-like cap. (The short jacket was called *jacquette* in French and *Schecke* or *Hänslein* in German.)

45 BURGUNDIAN FASHION *represented in Flemish Book Illustrations (Miniatures) of the 15th Century.*

Top Picture

Reception and banquet at the court of the Duke of Burgundy. Miniature from the *Geschichte des Karl Martell* (history of Charles Martel). Painted at Bruges 1470 by Loyset Liédet. The ladies on the left wearing the high conical Burgundian steeple cap *(hennin)* and long trailing gowns girdled under the breasts; the men wearing either the short jacket or long coat with padded sleeves *(mahoîtres)*, high or medium high hats with narrow brims, long pointed shoes without the wooden sandals attached (cf. plate 51).

Bottom Picture

Coronation ceremony with retinue. Miniature from Jean Mansel's *Fleur des histoires*, painted about 1425–1435 by the so-called *Mansel Master*. Most of the women wear the high head-dress made of kerchiefs and drawn out at the sides to the form of a pair of bull's horns wide veil, and a long fur trimmed outer garment draped in such a way as to expose the gown beneath. Short low-necked bodice. The kneeling woman on the left as well as two others in the outer court wear, in place of the short low-necked bodice, an ermine jacket with pieces cut away under the arms and on the hips. These jackets were worn by princesses, only on ceremonial occasions and weddings, in the 15th century. (Photographs by Prof. Dr. Friedrich Winkler.)

46 BURGUNDY. HEAD-DRESS. *15th Century.*

1. Middle class woman with a large linen head-dress, covering the hair. According to R. van der Weyden.
2. Distinguished Italian merchant (representing his country in Bruges) wearing high Burgundian beaver hat, 1434, according to Jan van Eyck's double portrait of Arnolfini and his wife.
3. Burgomaster's wife from Bruges, 1480, in a medium high Burgundian cap with veil (so-called *hennin*). According to Memling.

4. Man with conical cap.
5. Learned man with hat made of a roll of material from which folds of cloth hang down (cf. 6 and 8). According to Quentin Massys.
6. Burgundian man of rank in the new-fashioned turban-hat. 1433. According to Jan van Eyck.
7. Duke Philip the Good of Burgundy (died 1467) with cropped hair giving the impression of a wig.
8. The same merchant Arnolfini in a hat made of a roll of stuff from which on one side the liripipe is hanging down and from the other a piece of material (cf. 5). According to Jan van Eyck. 1439.
9. Youth from Bruges with long curled hair falling down to his shoulders. According to Hans Memling. 1487.
10. The Count of Croy with his hair cut like 7. According to Hans Memling.

47 LATE MIDDLE AGES. FOOTWEAR *(Pointed shoes and wooden under-shoes).*

1. Pointed shoe with wooden under-shoe.
2. Pointed shoes with the point turned up and wooden under-shoes.
3 and 4. Pointed shoe in the museum of Colmar in Alsace (about 1460). (The under-shoe is a later and incorrect reconstruction).
5. Pointed shoe in addition to greaves and spurs.
6. Pointed shoe, part of the armour.
7. Ordinary wooden under-shoe, seen from above.
8. Pointed under-shoe. Side view.
9. Elongated flat under-shoe, side view.
10. Elongated under-shoe seen from above.
11. The same shoe seen from below.
12. Pointed boot of king James I. of Scotland.
13. Pointed boot with short under-shoe.
14. Short pointed shoe seen from below.
15. Pointed shoe.
16. Shoe as part of the armour, similar to 6.
17. Flat under-shoe showing the straps.
18. Thick under-shoe with wide strap in front. (According to originals and works by Hefner von Alteneck, Weiss, von Falke and Heyne). These pointed shoes (French: poulaine = prow) are already mentioned at the Synod of Reims 972, it is true but they only became fashionable in the 14th century, originating in France they were imitated in Burgundy, from there went to Germany, England and Scotland. During the whole of the 15th century they were considered a requisite of distinguished costume. The points were sometimes turned up or held up by bands or chains. The wooden under-shoes worn as a protection against the dirt and mud of the unpaved streets were mostly raised by thick heels. We hear from a chronicle of 1480 that the fashion of the pointed shoe disappeared about this time and that shoes with broad toes came into fashion which after 1500 remained in use for about a generation.

48 ITALY. EARLY RENAISSANCE. *1485–90 according to Mural Paintings by Domenico Ghirlandaio.*

Top Picture

A Florentine woman of rank (Ludovica Tornabuoni) and her retinue visiting a woman in childbed. *Birth of Mary*, mural painting by Domenico Ghirlandaio, choir chapel of Santa Maria Novella, Florence (left wall) 1486–90.

Bottom Picture

Birth of John the Baptist. Mural painting by Ghirlandaio (as above, right wall).
Both pictures show characteristic costumes of Florentine women and girls of different classes towards the end of the Early Italian Renaissance.

49 GERMAN KNIGHTS' *apparel about 1500–1515.*

1. Knights riding to take part in tilting, i. e. display of fighting by several combatants. Plate harness with overlapping pieces at the joints. Lances with blunt points. They were not manipulated by the hand alone but they were supported by two hooks, attached to the armour, one holding the lance from below and the one in front from above to keep it in a horizontal position. The horses, too, (strong stallions) had plates of armour on their heads. In addition, there were the magnificent tournament trappings, often embroidered with symbolical pictures and letters. The shape of the surcoat with long wide skirts corresponds to men's fashion about 1500. (From the tourney book by Hans Burgkmair, the Younger; formerly in the possession of the Princes of Hohenzollern.)

Bottom Picture

Tournament with pointed lances. Knights jousting. On the left Duke William IV. of Bavaria (died 1550), on the right Ritter von Egloffstein. (According to the tourney book of Duke William IV. of Bavaria.) Original miniatures in the Bavarian State Library, Munich about 1515.

50 FRANCE. *First Half of the 15th Century.*

Top Group

1–4. Young men of rank hawking; 1 and 2 wearing wide and long fur-trimmed girdled coats, open in front over short *pourpoint* or *jacquette*, small beret with ostrich feather over the tight fitting cap *(calotte)*. 3 and 4 wearing short skirted coats, conical hats with narrow brim, tight hose and soles attached under the feet.
5 and 6. Youths wearing short fur-trimmed jackets with slits for the arms, exposing the long sleeves of the tunic. Soft pointed shoes, 5 with under-shoes, high heeled wooden soles as a protection against the mud in the streets.

Centre Group

7. Similar to 1 and 2 with specially long sleeves.
8 and 9. Elderly men in long gowns (slipped over the head).

10. Lady wearing the sleeveless surcoat slipped over the head over the wide-sleeved outer garment, showing the narrow sleeves of the undergarment.
11. Lady wearing a veiled coif drawn out into two points at the sides and a short-sleeved outer garment over the patterned under-garment which has wide sleeves sewn onto it.
12. Princess wearing a low-necked trailing and girdled outer garment over the long-sleeved undergarment.

Bottom Group

13–17. French ladies of rank in long trailing gowns some of them with girdle under the breasts (14). In the low-cut neck a small stomacher is inserted (14–17). Figs. 13 and 16 wear the new fashioned short fur-trimmed surcoat which is open in front. They wear various shapes of the characteristic *hennin* (the Burgundian steeple cap with veils floating from it).

51 FRANCE. *(Charles VIII., 1483–98, Louis XII., 1498–1515).*

Top Group

1. Lady wearing a somewhat shorter garment over a trailing under-garment and a head-dress in the Italian style covering ears and nape.
2. Man of rank in hunting costume with a horn hanging from a belt and wearing a beret, a knee-length coat with turned up cuffs and richly decorated borders. The shoes are slightly pointed (forming the transition to the broad toes of the 16th century).
3. Queen with a long trailing outer garment with slits for the arms and a veil falling down from her head.

4 and 5. Ladies in waiting wearing draped outer garments with low cut neck exposing the fine Frisian linen. The woman on the right wears a head-dress covering the nape with a sort of roll on top.

Centre Group

6 and 7. King in a long sleeveless fur-trimmed mantle over the long pleated skirted doublet, close-fitting cap under the beret. Shoes with broad toes. Behind him the squire carrying his sword (6) wearing an outer garment which is fastened up at the front.

8. Man of rank, sitting with a flute. Mantle with long sleeves hanging down to the knees. Medium length hair. Beret.
9. Lady of rank in a trailing gown with long wide hanging sleeves with slits for the arms, showing the sleeves of the undergarment. Velvet turban-like cap fastened under the chin.
10. Man in a ceremonial costume: under-garment with scarlet sleeves, over it long sleeveless trailing gown, slashed open at the sides and fastened by means of ribbons. Red chain round his neck made of tassels. Medium length hair, cut straight over the forehead. Flat broad shoes.

Bottom Group

11. Lady in mourning. Hood-like veil with pleated kerchief in front, so-called barbette. Long fur-lined gown.
12. Old man wearing wide mantle with cape-like collar. Berte with ostrich feather. Wide shoes with slits (about 1510).
13. Messenger with sealed letter. Coat as worn by heralds (shape of the dalmatica) with embroidered heraldic designs. The staff is the emblem of the messenger.

14 and 15. Distinguished couple wearing garments similar to 4 and 10.

52 BURGUNDIAN FASHION. *1425–90.*

Top Group

1 and 2. Courtiers about 1470 wearing a long *houppelande*, i. e. the long ceremonial girdled garment, open in front mostly with long sleeves and padded shoulders *(mahoîtres)*. High padded conical caps.

3 and 4. Ladies of the court, in long trailing gowns with high girdles and low cut neck. They wear the high Burgundian caps (steeple caps) with veils or fine linen kerchiefs forming an elaborate decoration (3). The under-garment *(cotte)* can hardly be seen.

5. Young Burgundian Duke (Charles the Bold) wearing a medium-length girdled outer coat over the short doublet *(pourpoint)* with collar and long sleeves. Fur beret with ostrich feather.

Centre Group

6. Queen Charlotte (of Savoy), consort of Louis XII. of France, wearing a Burgundian costume with steeple cap *(hennin*, cf. 9).
7. Young courtier wearing long fur-trimmed *houppelande* open in front with low cut neck (cf. 1 and 2). Attached to his girdle is the bag for alms *(aumônière)*.
8. Duke Philip the Good (died 1467) wearing the costume of the Grand Master of the *Order of the Golden Fleece*. The characteristic liripipe is hanging down from the cap.

9 and 10. Archduke Maximilian of Austria (later Emperor Maximilian I) and his betrothed, Maria of Burgundy, daughter of Charles the Bold. 1477. (According to a drawing in the Germanische Museum, Nuremberg). Maximilian wearing the *houppelande* open in front over the laced jacket. Shoes with broad toes, no longer the pointed shoes. Maria is wearing the well-known Burgundian costume.

Bottom Group

11. Young man (about 1425) in a half-length jacket with skirt, consisting of four overlapping pieces which are jagged at the edges and embroidered with gold. Out of the sleeves, at the wrists, fall long white jagged linen streamers. The fashion of jagging (i. e. indenting the borders) spread especially from Burgundy at the beginning of the 15th century. His shoulders are covered by a red velvet cape. He wears a wide-brimmed hat made of material with feathers and tightly sewn hose on his legs, as well as wooden undershoes (cf. plate 50). His hair is cut short round the head giving the impression of a cap.
12. Lady in a long trailing girdled gown. On her head a gold-bordered piece of cloth, a flat bag fixed on top of the cap (similar to the kerchief of Italian peasant woman in modern times).
13. Man going hawking, wearing the heavy sleeveless *hoike* (bellshaped coat) which is slashed open at the sides and ornamented with jagging. It is made of velvet and lined

with fur. The gauntlet for hawking, made of stag-leather, has large cuffs. Gaiters round the calves. Pointed shoes. Cap made of a bag and a piece of cloth hanging down, both jagged.

14. Duke Philip the Good of Burgundy. Padded cap with long liripipe. The ringed mail-coat can be seen at the neck under the plates of the armour. Fur-trimmed surcoat and cape round his shoulders are decorated with armorial designs.
15. Young man of rank wearing fur-trimmed *hoike* with wide sleeves fastened on the left shoulder with three jags by means of three buttons. When unbottoned the garment can be slipped over the head. The lower part of the legs is covered by a kind of gaiters. Hair cut straight in front (cf. 11).

ITALIAN EARLY RENAISSANCE. *14th Century* 53

Top Group

1 and 2. Italian princes. 1. wearing a long tunic buttoned down the middle and along the sleeves with lined cloak. 2. wearing a short close-fitting sleeved doublet with a girdle round the lower part. This short doublet, fashionable in Burgundy and France since 1380, exposes the long hose. Shoulder mantle buttoned on the right shoulder according to older fashions. (From the Florentine painting of the *Adoration of the Kings*, about 1375 to 1400, formerly Berlin, Kaiser Friedrich Museum.)

3 and 4. Queen and princess. Back part of the head and the neck covered by the so-called *Rise* made of linen. Short-sleeved outer garment with ermine trimming over the long-sleeved under-garment. (According to a miniature, Naples 1352).

5 and 6. Lady (6) with servant (5) both wearing a high-girdled coloured outer garment with semi-long wide sleeves over a longer under-garment. The lady wears a wide cloak over it. (According to Giotto's frescoes in the Capella dell'Arena at Padua about 1305–8).

Centre Group

7. Municipal mercenary wearing a short girdled coat with sleeves and a basinet.
8. Man of rank wearing a cloth hat with the ends of the cloth capuccio sticking out. Underneath a white cap covering the cheeks. Long wide mantle with wide sleeves (the costume of learned men) about 1350.

9 and 10. People of rank in a short girdled tight coat with hanging sleeves and a hood which was worn with the liripipe (originally only worn by lower-class people, in German called *Gugel*) about 1350.

11. Lady about 1320 wearing a richly draped outer garment with wide sleeves over the trailing tunic with buttoned sleeves and a narrow high collar which is sewn on. Veil-like kerchief.

12 and 13. Man of rank (side and front views) about 1320. Under-garment reaching down to the knees. Right: open mantle with a hood sewn on, decorated with a long liripipe.

Bottom Group

14–16. Noble ladies about 1340 wearing long trailing gowns with narrow braid trimming around the neck. 15 and 16 wear an outer garment with wide or hanging sleeves over the long-sleeved under-garment. Over the fine plaited hair 14 wears a round cap with the ends of the pleated cloth standing up, 16 wears a draped veil with lappets.

17. Musician (knight) in a long coat (slashed open at the sides) over a tight-sleeved under-garment. The garland of the Minnesingers on his head.
18. Young lady of rank wearing a medium-length sleeveless outer-garment over the long tunic with long and tight-fitting sleeves. Plaits arranged like garlands on the head.
19. Citizen in a long garment and a shorter outer garment (like 18) slit at the sides with a hole for the neck. Cap over the linen cap with lappets.
20. Ordinary citizen in a short girdled coat and cap, the cloth ends hanging down.
21. Gentleman about 1370 wearing a fastened-up cloth coat with jagged seam and hood with collar attached on to the coat. According to small sculptures and paintings of the 14th century, partly according to frescoes of the Campo-santo at Pisa.

ITALIAN EARLY RENAISSANCE *about 1425–80.* 54

Top Group

1–4. Heralds in short outer garments, some with girdles over a shorter jacket recognizable only by the tight sleeves.

5. Man of rank (king) in a long coat with hanging sleeves.
6. Youth in a short quilted garment with wide sleeves decorated with emblems.

7 and 8. Youths in dark mantles, on their heads caps made by pieces of cloth wound round the head and with liripipe according to the fashion of the Burgundian turban caps.

Centre Group

9. Falcon-bearer wearing a girdled mantle slashed open at the sides which is slipped over the head, so-called giubberello (cf. fig. 1).
10. Very short jacket with sleeves cut wide on top. Outer garment (like 9).

11–15. Group of soldiers. 11 and 14 officers wearing surcoat (cut like 1 and 2) with short sleeves over the plate armour. The soldiers in short jackets some with mantles. Helmets; 11 iron hat, 13 conical pointed basinet with chin-strap, 14 and 15 flat iron caps. 1–8 from Masaccio's (Florence) paintings *Birth of the Virgin* and *Adoration of the Kings.* 11–15 from the *Martyrdom of St. Peter and John the Baptist* by the same artist (about 1425). 9 according to Vittore Pisano's (called Pisanello) *Adoration of the three Kings*, 10 according to Domenico Veneziano, both about 1450.

Bottom Group

16. Duke of Mantua in a girdled mantle (like 9) over short jacket with slit sleeves. Brimless cap (according to Mantegna's frescoes in the castle of Mantua about 1475).

17. Italian knight wearing wide brimmed straw-hat and plate armour over the middle part of which the feather or fur-trimmed surcoat is worn (according to Pisanello's painting: *St. Anthony and St. George* about 1450).

18 and 19. Men's costume from Viterbo. Fez-like caps with or without brim, light sleeveless mantle (similar to 9), the one of the youth on the right is open in front. Slit sleeves with tags (according to Lorenzo da Viterbo's *Marriage of the Virgin*, fresco 1469).

20 and 21. Venetian men's costume made of magnificent material. 20: Fur-trimmed mantle, ambassador's chain, bracelet. 21: Magnificent richly ornamented pleated coat with girdle *(giubbone)* and hanging sleeves. Large hat with fur-brim. Hair falling down to the shoulders.

55 NORTHERN ITALY. EARLY RENAISSANCE *(1440–90) under the Influence of Burgundian Fashion.*

Top Group

1 and 2. Elegant Veronese youths about 1440.

1. In a simple mantle, the *giubberello* in the shape of a *poncho* slit at the sides and without girdle.
2. Wearing a short pleated and quilted jacket with wide winglike sleeves. He wears the originally Burgundian cap which is made of material draped round the head. (1 and 2 according to Pisanello's *Adoration of the three holy Kings*.
3. A representation of a scholar wearing a white fur beret with liripipe.
4. Venetian woman about 1470 wearing an outer garment with slit sleeves, a low neck, double roll cap with veil.
5. Young man with spurs, perhaps a messenger in a short coat trimmed with bells.

Centre Group

6–11. Lombard rich ceremonial costume (according to Vivarini's *Adoration of the three holy Kings*).

6. Groom.
7. Flautist wearing a jagged mantle (cf. Fig. 1: giubberello) over a short brown jacket with parti-coloured hose *(mi-parti)*.

8 and 11 wear the long bell-shaped, fur-lined surcoat *(tabarro)* with open wing-sleeves, partly jagged.

8. One of the kings, 9 and 11 distinguished companions of this king.
9. He wears a half-length jagged outer coat *(giubbone)* with a low belt. On his head the short liripipe *(mazocchio)*.
10. Herald.

Bottom Group

12–14. Venetian costume about 1490 (according to Carpaccio's *Ursula* series, Venice, Academy).

12 and 13. Page and falcon-bearer.

14. Podestà, i. e. burgomaster in a long, wide *houppelande* with wide fur-lined sleeves.

15 and 16. Venetian youths, members of a distinguished guild, the *Compagnia della Scalza* (meaning: stocking), i. e. a sort of *maître de plaisir:* 15 with a short jacket and parti-coloured hose. 16 wearing a long trailing mantle (according to Carpaccio's painting *The Wonder of the Cross*, Venice).

56 ITALY. EARLY RENAISSANCE. *1350 - 1500*

Top Group

1. Young florentine man about 1350 in a long girdled parti-coloured robe of former fashion (according to Taddeo Gaddi, Florence).
2. Hooded cloak over a short tunic with low belt. Close fitting hose and pointed shoes. 1370.
3. Long hooded cloak fastened by buttons.
4. Cloak with wide sleeves. The hood is attached to a special shoulder cape. The liripipe goes out of fashion before the end of the 14th century.
5. Head of the hospital at Siena wearing a long robe and a mantle made of watered silk. Beret (beretto) worn by officials. About 1375.

Centre Group

6. Florentine nobleman about 1400 in a cap shaped like a bag and a long girdled cloak with wide sleeves.
7. Gentleman wearing a short-sleeved cloak over a long-sleeved garment. Gloves with the cuffs extended to a bag. Cap made of a roll of material, the ends falling down onto the shoulders. According to a painting by Fra Angelico about 1450.
8. Lady about 1420 wearing a girdled outer garment with long wide hanging fur-trimmed sleeves. Round cap made of a roll of material over the hair which is arranged in a roll round the head.
9. Young man of rank about 1420. Girdled outer-garment with wide pleated and fur-lined sleeves. Hat decorated with a feather.

Bottom Group

10. Archer wearing small round cap with feather.

11–14. Venetian youths in different attire.

(10–14) according to paintings by Vittore Carpaccio about 1495.

57 ITALY. EARLY RENAISSANCE. *Head-dresses and Hair Styles.*

At the courtly time of the *minnesingers* Latin races preferred fair hair (as had the women of Imperial Rome, who wore the imported fair hair of the Germanic women) and this fashion was still fostered during the Renaissance from the 14th to the 16th centuries. This is specially apparent in Venetian portraits of women who took great pains to bleach their hair. Shaving the eyebrows and the hair of the forehead, sometimes up to the middle of the head in order to show *an egg-like moulded brow* was fashionable in the Middle Ages, and was especially brought to perfection in Italy in the 15th century.

1. Woman's head by Sandro Botticelli with yellow-brown curls and plaits entwined with pearls.

2. Maddalena Doni, née Strozzi. According to a painting by Raphael.
3. Woman's head. Painting by Piero della Francesca.
4 and 5. Venetian courtesans. Details from a painting by Vittore Carpaccio. Venice about 1505.
6. Piero de' Medici, father of Lorenzo (8), died 1469. After a medal.
7. Young woman. Painting by Domenico Veneziano about 1458–60.
8. Lorenzo de' Medici, son of Piero (6). After a medal.
9. Giuliano de' Medici, brother of Lorenzo (murdered in 1478 by the party of the Pazzi). Painting by Sandro Botticelli.
10. Angelo Doni. Painting by Raphael.
11. Self portrait of the Venetian painter Gentile Bellini.

GERMANY IN THE LATE MIDDLE AGES. *Costume of Craftsmen and Burghers* 58

Top Group

1–7. After drawings from the so-called *Mittelalterliche Hausbuch* (mediaeval housebook), an illuminated manuscript in the possession of the prince of Waldburg-Wolfegg (about 1480).
1. Copper-smith with turban-cap and wooden under-shoes under the pointed shoes.
2. Man of the lower classes wearing a round brimmed hat.
3. Woodcarver wearing short sleeveless outer jacket.
4 and 5. Peasant and peasant woman.
6 and 7. Young distinguished couple. She is wearing a trailing garment with laced bodice, he has a short shoulder mantle over a short sleeved jacket.

Centre Group

8. Wearing a long fur-lined gown open in front (German: *Schaube)* and a fur beret.
9. Distinguished burgher wearing a half length coat with skirts and long sleeves wide at the ends. Beret over tight-fitting cap, broad flat shoes.
10–13. People taking part in a ball, the women in long trailing garments. 10: With long trailing sleeves. 11: With Burgundian steeple cap; the youths: 12 in a short jacket laced by cords over the low-cut neck, pointed shoes; 13: In a long skirted coat with a low-cut neck. (After a copperplate by Israhel von Meckenem in Westphalia, died 1503.)

Bottom Group

14. North German peasant with spade and shepherd's staff. Sickle in his girdle. (According to a Lübeck woodcarving.)
15. Mercenary with halberd, armour and sallet (vessel-like helmet). According to a chronicle at Bern about 1485.
16. Executioner's assistant (with wooden logs) wearing pointed cap. (After woodcarvings by Michael Wohlgemuth.)
17. Jew with the yellow ring to mark his race. (According to woodcarvings by Michael Wohlgemuth.)
18. Archer (mercenary) wearing *iron hat.*

SPAIN IN THE MIDDLE AGES. *(Late 13th to 15th Centuries)* 59

Top Group

1 and 2. Burghers about 1275. Outer-garments with wide three-cornered sleeves with light border decoration. Hooded shoulder-capes.
3. Knight (caballero) about 1300. Shoulder cape with decorated border.
4. Lightly armed horseman in a sleeveless surcoat without girdle. Small leather-covered wooden shield studded with metal.
5. King about 1350 (Painting in the Alhambra, Granada).
6. Knight about 1375. Helmet with vizor, ringed coat of mail, parti-coloured doublet covering the loins and slit open at the sides, low-belt made of gold-plated pieces of metal. Light coloured morocco leather shoes.

Centre Group

7. Knight about 1375. Blue and white turban-cap, red hood with collar and long liripipe, white tight-fitting coat reaching to the loins. Low gold-plated girdle, yellow hose, shoes like 6.
8. Court lady wearing long red gown with blue sleeves and white sleeveless outer garment with gold braids. Necklace and earrings. On her head a garland.
9. Court lady wearing a white mantle lined with red material and the borders trimmed with gold braid over a white outer-garment. The under-garment is of reddish-violet colour. Bleached hair. 8 and 9 about 1300.
10. Man of rank about 1400 wearing high pointed hat and fur-trimmed cloak (houppelande).
11 and 12. Soldiers about 1400 wearing *brigantine* and over it a leather doublet. Iron gloves, round shield with hollow for the fist.

Bottom Group

13. Rodrigo de Lauria (died 1314).
14. Lady of rank about 1390. Doña Elvira de Ayala.
15. Spanish Countess 1353.
16. Lady about 1435.
17. Man of rank about 1430.
18. Don Alvara Perez de Guzman, Admiral of the kingdom of Castile. 1394. (13–18) according to *Iconografia Española.*

GERMANY *about 1500* 60

Top Group

1 and 2. Huntsmen.
3. Bag-piper.
4. Nuremberg citizen's wife
5. Young peasant.
6. Peasant girl.
7. Old peasant.

(4–7) according to Albrecht Dürer's paintings.

Centre Group

8–13. Peasants at the time of the Peasants' Revolt 1524–1525 (according to representations by Dürer, H. S. Beham and others).

Bottom Group

14–19. Vagrants (according to Hans Burgkmair's *Triumphzug Kaiser Maximilians* (The Triumph of Emperor Maximilian).

61 ITALY. RENAISSANCE *1520–30. According to Contemporary Paintings*

1. Picture of a young woman called *La Bella* by Francesco Mazzuoli, (called Parmigianino), about 1530. Naples National Museum.
2. Italian nobleman. Painting by Alessandro Bonvicino, called Moretto da Brescia, about 1525. London, National Gallery.
3. Italian nobleman. Painting by Moretto, 1526. London, National Gallery.
4. Woman and child. Painting by Paris Bordone, about 1525. Leningrad, Eremitage.

62 GERMANY AT THE TIME OF THE REFORMATION. *Head-dress (1500–50)*

1. The Emperor Maximilian I. According to Dürer's painting.
2. The Elector Frederick the Wise of Saxony, 1534. According to Dürer.
3. Ulrich von Hutten. 1520.
4. Bernhard Knipperdollinck, a draper and one of the heads of the Anabaptists at Münster, 1534.
5. Duke William IV. of Bavaria, painted in the year of his death, 1550.
6. Leonhard von Eck, 1475–1550, the efficient chancellor and statesman of Duke William IV. of Bavaria (He should not be confused with Johann Eck, who had a disputation with Luther). Engraving by B. Beham. 1527.
7. A 24-year-old member of the Augsburg patrician family of the Welsers, painted in 1533.
8. Sebastian Münster, the scholar and cosmographer who came from Ingelheim and lived in Basle 1489–1552. Painted by Christian Amberger.
9. Katharina von Bora, who married Luther in 1525. According to Cranach.

63 ENGLAND DURING THE REFORMATION PERIOD. *(Henry VIII., 1509–47).*

1. Edward, Prince of Wales, son of Jane Seymour, 15 months old. About 1538. New York. Mellon Collection.
2. Anne of Cleves, later Queen of England, 1530. Paris, Louvre.
3. King Edward VI. as a youth, about 1548. Windsor Castle. (cf. Plate 88).
4. Jane Seymour 1536. Vienna, Kunsthistorisches Museum.

1, 2 and 4 paintings by Hans Holbein, the Younger. 3 Painting by an unknown English painter about 1548, in Holbein's style.

64 SPANISH FASHION. *1550–80, according to Contemporary Paintings.*

1. Philip II. of Spain. Painting by Anthonis Mor. Althorp, Lord Spencer's Collection.
2. Isabella of Valois, Queen of Spain (third wife of Philip II). Painting by Pantoja de la Cruz. Madrid, Prado.
3. Don Carlos, Infante of Spain (son of Philip II.) Painting by Anthonis Mor. Formerly Cassel, Picture Gallery.
4. The Infante Don Diego of Spain (son of Philip II.) Painting by Sanchez Coello. Collection of the Earl of Northbrooke.

65 GERMANY AT THE REFORMATION PERIOD. *Citizen's Costume and Peasants, 1510–1550.*

1. Scholar of the University of Strasbourg. 1516.

2 and 3. Scholar with three distinguished students. 1512.

4. Peasant 1512.
5. Peasant from the Upper Rhine carrying the flag of liberty of the so-called *Bundschuhe* (laced shoes). 1520.
6. Wife of a patrician wearing high cap and pleated mantle (worn out-of-doors). 1516.
7. Couple, patricians from Münster in Westphalia during a wedding-dance. According to Aldegrever's series of copper plates: *Wedding-dancers* 1538.
8. Swabian peasant with hooded shoulder cape and short pleated skirt. 1521.
9. Mayor, member of a court martial. Upper Rhine. 1512.
10. University professor of law. 1549.
11. Merchant of Augsburg. 1539.
12. Patrician's wife from the Electorate of Saxony. 1550.
13. Horseman (servant from Augsburg). 1539.
14. Mercenary officer. 1549.

66 ITALY. RENAISSANCE. *Head-dress and Hair styles (1500–1550)*

Persons of the Renaissance with the typical head-dress and hair styles as well as the characteristic collar fashions of the period.

1. Self-portrait of Raphael (1482–1520)
2. According to Sebastiano del Piombo (1483–1547).
3. According to Francesco Franciabigio (Florentine painter 1482–1525).
4. Lady of the time of the new Duchy of Tuscany. According to Bronzino (1502–1572).
5. Person of rank according to a painting of northern Italy.
6. Venetian woman. According to Paris Bordone (1500–1570).
7. According to a painting by Girolamo Romanini (Brescia 1485–1566).
8. According to a picture by Lorenzo Lotto. (Venetian painter, about 1480–1556).
9. Pietro Aretino, famous and notorious author, ruthless literary money maker and libertine (1492–1557), came from Arezzo, but lived mainly in Venice. According to a painting by Titian.

ITALY. EARLY RENAISSANCE *1460–90* 67

Top Group

1–8. Participants in a betrothal celebration (Ferrara?). The women 1–3 wearing sleeveless girdled outer garments over long garments with a low-cut neck and long slightly slit sleeves. The betrothed wears her long hair falling down to the knees instead of a veil. The men 5–8 are wearing long cloaks reaching down to the ground and some of them girdled and with long hanging sleeves (8) and with a high collar (7 and 8). The bridegroom (4) has a shorter cloak with slit sleeves and a small cap on his half length curled hair, with the part over the forehead cut in a fringe. According to a picture painted by a Ferrara artist between 1460 and 70. Formerly in the Kaiser Friedrich Museum, Berlin.

Centre Group

9–13. Venetians about 1496. 9, 11–13 in long coats with wide sleeves (9) or with hanging sleeves (12 and 13) over long-sleeved tunics most of them buttoned up to the neck. Narrow-brimmed stiff hats worn over the tight-fitting caps. The youth (10) is wearing a short jacket (giubberello) with wide inserted sleeves open at the sides over a still shorter long-sleeved jacket. Parti-coloured hose *(mi-parti)* and flat leather soles. This striking hose points him out as a member of the *Compagnia della Calza* (Hose company), a group of young Venetian noblemen. (According to Gentile Bellini's painting of the procession on St. Mark's square, dated 1496. Venice Academy.)

Bottom Group

14. Italian youth with shield and spear in a girdled fur-edged giubberello with the medium length sleeves attached by laces. Parti-coloured hose and soft shoes.
15. Ferrara dandy wearing a somewhat longer fur-trimmed giubberello with trailing sleeves open at the top over a short jacket buttoned up to the neck. Arrow and hoop in his hands. (Part of the fresco by Franc. Cossa), about 1470 in the Palace, Ferrara.
16. Girls' costume at Ferrara: High-girdled trailing brocade gown with a V-neck. Small cap (From the same fresco).
17. Florentine Patrician woman about 1490 in the *giornea*, a sleeveless garment open at the sides and slipped over the head. The garment underneath with slit sleeves. Ingeniously plaited hair. (According to Domenico Ghirlandaio's fresco *The Visitation* at Florence, Santa Maria Novella.)

ITALIAN RENAISSANCE *about 1500* 68

Top Group

1–8. The Doge of Venice in ceremonial costume with his retinue.

1 and 3. Retinue of the Doge, 15th century.

2. Venetian Jew. 15th century.

4. Cushion-bearer in the Doge's public procession. About 1500.

5 and 6. Venetian Doge with canopy-bearer in a ceremonial procession about 1500.

7 and 8. Trumpeter in the Doge's procession. The shape of the Doge's cap *(il corno* or *beretta ducale)* was developed from the fisherman's cap (similar to the Phrygian cap) and was made of stiff brocade with a crown-like fillet.

Centre Group

9. Young man from Padua. 1508.
10. Recruiting officer wearing a turban. Milan 1505.
11. Venetian negro as a gondolier.
12. Youth from Siena. (According to Sodoma).
13. Venetian about 1505. (According to Giorgione).

Bottom Group

14–16. Young Florentines in short doublets slit in front; long tight-fitting hose, in front cod-piece.

17. The same. – The fashion of slashed and puffed trousers begins to appear.
18. Young student in a half-length coat fastened up to the low-cut neck.
19. Mercenary officer in parti-coloured costume.

GERMANY *under the Influence of Burgundian Fashion (15th Century)* 69

Top Group

1. Lady of rank wearing the Burgundian *hennin* (steeple hat draped with veils).
2. Girl wearing a brimmed conical hat.
3. Woman wearing *hennin* divided in the middle. (Bull's horns cap.)
4. Girl wearing a wide trailing outer garment (in German called *Tappert*) with wing-like sleeves and a jagged cap.
5. Merchant in a short *heuke* with long hanging sleeves and hat made of a thick turban-like roll of material. About 1407.
6. Man wearing a knee-length girdled coat with short sleeves over a long-sleeved short doublet.

Centre Group

7. Man wearing a tight-fitting jacket with baggy sleeves (in German called *Schecke*).
8. Knight.
9. Lower Rhenish costume.

10–12. Gentleman and youths in quilted jackets.

Bottom Group

13. Knight in armour.
14. Herald wearing high leather boots. The herald, as an official messenger, wears the armorial designs and colours of his master or his authorities on his coat.
15. Man of rank wearing a wide coat (German: *Tappert*).
16. Young knight with falcon.
17. Dandy.
18. Wife of an innkeeper.

70 GERMANY. *Mercenaries (1500–40). The Fashion of Slashes*

Mercenaries take the place of the technically antiquated knights and form the modern army towards the end of the 15th century. They are recruited from citizens and peasants but partly also from young impoverished knights.

Top and Centre Group

1–9. The characteristics of the costume are: the parti-coloured costume (so-called *mi-parti*), the slashings on sleeves, doublet and trousers. The beret is decorated with feathers which attained their largest size about 1525–30. Leather doublet, mantle thrown round the shoulders, wide, flat shoes. About 1520 the costume becomes more conspicuous with brighter colours; slashes and puffs increase. Weapons: long pike, partisan and halberds and straight or S-shaped parrying rod. The superiority of fire-arms soon led to the use of the arquebus and musket.

Bottom Group

10. Standard-bearer of the town of Basle about 1520.
11. Mercenary wearing costume with profuse slashing about 1530.
12. Captain of the mercenaries wearing a long skirted coat and a wide beret with feathers.
13. Mayor of the court-martial about 1530, a man versed in the law with the staff of the regiment.

71 GERMANY. *Mercenaries (1520–60). The Wide Trunk-hose*

Top Group

1 and 2. Executioner's assistants.

3. Executioner or *free man* with a red feather on his beret.
4. So-called *harlot's sergeant* who had to see to the sutler-women and soldiers' wives among the camp-followers.
5. His wife, a sutler-woman.

Centre Group

6–13. Shows the later costume with the wide bag-like hose from about 1540 on.

6. Provost, the lower police judge and executive. Wide baggy trunk-hose and short Spanish cape. High hat.

7 and 8. Drummers wearing long wide baggy trunk-hose and big hats.

9. Standard-bearer.
10. Pikeman.

Bottom Group

11. Soldier who receives double pay with arquebus. Richly incised helmet in the shape of a morion *(Marianus)*.
12. Executioner with a red feather.
13. Armoured soldier who receives double pay, wearing pointed basinet (pear-shaped helmet).

14 and 15. Pikemen with the pike (formerly called spear). The soldiers who were armoured and those armed with musket or arquebus were entitled to double pay.

72 GERMANY DURING THE REFORMATION PERIOD. *(1500–30)*

Top Group

1, 3 and 4. Nuremberg middle class women about 1500 according to the well-known watercolours by Albrecht Dürer, from the Albertina, Vienna, dated 1500, with the characteristic explanations of 1: *Thus one goes to church in Nuremberg*; of 2: *Thus one walks about at home*, of 4: *Thus the Nuremberg women go dancing.* No. 2 represents (in the same series of Dürer's costume studies) a Venetian woman of 1495 who in contradistinction to the Nuremberg women shows the new fashion of northern Italy: short bodice with wide bands across the low-cut neck. The damask under-skirt attached to the bodice is covered by a skirt slashed open and fastened by two large buttons over the stomach. The false sleeves are laced to the bodice and consist of several parts exposing the fine pleated blouse.

Centre Group

5–8. Costume of Basle middle-class women about 1530, according to the drawings in Indian ink by Hans Holbein the Younger in the museum, Basle. Bodice with long trailing skirt falling down in folds. Underneath the bodice-like blouse and under-skirt. Low cut neck or blouse with pleated collar inserted. 7. Long sleeves with puffs, elongated ruffles or velvet cuffs round the wrists. 5–7. Wear small white embroidered caps covering the hair. 8. Has a large beret decorated with feathers over the hair net. 6. Wears over the low-cut neck the new-fashioned *goller*, a short shoulder cape with the lapel turned up. Characteristic is the girdle with sewing material, keys, knife and fork, pocket, etc., hanging down from it.

Bottom Group

9. Young man about 1500 in a short doublet with slashed sleeves, a low-cut neck exposing the shirt and laced by bands. Slashed breeches, long mantle thrown over the shoulders. Slightly pointed flat shoes (transition to the broad shoes), slashed plate-like beret. Long loose hair.
10. Old man of rank wearing the characteristic fur-trimmed long sleeveless coat (in German: *Schaube*) over the skirted doublet with wide baggy sleeves. Half-length hair with a fringe (called *Kolbe* in German). Broad flat shoes.
11. Man of rank wearing a short fur-trimmed coat *(Schaube)* and cap. Spade beard.
12. Ceremonial costume of the new Protestant pastors (according to a picture of Dr. Martin Luther by Lucas Cranach the Elder). A composition of the black Augustinian cowl and the gown *(Schaube)* of the university men (Doctores). Broad soft closed shoes.
13. Patrician horseman about 1530. Short doublet with slashed and puffed sleeves and a skirt attached. Laced leather leggings. Slit shoes. Beret-like cap with peak over eyes.

GERMANY UNDER THE INFLUENCE OF SPANISH FASHION *(1550–1600)*. 73

Top Group

1. Gentleman in Spanish costume about 1595 wearing short padded trunk-hose.
2. Gentleman (1590) wearing long padded breeches.
3. Gentleman from Görlitz (1591) with only slightly padded long breeches.

Centre Group

4–7. Betrothal ceremony about 1585. 4 in a genuine Spanish costume, 5 wearing breeches according to German fashion but with padded jerkin (in German: *Gänsebauch* – goose stomach); the old gentleman (7) is dressed according to the older fashion with German trunk hose and a large bow in front to hide the cod-piece. But he wears the short Spanish cape and high hat instead of a beret. The shoes are still broad. Similar to the shape called cow's mouth *(Kuhmaul)* about 1520–1530. The betrothed (6) is wearing two stiff Spanish skirts on a stiff under-skirt and a stiff bodice. Close-fitting cap with ostrich feathers.

8. Gentleman in dark Spanish costume: a longish coat and breeches with knee-bands. Tight-fitting soft pointed shoes.

1–8 According to original paintings from contemporary genealogical registers formerly in the department of the Lipperheide costume library of the State Art Library.

Bottom Group

9 and 10. Duke Albrecht V. of Bavaria (1550–1579) and his consort Duchess Anna in the then new-fashioned Spanish costume. According to pictures by Hans Mielich, the Bavarian court painter.

11. Master goldsmith about 1560 wearing the short Spanish cape and the German trunk-hose as well as a high fur-cap,
12. German merchant in German costume; a knee-length coat. soft ruff, cap with ear-lappets.
13. German nobleman in Spanish costume.

SPAIN AND PORTUGAL *1500–1540. Spanish Moors, 15th Century* 74

Top Group

1–7. Spaniards.

1. Figure and armour in the Armeria Real (armoury at Madrid).
   Supposed to be Charles V. armour: iron hat, ringed coat of mail covered by plate armour, round shield, velvet surcoat with skirt and high tight-fitting leather stockings.
2. A later development of armour as compared with 1(Armeria Real).
3. Fernando Cortez according to a painting in Madrid.

4, 5, 7. Soldiers of Cortez from contemporary paintings in Mexico.

6. Costume of Christopher Columbus.

Centre Group

8–11. Portuguese.

8. Vasco da Gama.
9. Alfonso d'Albuquerque.
10. Nuno da Cunha. 1487–1539.

Bottom Group

11. Pedro de Mascarenhas (discoverer of the Mascarene Islands) as a captive in chains. (8–11 according to Manuscripts and old pictures from S. Ruge's *Zeitalter der Entdeckungen.*)

12–18. Spanish Moors of the 15th century.

12. Huntsman with hunting spear. Cloth coat with sleeves. Hooded cape. Yellow leather shoes over red hose made of soft Cordovan leather.
13. Soldier with iron ringed coat of mail, plate armour, shield with rounded corners and a straight sword.
14. Man wearing turban wound round the head in a simple way.
15. Upper middle-class citizen wearing a sleeved coat, long baggy trousers, mantle, soft shoes and turban and carrying a leather bag.
16. Man with conical embroidered cap.
17. Better class Moorish woman wearing long baggy trousers, pleated garment, white mantle and decorated shoes.
18. Common man wearing a garment with half-long sleeves and wide breeches down to the knees. (According to paintings and sculptured figures in the Alhambra, Granada.)

FRANCE AT THE TIME OF THE RENAISSANCE *1500–75. (Francis I. and Henry II.)* 75

Top Group

1. French court costume about 1505, still under the influence of Italian fashion before 1500 (Charles d'Amboise died 1511).
2. Costume of French noblemen imitating to some extent the German mercenaries' costume but more refined and less spectacular as far as the slashing and colours are concerned. (Duke Claude de Guise about 1525.)
3. King Francis I. of France (1515–47) wearing short doublet, short trunk-hose, short girdled fur-trimmed jacket, about 1538–39.
4. French nobleman about 1540 wearing a short V-necked coat with skirt and elbow length sleeves, in addition short, padded and slashed trunk-hose and brimmed Spanish hat. (François de la Tremouille, died 1541.)
5. Scotsman in the bodyguard of Francis I. wearing coat with skirt, beret and carrying halberd.

Centre Group

6 and 7. Ladies at the court of King Francis I. in long trailing outer garments with fur-lining and fur cuffs over the equally long under-garments with a square-cut neck. Caps from which falls a piece of cloth.

8. French nobleman about 1550 wearing a knee-length fur-trimmed and sleeved coat. Shirt buttoned up to the chin with small ruff. Small beret.
9. King Anton of Navarra (died 1572, father of the French King Henry IV.) wearing Spanish costume about 1560. Cape with up-turned collar.
10. King Henry II. of France (1547–59) in Spanish costume.

Bottom Group

11. French citizen in a short mantle with folds (resembling the German *Schaube*) with the collar turned up.

12. French citizen with mantle thrown over his shoulders and padded Spanish cap (called *tocque*).
13. Nobleman with a narrow-brimmed conical hat.
14. Lady in out-door costume with the outer garment draped in folds. Tocque (hat) decorated with a long veil.
15. Maid of honour of Queen Catherine de Medici, widow of Henry II. of France.

76 FRANCE. SPANISH FASHION *1560–90 (Charles IX.)*

Top Group

1. Chancellor in ceremonial costume (long wide robe with fur-collar i. e. shoulder cape and small stiff beret).
2. King Charles IX. (1560–74) wearing a round carefully ironed ruff, short sleeved and padded doublet. Short padded trunk-hose, small Spanish mantle, tocque (a shortened beret), tight-fitting cotton hose. (Mechanical stocking knitting was not invented till 1589 by the Englishman William Lee.)
3. Maid of honour. Conical Spanish hooped petticoat. Over the hoop arrangement two garments, the outer one open in front. Neck ruff, cap-like head gear.
4. Officer wearing plate armour over the doublet with hanging sleeves. Helmet *(Morion)* on his head.
5. Arquebusier.

Centre Group

6. Soldier, 1562 with a curved-bladed sword and dagger.
7. Officer, 1562.
8. Arquebusier, 1562.
9. Citizen, 1562.
10. Chamber maid from the provinces, district of Saumur. Cap according to the Anjou costume. Outer skirt slit open in front. The sleeves of the bodice decorated with velvet cuffs.
11. Wine hawker in Paris 1586 as advertiser for his inn.

Bottom Group

12. Street hawker selling shoe polish, Paris 1586, with leather bag and earthenware jug.
13. Peasant woman from Saumur in outdoor attire. White petticoat, blue outer garment, black apron.
14. Peasant from Saumur going to the weekly market.
15. Servant girl carrying pails of water, Paris 1590.
16. Porter, Paris 1590.
17. Paris citizen wearing long cape-like mantle (with velvet collar) 1590.

77 SPANISH FASHION IN FRANCE. *1575–90 (Henry III.)*

Top Group

1. King Henry III. (1574–89) in the costume of the Order of the Holy Ghost (Saint Esprit) founded by him in 1578.
2. His consort, Queen Louise. The former conical shape of female costume now disappears in favour of a more accentuated waist line. The low-cut neck appears in contradistinction to the Spanish fashion. Lace collars are arranged fan-like round the neck.
3. Courtier with the ribbon and cross of the Order of the Holy Ghost (Saint Esprit).
4. Lawyer with a beret with a pompon in a long gown with soft collar. *(Golilla.)*
5. Huguenot musketeer.

Centre Group

6–7. Noble ladies about 1500. Barrel-shaped skirts and the hoop arrangements *(Vertugade* or *vertugalle)* underneath. Over the outer garment there is a frill attached covering the hips. Slashed and puffed sleeves.
8. The queen's page.
9. Footman in livery at the royal court.
10. Nobleman's footman.
11. Servant or housekeeper out shopping.

Bottom Group

12. So-called *Mignon* in dandy's costume (one of the feeble and effeminate King's favourites, who surrounded and influenced him).
13. French admiral.
14. Duke Louis of Nevers from the house of Gonzaga.
15. French nobleman.
16. *Gentilhomme de la Compagnie* (Gentleman of the bodyguard, 1581).

78 ITALY UNDER THE INFLUENCE OF SPANISH FASHION. *1590–1610*

Top Group

1. Roman courtesan. 1590.
2. Respectable unmarried Venetian woman of rank in outdoor attire hiding head and part of body.
3. Venetian courtesan in a garment made of heavy silk damask with a lace collar standing up fan-like and a handkerchief *(fazoletto).*
4. The same woman (the front part of the dress being removed) wearing breeches, stockings with gore and stilt-shoes (wood with leatherwork or painting). These stilt shoes *(zoccoli)* were also worn by respectable women. Hair arranged in the shape of a half-moon.
5. Lady from Ferrara, the short sleeves padded to form a roll on the shoulder. The outer garment slashed open in front. Feather fan. 1590.

Centre Group

6. Venetian lady. 1610.
7. Old Venetian man of rank. 1610.
8. Venetian gentleman dressed in Spanish fashion. 1610.
9. Venetian lady. Outer garment with hanging sleeves. 1605.
10. Young Venetian *Nobile.* 1605 (Spanish fashion).
According to costume books of the 16th century.

Bottom Group

11–15. Milan ladies and gentlemen performing court dances. 1604.

FRANCE. LATE SPANISH FASHION. *1600–40 (Henry IV. and Marie de Medici)* 79

Top Group

1. King Henry IV. of France (1589–1610). He never wore the beard called *Henriquatre*, but a full short beard. Stiff wheel-like ruff, trunk-hose.
2. Nobleman with pointed beard, flat collar, perhaps in imitation of the collar of the Walloon guards of the 16th century. Stiff short padded trunk-hose.
3. Nobleman with wheel-like ruff, ribbons on knees and shoes, slashed bag-like breeches.
4. Henry IV. in a stiff Spanish hat and short padded trunkhose.
5. Leader of the mercenaries with feather hat, leather doublet and leggings covering the whole legs.

Centre Group

6 and 7. Marie de Medici, wife and widow of Henry IV. shown in different shapes of the Spanish hoop-petticoat, stiff ruff and fan-like high lace collar.

8 and 9. Noblemen in the reign of Louis XIII. (1610–43). The ruff disappears in favour of a flat fine pleated collar. The hair is worn longer. The high horsemen's riding boots come into fashion.

10. Citizens about 1610.

Bottom Group

11. French nobleman *(gentilhomme)*. 1630.
12. The same. 1635.

13 and 14. The same 1635–40.

15 and 16. People of rank in outdoor costume. 1635.

(11–16. According to engravings by Abraham Bosse, died 1678).

SPAIN *in the 16th and 17th Centuries. (Spanish Fashion from 1540–1660)* 80

Top Group

1–10. Times of Charles V. and Philip II. (1540–90).

1. Captain of the Spanish infantry.
2. Spanish soldier.
3. Armour worn at military parades about 1580.
4. The earlier Spanish costume about 1530 (The Emperor Charles V., King of Spain, according to a painting by Titian about 1533. Madrid, Prado).
5. Spaniard of rank about 1550.

Centre Group

6. Spanish Queen (Isabella of Valois, third wife of King Philip II., married in 1559) about 1565.
7. King Philip II. of Spain (1555–98) as a young prince, according to a painting by Titian 1550–51.
8. Lady of rank (the Infanta Isabella Clara Eugenia).
9. Don Juan d'Austria, illegitimate son of Charles V. and half-brother to Philip II. (the victor in the naval battle of Lepanto against the Turks, 1571). According to a painting of 1572.
10. Spanish nobleman and knight of the Order of Santiago (red sword on a black mantle).

1–10. According to contemporary pictures and costume of the Armeria Real at Madrid.

Bottom Group

11–13. Time of Philip IV. (1621–65).

11. King Philip IV. of Spain (1621–65) painted 1644.
12. Infant Balthasar Carlos in hunting costume about 1635.
13. Infant Don Carlos about 1626.
14. Queen Maria Anna of Austria, second wife of Philip IV., painted 1658–60.
15. Infanta Margareta, about 1660.

11–15. According to paintings by Diego Velasquez (1599–1660).

RUSSIA. *16th and 17th Centuries* 81

Top Group

1 and 5. Two warriors of the 16th century. A ringed coat of mail strengthened with plates and worn over the tunic. Helmets with guards over the forehead and with ringed mail attached (1) used as ear guards (5). Shields made of chased metal. Sword, halberd (battle-axe) (1) and mace (5).

2 and 4. Boyar women in ceremonial dress from Torzhok. (The Boyars, meaning fighters, were formerly warriors in the retinue of princes; later on they became the leading aristocracy). The garment made of velvet and brocade. The high head-dress draped with large, fine veils. Torzhok in the Government of Tver is a famous centre of embroidery and lace handicraft.

3. Tsarina (mother of Peter the Great, died 1694) in a gold-brocade garment covered by a mantle of fur-trimmed silk. On her head a narrow pleated cap covered by a fur-cap with hood.

Centre Group

6. Boyar in military costume about 1600.
7. Tsar wearing in-door costume about 1550.

8 and 9. Boyars, 16th century.

10. Boyar, 17th century.

Bottom Group

11 and 12. Cossack of rank in a coat of honour.

13. Tsar in coronation robes, with a conical fur-trimmed gold cap to which the small crown is attached.
14. Boyar (Prince Repnin).
15. Boyar, 17th century.

POLAND, HUNGARY AND UKRAINE. *16th–17th Centuries* 82

Top Group

1. Great hetman, commander-in-chief of the Polish army, about 1600 (According to a picture of the great hetman Stanislaus Solkiewski, died 1620).
2. Young Polish noble lady wearing the national beret.
3. Marshall of Lithuania (end of 16th century). *Szuba* (long coat) taken in at the waist. Ornamental shoes made of yellow morocco leather. The *szuba* is usually a fur-lined coat with a turn-down collar.

4. Polish nobleman, end of the 17th century.
5. Heyduck, old Hungarian warrior used to guard the frontiers against the Turks. Later on also the name of Hungarian foot-soldiers and servants of the magnates and town administrators.
6. Polish peasant, end of 17th century.

Centre Group

7. Armed Polish nobleman.
8. Armed Polish lancer.
9. Polish nobleman about 1580. Over his coat he wears the *Bekièsche.* The decorative fastening by buttons and laces is influenced by Hungarian costume.
10. Polish nobleman.

11 and 12. Magyar couple of rank (end of 17th century).

Bottom Group

13. Peasant from the Cracow district.
14. Polish nobleman.
15 Peasant girl from the Ukraine.

16 and 17. Peasants from the Ukraine.

83 GERMANY

Reformation and Spanish Fashion as represented in paintings by Lucas Cranach, Father and Son (1514–64)

1. Prince Christian I., son of the Elector August of Saxony, at the age of four. Painting by Lucas Cranach the Younger. 1564, Moritzburg near Dresden.
2. Prince Alexander, son of the same elector, as a ten-year old boy. Painting by Lucas Cranach the Younger. 1564. Formerly Dresden Museum.
3. Prince Moritz of Saxony. Painting by Lucas Cranach the Elder. 1526. Darmstadt, formerly in the possession of the Great Duke of Hesse.
4. Margrave George Frederick of Ansbach-Bayreuth, painting by Lucas Cranach the Younger. 1564. Formerly Berlin, State Castles.
5. Duchess Katharina, consort of Duke Henry the Pious of Saxony. Part of the painting by Lucas Cranach the Elder. 1514. Formerly Dresden Gemälde Galerie. According to photographs in the Kaiser Friedrich Museum, Berlin.

84 COSTUME OF GERMAN CITIZENS *about 1560–80*

Top Group

1. Craftsman's wife from Dantzig.
2. Maid-servant from Dantzig using a wooden carrier (cut out for the neck) with two chains and hooks for the water pails.
3. Wife of a distinguished citizen from Cologne.
4. Craftsman's wife from Cologne.
5. Wife of a distinguished citizen from Lübeck.

Centre Group

6. Nuremberg woman with a small *Schaube*, i. e. shoulder cape.
7. Nuremberg maid-servant.
8. Patrician's wife from Nuremberg going to a wedding.
9. Craftsman's wife from Augsburg.
10. Daughter of a patrician from Augsburg.

1–10. From *Trachtenbuch* by Weigel 1577. Woodcuts by Jost Amman.

Bottom Group

11–13. Men at the age of 20, 30 and 40 years in German Costume, i. e. slashed sleeves and trunk-hose about 1560–80.

14. Horse-cart driver from Franconia wearing wide high boots which can either be laced to the doublet or let down. According to Amman.
15. Nuremberg burgher wearing Spanish holiday attire.

85 MILITARY COSTUME. EUROPE. *End of 16th Century*

Top Group

1. Spanish soldier, 1555.
2. Musketeer about 1590 with gun-powder bag hanging from the belt.
3. Captain, 1590.
4. Higher officer with gold-inlaid breast plate armour slightly indicating the cod piece (padded front part) without hip plates. 1590.
5. Musketeer with pouch-belt, from which hang wooden boxes or leather pouches containing ammunition. Light helmet *(morion)*. Gun-powder bottle attached to the belt. 1590.

Centre Group

6. Standard-bearer during the war in the Netherlands with the fashionable cod piece (padded front part).
7. Musketeer.
8. Captain.
9. Standard-bearer (6–9) according to engravings by Hendrik Goltzius, Haarlem 1585–87.

Bottom Group

10–13. French soldiers about 1581.

10: Pikeman; 11: Musketeer; 12: Halberdier; 13: Arquebusier.

86 GERMANY. *Head-dress (Spanish Fashion) 1550–1600*

1. Duke Maurice of Saxony, died 1553. Small beret. Forked beard.
2. Otto Heinrich, Elector Palatine, died 1559. Painted by B. Beham.
3. Calvin, Geneva Reformer (died 1564). Tight flat beret over skull cap reaching to the ears.
4. Lady with small *tocque* over caul.
5. Duke William of Jülich, 1566. According to a memorial coin. Ruff under the ring collar.
6. Philippine Welser, 1527–1580. High collar and ruff. Painting in Ambras Castle.

7. The famous goldsmith W. Jamnitzer from Nuremberg, 1568 wearing a fur-trimmed high cap.
8. Merchant from the Meissen district. According to Jost Amman. Ruff. Long pointed beard.
9. William of Orange, the hero of the Netherlands (by birth a German prince of Nassau). According to a painting. Pointed beard, Spanish hat. Double ruff.
10. The French Admiral Coligny. Added to this plate by the artist for the sake of comparison.
11–15. Heads from Jost Amman's woodcuts about 1570–80.
16–18. Heads from a woodcut representing the Nuremberg rifle association. 1592.

GERMANY, HOLLAND, FRANCE. *Costume during the Thirty-Years' War (about 1630–35)* 87

1. and 5. So-called *alla modo* costume. Germany 1629. According to alla-modo pamphlets. 1. *How a German gentleman should be dressed.* 5. *Gentlemen's alla modo costume and ladies' oddities.*
2. French nobleman greeting someone.
3. Lady playing the spinet.
4. Woman from Cologne. 2–4 according to etchings by Wenzel Hollar, about 1635–40.

ENGLAND. SPANISH FASHION. *(Time of Queen Elizabeth I., According to Contemporary Paintings)* 88

1. Queen Elizabeth I. of England (1558–1603). Painting by an unknown artist. Chatsworth. Collection of the Duke of Devonshire.
2. King Edward VI. of England (1547–1553). Painting by Anthonis Mor. Paris, Louvre (cf. plate 63: England at the Reformation period).
3. James I., King of England and Scotland (1603–25). Painting by a Flemish master. Madrid. National Museum.
4. Mary, Queen of Scots (died 1587). Painting by Frederigo Zuccaro, Chatsworth, Collection of the Duke of Devonshire.

SPANISH COURT COSTUME *about 1630–60. According to Paintings by Diego Velasquez* 89

1. King Philip IV. 1632–35. London, National Gallery.
2. Infanta Maria, Queen of Hungary. 1630. Formerly Berlin, Kaiser Friedrich Museum.
3. Prince Balthasar Carlos about 1639. Vienna, Kunsthistorisches Museum.
4. Infanta Margherita. 1656. Vienna. Kunsthistorisches Museum.

TURKEY. *16th and 17th Centuries* 90

Top Group

1. Turk of rank with the title of Emir held by all direct descendants of Mohammed and some others. Kaftan with scarf worn as a girdle. Coat with long hanging sleeves. Large turban.
2. Commander-in-chief of the janissaries. Brocade garment covered by a sleeveless mantle. High pointed cap of the highest dignitaries, with large turban. Braids for lacing the outer garments are as much in use in Turkish costume as with that of the neighbouring peoples: Magyars and Poles.
3. Cook. Wide baggy breeches as worn by male and female persons; the coat shortened by tucking up as is done with the coats of marching troops. Cap with border decoration.
4. Medical man (Jew) with *tarbush*, so-called Fez.
5. Janissary of the body-guard of the sultan with a high flat-topped cap, a piece of cloth hanging down from it at the back and large feather decoration; the border over the forehead decorated with a wide gold band.

Centre Group

6. Turkish woman in out-door costume. Low decorated *tarbush* (Fez). The women's outfit of this time consists of baggy trousers, cotton or silk undergarment and one or two outer garments. Soft slightly turned-up leather shoes.
7. Middle class Turkish woman at home. Tarbush with turban. Garment covered by a fine, knee-length outer garment, scarf used as girdle.
8. Turkish woman of rank at home. Tarbush draped with a veil, necklaces, woven dress, scarf-girdle, trousers, the naked feet on high wooden sandals.
9. Arabian merchant.
10. Woman of rank from Pera, the residential part occupied by the Franks (Europeans) in Constantinople.

1–10. According to *Raiss und Schiffahrt in die Türkey* by N. Nicolai. 1576.

Bottom Group

11. Lady in out-door dress.
12. Woman of the seraglio.
13. Turkish lady in in-door attire.
14. Imam; leader of the prayers in the mosques. Costume: long outer garment and white turban.
15. Wandering dervish, member of the *Calenderi*, a special order of the dervishes, which requires ceaseless wandering from their members.

11–15. According to pictures of the 17th century.

TURKEY. *17th Century. Costume at the Sultan's Court represented on Miniatures* 91

Top Group

1. Mufti, i. e. judge who studied the secular law and that of the Koran.
2. The Sultan's personal physician having in his left hand a chain (similar to the rosary) favoured in the Balkans but only used for distraction.
3. The sultan's turban-bearer.

4. The sultan's chief wife.
5. Woman smoking a pipe.

Centre Group

6. High officer of the archers.
7. Archer of the janissaries.
8. Officer of the sipahi or spahi (cavalry).
9. Officer of the Egyptian-Ottoman troops.
10. Janissary from Barbary (North Africa).

Bottom Group

11. Orderly officer of the sultan.
12. Bread-carrier for the advance guard of the army.
13. Officer of the Deli (the word meaning fool; fool-hardy); they were the storm-troops of the armies, mostly stimulated by opium. (Body-guard of the great viziers.)
14. Privy Chamberlain of the sultan.
15. Woman fan-bearer to the mother of the sultan. Her cushion-like cap resembles the head-dress of the Turk peoples in Central Asia. (Mostly according to a Turkish miniature manuscript of the 17th century, formerly in the Lipperheide department of the Staatliche Kunstbibliothek, Berlin.)

92 EUROPE. MILITARY COSTUME *1600–50*

Top Group

1 and 2. Musketeers, 1609. Over the doublet the bandolier (worn from the left shoulder to the right hip) with the bullets in little wooden boxes.

3 and 4. Pikemen. Breast plates with loin-plates attached to them in front.

5. Captain, 1613 with partisan, the weapon of the pikemen's officers. Chest and arms protected by armour underneath. Brocade doublet with skirts.

Centre Group

6. Wallenstein.
7. The Elector Johann Georg I. of Saxony. 1631.
8. The Swedish King Gustavus Adolphus in war costume.
9. Officer about 1635.
10. High officer, 1632.

Bottom Group

11. Musketeer with forked rest for the arquebus.
12. Lancer with the old vizor-helmet. 1635.
13. Cuirassier 1640.
14. Captain 1640.
15. Dutch captain of the rifle-men with sash and pike. 1648.

93 FRANCE AT THE TIME OF LOUIS XIV. *1650–1700*

Top Group

1. Man of rank about 1670 with sword and stick. Large wig, large felt hat with feathers, neck-cloth (called *steenkerke* since 1692). Outer coat *justaucorps* with large cuffs and galloons. Wide pleated breeches giving the impression of a skirt, hose decorated with ribbons at the knees. Shoes with latchets, buckles and red heels.

2 and 5. Officers.

3 and 4. A marshal's wife in a widow's costume and her page.

6. Lady about 1675 in a long trailing outer garment (manteau) draped in folds over a trailing under-garment (robe). Wide cut neck with lace trimming. Hat decorated with ribbons.
7. King Louis XIV. about 1660. White decorative shirt, short waistcoat, mantle, short skirt showing lace breeches (Rhinegrave breeches). Buckled shoes.
8. The same about 1670.

9 and 10. Men of rank. 1664.

11. Man of rank in the earlier costume about 1660. High hat. Wide riding boots richly lined with lace.

12 and 13. Ladies wearing the costume of about 1680–1700. High stiff cap of frilled linen *(fontage)* with veil, trailing outer garment *(manteau)* with baggy folds at the back, laced bodice *(planchette*, German *Blankscheit*), flounced skirt (12) or with cross stripes (13). The outer garment with semi-long sleeves and linen cuffs opens in front over the skirt.

14. Man in a dressing-gown with turban-like night cap.
15. Louis XIV. about 1700 with a later development of a coat (*justaucorps*, cf. 1) with wide cuffs and large pockets. Underneath a jacket of the same length with sleeves. Large ceremonial wig (Allonge wig). The large brimmed hat is turned up to form a three-cornered hat.
16. Duke Philip of Orléans *(Monsieur)* brother of the king (about 1690–1700).

94 FRANCE. RÉGENCE AND ROCOCO *about 1700–40*

Theatre and Dancers.

Top Group

1–6. According to paintings by Antoine Watteau about 1710–15.

1 and 2. Pierrots of the Italian Commedia dell'arte (cf. pl. 103) from which the comic characters and buffoons originate. Pierrot (or Pierre: stupid Peter) is originally the type of the deceived fool. He appears on the stage of the Italian comedy in Paris at the end of the 17th century, adopting the outfit of Pullicinello, (Pulcinella or Polichinelle).

3. Arlecchino, Arlequin, harlequin in coloured-patched attire (jacket with sleeves, long trousers, bearded mask).
4. Lady of *Crispin* (from the painting by A. Watteau, *L'amour français*).
5. Crispin (Crispino) a French imitation of the harlequin, an impudent and witty valet, appearing about 1600 for the first time. Black (Spanish) costume with mantle, high leggings, leather cap, round hat, wide yellow leather belt, rapier. Title hero of many French comedies, ceasing to appear after 1750.

6. *L'indifférent* (Who is indifferent to his surroundings; melancholy figure on the stage according to a painting by Watteau).

Centre Group

7–11. The dancer Camargo according to a painting by Nicolas Lancret, about 1740.

Bottom Group

12–17. The *moulinet* (group-dance). According to the same artist, about 1740.
Examples of the shepherd dances and scenes in high society of the Rococo.

GERMANY. *1625–75. Citizen's Costume, partly under French Influence* 95

Top Group

1. Nuremberg merchant, south German costume about 1626.
2. Jew of the same period with the yellow ring, which Jews were compelled to have on their coat.
3. South German burgher of the same period in travelling attire.
4. Man of rank belonging to the social class privileged to wear a sword. Same period.
5. Man of rank from Cologne, about 1630–35.

Centre Group

6. Cart driver about 1650.
7. Merchant from Hamburg of the same period.
8 and 9. Germans of rank. They wear the French petticoat breeches (*rhinegraves*, cf. explanation of plate 97). About 1670.
10. Burgher about 1675.
According to contemporary engravings.

Bottom Group

11. Augsburg woman in mourning.
12. Artisan's daughter from Strasbourg in wedding attire.
13. Wife of a physician in Strasbourg wearing a skirt with hip frill.
14. Maid servant from Strasbourg.
15. Citizen's wife from Strasbourg wearing special costume for the Holy Communion.
16. Citizen's wife from Strasbourg.
11–16. According to etchings by Wenzel Hollar about 1640–44.

THE NETHERLANDS AND ENGLAND. *17th Century. Contemporary Paintings* 96

1. The family von Hutten; Painting by Cornelis de Vos, Antwerp about 1610. Formerly Munich, Alte Pinakothek.
2. Picture of Helene Fourment (Rubens' second wife) as a bride. Painting by Peter Paul Rubens. 1630. Formerly Munich, Alte Pinakothek.
3. Portrait of Thomas Wharton. Painting by Anthony van Dyck. Leningrad. Eremitage.

THE NETHERLANDS. *1650–1680, partly under French Influence* 97

Top Group

1–5. Dutch citizen's costume about 1650–60 according to paintings by de Keyser, Terborch and Metsu.
1. Councillor offering a drink of honour.
2. Member of a rifle-association (or officer) in a short cuirass eating his breakfast.
3. Daughter of a distinguished citizen wearing silk dress with short cape.
4. Physician dressed in a doctor's gown.
5. Trumpeter of a troop of horsemen.

Centre Group

6–13. Types of Dutch citizens about 1675–80.
6. High officer wearing high open boots with heels.
7. Cavalier wearing the Rhinegrave breeches or petticoat breeches in French called *rhingraves*, which are said to have been invented by a Rhinegrave of Salm. (The officer No. 6 wears them gathered by a cord and tucked into his wide horseman's boots).
8. Lady in out-door garments (draped outer garment with a low stiff bodice).
9. Cavalier bowing and wearing wide baggy breeches (resembling plus-fours) and shoes with heels.

Bottom Group

10 and 11. Female skaters with masks for protecting the skin, fur cape and long tube-shaped velvet muffs.
12. Male skater playing ice-hockey.
13. Cavalier with Rhinegrave breeches (petticoat breeches) and wig. Heeled shoes with long, narrow bows. According to the series of engravings by Romeyn de Hooghe: *Figures à la mode* about 1675–80.

THE NETHERLANDS. *Ruffs and Collars, Hair and Beard Styles of the 17th Century* 98

1. Wide, pleated lace collar falling down over chest and back. (According to a picture by Rembrandt 1693).
2. Cape-like collar trimmed with lace and cut away in front exposing the jagged shirt. (According to a Rembrandt picture of 1644).
3. Starched wheel collar made of fine linen and crimped with a crimping iron. (According to a picture by Rembrandt about 1642). The wheel collars appeared first after the middle of the 16th century, at first increasing in size, later on slowly decreasing in width. They were often worn in two or three layers on top of each other. At about 1630 they went more or less out of fashion and were only worn by older people. Today they are still worn with the official dress of Protestant preachers of some German districts and the Hamburg senators.
4. The Emperor Ferdinand II. about 1625 wearing the wheel ruff, crop head and small pointed beard.
5. The Elector Maximilian I. of Bavaria about 1635. The large wheel ruff has been replaced by a simple linen collar leaving the chin free so that a fuller beard can be worn again.
6. King Christian IV. of Denmark about 1640 wearing a plait of hair hanging down from one side, a short-lived dandy

fashion originating from the time of the wheel ruff. (Painting in the palace of Rosenborg, Copenhagen.)

7. King Charles I. of England 1632 according to a portrait by A. van Dyck. The hair falls down freely and untrimmed and has not assumed the shape of a wig like 17. The beard, too, looks natural and little trimmed.

8–14. French head-dress and hair styles of the 17th century.

8. Rubens' first wife, Isabella Brant (1609–10). She wears a cap under her hat. This hat, really a male head-dress, was then not usually worn by better class women.

9 and 10. Mother and daughter (from a painting by Franz Hals about 1645). The mother still wears the wheel ruff, the daughter has a soft linen collar with lace, falling down on breast and shoulders.

11. Marie Luise of Taxis according to a picture by van Dyck. Hair style influenced by French fashion, about 1630.

12. English woman about 1645 not showing any foreign influence in her way of dressing. (According to an etching by W. Hollar.)

13. Dutch woman showing the hair style of 1660. (According to a painting by Terborch.)

14. Dutch woman about 1675 (according to a painting by Vermeer van Delft.)

15. Duke Ernst of Mansfeld (about 1625–30). The hair is worn longer after the disappearance of the wheel ruff.

16. Shows the transition from the stiff crimped wheel ruff to the simple turn down collar. The shape of the round ruff is still preserved, but the collar does not fit so tightly round the neck and the stiff pleats are abolished. Nevertheless, there are still several ruffs on top of each other. (According to a picture by E. Pickenoy 1627.)

17. Bernhard of Weimar about 1635. The hair becomes more predominant and longer, the beard smaller.

18. Starched and crimped wheel ruff consisting of three layers on top of each other. (According to a picture by P. Codde 1627.)

99 ENGLAND *about 1640. According to etchings by Wenzel Hollar*

Top Group

1, 2 and 4. English ladies of rank with low-necked lace turn down collars (cf. plate 98: ruffs). Wide pleated skirts (without farthingales as in the late Spanish fashion). Short jacket with skirts and short sleeves with lace cuffs. Feather fan or pleated felt fan.

3. English lady of rank in a winter out-door costume with outer jacket, hoodlike cap, face mask (worn to protect the skin against the weather) and muff. The mask originated in France and became fashionable not only as a protection but also as a sign of good manners and renouncement of vanity (for instance at church processions); it was much used in Northern Italy, not only at Carnival.

Centre Group

5. Citizen's wife from London with broad-brimmed soft felt hat and draped outer skirt.

6. Wife of the Lord Mayor of London with broad-brimmed high stiff hat and the old-fashioned wide Spanish ruff (a sign of her official rank, similar to some ceremonial costume in England and Hamburg in present times). Laced bodice.

7. Citizen's daughter with fastened turn-down collar, apron and linen cap.

8. Craftsman's wife.

9. Citizen's wife (cf. 5) with apron. Wooden sandals under the shoes as protection against the dirt of the street.

Bottom Group

10, 11, 13, 14. English ladies of rank (14 again with a face mask).

12. Wife of a rich merchant.

100 FRANCE. *Fashions at the Court of Versailles according to Contemporary Engravings, about 1700*

Fashions at the court of Versailles after contemporary engravings. Paris about 1700.

1. *Dame de qualité en déshabillé* (Lady of rank in dressing gown). Engraving by Trouvain about 1700.
2. Lady and gentleman at court. Mezzotint by J. Gole about 1700.
3. François Louis, Prince of Bourbon. Engraving by Peter Schenck, Amsterdam about 1700.
4. *Dame de qualité en habit d'été.* (Lady of rank in summer costume). Coloured mezzotint, Paris about 1695. The men wear the large ceremonial wig, long outer coat *(justaucorps)* with rich braid trimming and large cuffs, kerchief *(steenkerke)*, sash, felt hat with turned up brim and feather decoration, ankle shoes with red heels, tight breeches *(culottes)*. Gored stockings. The women are wearing a high stiff linen cap *(fontange)* and beauty-patches *(mouches)*, a trailing outer garment *(manteau)* over a bell-shaped skirt *(robe)*, small apron, stiff bodice *(planchette)*.

101 FRANCE AT THE TIME OF LOUIS XIV. *1695–1700*

Cavaliers and ladies of Paris society. According to engravings by Sebastian Le Clerc from the series: *Divers costumes français du Règne de Louis XIV.* Paris about 1695–1700. This plate demonstrates the costume of the courtiers at Versailles, which is characterized by the ceremonial wig of the men and the fontange caps of the women.

102 FRANCE. TIME OF THE RÉGENCE *about 1715–20*

1–4 and 6. Parisian cavaliers.
5 and 9. Parisian women of rank.
7. Woman from Valenciennes.
8. Girl from Paris. Etchings by Antoine Watteau from the series *Figures de Modes.* Paris 1715–20. This plate shows the transition from the stiff Versailles court dress (about 1700) to the more comfortable and natural costume of the time of the *Régence.*

ITALIAN COMEDY IN PARIS *about 1730* 103

Some of the typical characters of the Italian Impromptu Theatre (Commedia dell'arte).

1. Scaramuccio Napolitano (the bragging coward).
2. Tartaglia (the comical stutterer from Naples).
3. Dottore (the avaricious, jealous scholar or lawyer).
4. Arlecchino (harlequin).
5. Pierrot (stupid Peter).
6. Pantalone (the old comical Venetian merchant).
7. Pulcinella Napoletano (Polichinelle), the predecessor of the circus clown with fat belly and hunchback.
8. Scapino (Scapin) the former *Zanne*, by Giovanni, the disorderly sly servant or peasant lout.
9. Capitano Espagnole, the boasting Spanish captain. According to engravings by Joullain in Louis Riccoboni: *Histoire du Théâtre Italien.* Paris 1728.

HOLLAND AND ENGLAND. ROCOCO *about 1740–50* 104

1. Dutch smoker's club. Picture in coloured crayons by Cornelis Troost 1740. The Hague. Picture Gallery.
2. Family group. Painting by William Hogarth about 1740. London, National Gallery.
3. Mariage à la mode (breakfast scene). Painting by William Hogarth 1745. London, National Gallery.

FRANCE AND GERMANY. ROCOCO *about 1730–60* 105

1. Louis, prince of France (son of Louis XV.). Painting by Louis Tocqué about 1739. Paris, Louvre.
2. Princess Sophie of Prussia and Margrave William of Brandenburg Schwedt. Painting by Antoine Pesne. 1734. Formerly Berlin, Hohenzollernmuseum.
3. Madame Adelaide of France, daughter of Louis XV. Painting by J. M. Nattier, the Younger. 1745. Paris, Louvre.
4. Madame de Pompadour. Painting by François Boucher. 1757. Paris. Rothschild collection.

ITALY. ROCOCO. *Venice about 1750* 106

1. Preparation for a masked ball.
2. Dancing lesson.
3. Dressing in the morning.
4. Levée of a Venetian woman of rank. Engravings by G. Flipart after paintings by Pietro Longhi, Venice about 1750.

FRANCE. ROCOCO. *Paris Street Life about 1740* 107

(According to *Cris de Paris* - Paris Street Criers - drawn by Bouchardon, engraved by Caylus)

Top Group

1. Chimney-sweep as street-crier.
2. Copper-smith and tinker from the Auvergne.
3. Female hawker with fresh walnuts.
4. Tradesman with lanterns.
5. Dealer in hare-skins.

Centre Group

6. Man dealing in mouse-traps.
7. Flower seller with bouquets of carnations.
8. Female street-sweeper.
9. Dealer in lottery tickets carrying the winning lists with him to attract buyers.
10. Woman buying old hats.

Bottom Group

11. Man selling knives and scissors.
12. Itinerant musician with large drum and flute.
13. Street musician with primitive barrel-organ.
14. Girl with *laterna magica* and barrel-organ. *(La petite Marmotte.)*

STREET LIFE IN VIENNA AND VENICE. *1770–90* 108

1–12. Viennese street life and street-criers about 1775. (According to Chr. Brand: *Kaufruf in Wien.* 1775.)

Top Group

1. Flower girl.
2. Girl selling honey and fruit.
3. Viennese chamber maid.
4. Female lemon vendor.
5. Laundress.
6. Man carrying cakes.
7. Man dealing in wooden utensils.

Centre Group

8. Jew selling second-hand goods.
9. Bay leaf hawker.
10. Man selling engravings.
11. Woman selling hats.
12. Casual worker.

Bottom Group

13–17. Street life in Italy about 1785. (According to Venetian engravings by Zamponi.)

13. Street crier selling fish *frutta di mare* and candied fruit. He wears a knitted woollen cap.
14. Theatre attendant at the Venice theatre.

15 and 16. Rag-picker and buyer of old goods.

17. Street crier.

109 FRANCE. LATE ROCOCO. *1776*

1. Maternal joy.
2. The rendezvous in Marly.
3. The grand toilette.
4. Taking leave. Engravings by various artists, after drawings by J. M. Moreau, the Younger, from the series: *Monument du Costume* ,Paris 1776 and following years. State Art Library.

110 ENGLAND. *1770–1800*

Top Group

1. Mrs. Carnach. According to a painting by Reynolds.
2. Mrs. Beaufoy. Costume about 1775. According to a painting by Gainsborough.
3. Mrs. Graham. According to a painting by Gainsborough.
4. The Duchess of Cumberland. 1783. After an engraving.

Centre Group

5–9. English fashions about 1770–95.

8. The London actress Elizabeth Farren, later the wife of Lord Derby. According to a picture by Lawrence, 1792, engraved by Bartolozzi.

Bottom Group

10–15. English fashions at the court of St. James about 1795 to 1800. According to aquatints by Nikolaus Heideloff in *Gallery of Fashion.*

111 FRANCE. LATE ROCOCO. *Women's Hair Styles. 1770–90*

After 1750 the flat and graceful hair style gradually rises upward so that the towering head-dress reaches its summit after 1770. The place of the *friseur* (who curls the hair) is taken by the *coiffeur* who works the former *coiffe* (cap) into the hair (in the shape of ribbons and decorations).

1. Madame Adelaide, daughter of Louis XV. (cf. plate 105). A transition from the low to the high hair style about 1755–60. Hair style with lace cap *(coiffe)*.

2 and 3. Rising toupets *(toupets croissants)*. *Toupet* is the name for the hair style which is attained by combing (brushing) the hair straight up from the forehead. According to Chodowiecki's engravings in an almanac.

4. Woman wearing *dormeuse* (night cap), a large cap worn as a *négligé* at home or by elderly women about 1780. *Négligé* meant free and easy attire in contradistinction to *grande toilette* (evening gown).
5. *Hérisson* (hedgehog) with a *coiffe* or cap on top.
6. *Coiffure à la belle poulaine* (prow of a ship) 1778. Besides such ships artificial flowers, fruit baskets, cornfields, etc., were fastened on top of the hair.
7. *Coiffure en bandeau d'amour* (love bands) about 1780.
8. *Tocque lisse avec trois boucles détachées* (Plain tocque with three detached curls). All that remained of the original tocque (the tight fitting beret of the Spanish fashion is the narrow cord).
9. *Hérisson avec trois boucles détachées* (cf. 8).
10. *Chien couchant avec un pouf* (lying dog with a large pad of hair).
11. *Coiffure en crochets avec une échelle de boucles* (with curls arranged like a ladder).
12. Loose floating hair with large brimmed hat, so-called *merveilleuse* about 1795 (cf. plates 116 and 117).
13. Woman's hair style with Phrygian cap (revolutionary cap). 1790. Transition from the artificial to the loose hair style.
14. Large felt hat with ostrich feathers on a curly wig, about 1785.
15. Queen Marie Antoinette in a high *coiffure* with turban cap and feathers, about 1780.
16. Large *dormeuse* (cf. 4) on a high *coiffure* about 1780.

112 GERMANY AND AUSTRIA. *China Figures. 1750–75*

Costume according to contemporary china figures.

1. Ballet dancer, 1760 (China figure from Höchst).
2. Shepherd and shepherdess (Frankenthal).
3. Dancing girl. 1760 (Höchst).
4. Viennese woman cutting wood with an axe. 1750–60.
5. Shepherdess (Vienna).
6. Cavalier, 1760–65 (Nymphenburg).
7. Itinerant hawker, 1750 (Meissen).
8. Huntsman in a nobleman's service, 1750. Fayence from Strasbourg.
9. Huntsman of rank, 1750 (Meissen).

113 FRANCE. ROCOCO. *1730–75*

Top Group

1. Lady wearing the so-called *contouche* made of taffeta or silk (1730) which replaced the outer garment of the evening dress (either *manteau* or *grande robe*) from about 1720. It was fitted to the body at the shoulders only and flowed loosely down over the under-garments with the farthingale *(panier)*. On the back an inserted fold (Watteau fold) ran down from the nape to the seam.
2. Costume of Queen Maria Leszczynska, consort of King Louis XV. of France. 1747. Rich white silk garment with gold embroidery, blue velvet ermine-lined coat with gold lilies. Folding fan, not open here. (According to a picture by Van Loo.)
3. Dancing master 1745 wearing the artificially stiffened coat with a contrasting long stiff waistcoat sticking out. (According to a painting by Chardin.)

Centre Group

4–8. Typical figures of 1755. Gentleman, ladies and two *abbés* (ecclesiastics). The outer garments of the ladies are open in front to display the petticoat decorated with frills of delicate pleated material. Small white silk or satin slippers. The gentleman with sword and three-cornered cocked hat. (According to an engraving by G. de. St. Aubin.)

Bottom Group

9–13. Scenes from contemporary French representations about 1760–1775.

9. Lady's maid with a tray, chocolate and letters. (From: *Le Bain* – the bath).

10–12. Cavalier with sword and three-cornered cocked hat and two ladies in hoop-petticoats with trailing outer garments and pointed bodice. High-heeled slippers. (From: *Promenade du soir* – Evening walk.)

13. Lady's maid in a gathered *contouche* with folds at the back (so-called *négligé* attire). High-heeled slippers and small cap (From: *The Wakening*).

FRANCE. LATE ROCOCO. *1775–85* 114

Top Group

1. Lady wearing the wrap-like gathered outer garment with stiff bodice (the so-called *contouche* or *robe ronde* over the short hoop-petticoat), cap tied under the chin on a high *coiffure*.
2. Lady wearing hood-like cap, trailing coat and petticoat without hoops.
3. Back view of a lady in a hoop-petticoat and *caraco* jacket with skirts and short folds on the back. High elaborate hair style.
4. Gentleman wearing cloth tailcoat, short waistcoat, breeches *(culottes)* and gored stockings. Round semi-stiff flat hat according to English fashion, lace frill on the front of the shirt *(jabot)*.
5. Gentleman in a long riding coat (*redingote:* derived from the English word) and stiff two-cornered cocked hat, high neck-cloth, 4 and 5 buckle shoes.

Centre Group

6. Gentleman in the earlier court dress (*justaucorps* – cf. France about 1700) with rather long waistcoat, two-cornered cocked hat in his hand and the sword at his left hip.
7. Courtier with the three-cornered cocked hat under his left arm. Silk sash or *Bandelier*. Stockings with gussets.

8–10. Parisian ladies in indoor dress. High coiffures with caps on top. Coat of various lengths over the round or oval hoop-petticoat.

Bottom Group

11–13. Ladies of the period about 1777–78. .The garments decorated with elaborate frills of silk ribbon (in the rococo style) or flower garlands, bows and lace.

12. *Grande robe* about 1780 decorated in the simpler style of Louis XVI. Lace ruffles, small upright lace collar in the so-called Medici-style. Pearl necklace, high *coiffure à la victoire*.

FRANCE. *1780–89 (Late Rococo)* 115

Top Group

1. Woman in out-door attire. Cap or bonnet, fastened with a ribbon. (This head dress was called *à la laitière:* in the fashion of the dairy maid). Fur-trimmed satin wrapper. Hoop-petticoat shortened for wearing out of doors, with *caraco* or *polonaise* (short jacket) made of the same material. Example of greater simplicity in the fashion of the country woman or burgher's wife as a reaction against the over-decorated, extravagant court fashion. The muff appeared about 1680, disappeared during the period of the Revolution and Empire.
2. Lady with large hat decorated with ribbons. Long *caraco* over ankle-length hoop-petticoat. Low neck.
3. Lady about 1783–84 in a ceremonial costume with large hoop-petticoat. *Coiffure à la Montgolfier* (i. e. named after the newly invented air balloon). According to an English engraving.
4. Woman wearing the so-called *dormeuse* (originally night-cap) fichu (breast kerchief) *en marmotte* (marmot) short hoop-petticoat with *polonaise* (jacket) to match.

Centre Group

5. Costume dating May 1786. Coat and waist-coat made of striped velvet. Black silk breeches *(culottes)*, white silk stockings.
6. Costume dating May 1786. Riding outfit in imitation of the English riding-coat; in French called *redingote.* Round English hat. Buck-skin breeches. Jack boots.
7. Costume of November 1785. Outer garment *à la Lévite* open in front; at first reaching down to the calves, later becoming a trailing garment. It was fastened up over the waist by means of bows, buttons or a sash. A *fichu* over under-garment and *lévite.*
8. Costume dating January 1786. *Robe à la Turque*, the older ceremonial garment. Large satin hat with ribbons and feathers.
9. Costume dated December 1785. Déshabillé garment, called *Pierrot.* Decorated cap, fichu (breast kerchief), short caraco (skirted jacket). Hoop-petticoat.

Bottom Group

10–14. Winter costumes 1788–89.

PARIS FASHION. *1790–95. Revolution and Directory* 116

Top Group

1. Gentleman in a silk tail-coat *à la française* 1790. Short waist-coat with fobs hanging down.
2. Lady with a stiff gray silk hat trimmed with silver braid. February 1790.

3 and 4. Ladies in December 1790.

5. Woman wearing cap under a round conical hat with feathers. September 1791.
6. Gentleman in a cloth tail-coat with silk waist-coat and round silk hat with tricolour ribbons. Short waist-coat with hanging down fobs.

Centre Group

7. Woman in 1791.
8. Woman in July 1792.
9. Man with open tail-coat, the front of which is partly cut away, and a round hat. August 1791.
10. Woman in a tricolour costume with cap.

11. Woman wearing silk dress and conical straw hat.
12. Woman with skirted jacket, short waist-coat, hat with *tricolour* ribbon, all in a man's style.

Bottom Group

13 and 14. Man and woman in 1795. (*Merveilleuse* and *Incroyable.*)

15. *Merveilleuse* partly suggesting antique pattern. 1795.
16. Citizeness 1795.
17 and 18. So-called *Muscadins* similar to the *Incroyables.* Dandies of the Revolutionary Period. Nouveaux riches and profiteers of the Revolution.

117 FRENCH REVOLUTION, DIRECTORY AND CONSULATE. *1790–1803*

Top Group

1. Member of the Paris revolutionary municipal council.
2. Model costume of the *Liberté* and the revolutionary women. (According to contemporary patterns of 1792–94). – The acute phase of the Revolution ended in July 1794, *Thermidor.*
3. Official employed at the Temple (the state prison where among others King Louis XVI. was kept a prisoner till his execution).

Centre Group

4. Member of the Jacobin Club.

1–4. Wear the Phrygian cap which had been declared an emblem of the people's government. The Jacobin (4) has a fillet attached to it with the inscription: *surveillance* (watching).

5–10. Some characteristic hair styles, head-dresses and neck cloths.
5. Charlotte Corday who assassinated Marat.
6. Marat.
7. Danton.
8. Henriot, 1783. Commander of the Paris National Guard The cockade fixed to the ship-shaped hat.
9. Robespierre.
10. Tallien.

Bottom Group

11 and 12. Ladies wearing antique garments fashionable at the time of the Consulate about 1800. *(Mode à la grecque.)*

13–16. *Merveilleuses* (women) and *Incroyables* (men).

118 GERMANY AND FRANCE. *Uniforms (1680–1790)*

Top Group

1–5. Germany.
1. Musketeer with doublet and pouch belt.
2. Officer about 1685.
3. Grenadier.
4. Corporal of the infantry.
5. Musketeer about 1690.

Centre Group

6–13. France.
6. Royal *garde de la porte* (guard at the gate) 1757.
7. Officer of the body guard of the royal family. 1745.
8. Dragoon 1724.

Bottom Group

9. Officer of the Swiss Guards in ordinary uniform. 1757.
10. Soldier of the French guards in ceremonial uniform. 1757.
11. Officer of the French guards in ordinary uniform. 1757.
12. Staff officer in ordinary uniform.
13. Corporal of the fusiliers in ceremonial uniform. 1786.

119 ENGLAND AND FRANCE. *1800–30. French Empire and English Regency*

Top Group

1–6. England 1800–1813.
1. Man in the national English tail-coat with high top hat, buck-skin breeches and jack-boots. (After a fashion engraving of 1801.)
2. Lady in ankle-length high-girdled tunic and short sleeves over a petticoat with bodice. Flat sandals. 1807.
3. Open mantle with stand-up collar. Pot-shaped hat trimmed with feather. 1809.
4. Long outer garment (open at the bottom) over the tunic. Shoulder cape with fringes. 1809.
5. Short bell-shaped garment with jagged seam and a richly decorated bodice. Low wide neck. 1813.
6. Lady in winter costume. Long cloth garment, short fur-trimmed Spencer jacket with fur collar. Fur muff and hat. 1813.

2–6. Repository of Art. London.

Centre Group

7–18. Paris Fashion 1814–30.

7–10. Fashionably dressed women 1814–15. (According to the series of engravings in *Incroyables et Merveilleuses* by Lanté after drawings by Horace Vernet.)

11. Lady in a bell-shaped flounced petticoat, short Spencer jacket with long sleeves (rather more a blouse without skirts) high lace ruffle round neck. Feathered hat. Fashion engraving. January 1828.
12. Man in a cloth tail-coat (out-door attire). Short waist-coat, neck-tie, high top hat with slightly turned up brim, striped trousers tapering towards the ankles, fastened with straps under the shoes. May 1823.

Bottom Group

13. Women wearing a dress fastened up to the neck with long sleeves puffed at the shoulders, high neck ruffle, large sun-bonnet, fur stole. December 1823.
14. Dandy wearing his tail-coat buttoned up and a wide open mantle with flounces round the shoulders. According to a picture by Ingres. 1823.

15 and 16. Women in 1830.

17 and 18. Well-dressed Parisian couple in 1831.

15–18. According to fashion pictures by Gavarni.

GERMANY. *1815–35.* BIEDERMEIER — 120

Top Group

1. So-called German costume (Teutsche Tracht) 1815 with a wide turned-up collar, puffed sleeves, stiff hat with feathers.
2. Lady's riding habit 1816.
3. Man wearing riding dress (tail-coat and breeches), with buttoned-up leggings. Small top hat with narrow brim. 1815.
4. Lady wearing evening gown reaching down to the calves and ending in bows. High girdle. Beginning of 1817.
5. Summer dress 1819. Feather hat. Low neck with lace collar.
6. Summer attire. Sun-hat, bell-shaped mantle with long cuffs. Narrow lace drawers showing beneath the dress.

Centre Group

7 and 8. Men in 1819. Trousers exposing part of the gaiters (7) or the striped stockings (8).
9. Woman in 1826.
10 and 11. Costume in 1829. Out-door attire.
12. Lady in evening gown, 1832, with full skirt, ample ribbon decoration. Lace stole. Hair arranged in curls.

Bottom Group

13–17. Fashions at Frankfurt on the Main, November/December 1834. (From: *Journal des Dames*, Frankfurt/Main.)

EUROPE. *Uniforms. 1795–1815. Revolution to the Bourbon Restoration* — 121

Top Group

1–7. Prussian military men. 1806–13.
1. Cuirassier in the regiment *von Holtzendorf*. 1806.
2. Infantry staff officer. 1806.
3. Grenadier of the 1st battalion of the body-guard 1806.
4. Musketeer (drummer) the King's regiment. 1806.
5. Lancer (uhlan) in the guards. 1810.
6. Fusilier. 1810.
7. Horseman of the Silesian Cuirassier regiment. 1813.

Centre Group

8–14. England, Russia, Austria, Denmark. 1802–15.
8. English sailor. 1814.
9. Imperial Russian grenadier. 1802.
10. Russian infantry general. 1813.
11. Russian artillery officer. 1813.
12. Officer of the Austrian riflemen. 1813.
13. Soldier in the Danish body-guard. 1805.
14. Cossack. 1813.

Bottom Group

15–21. France. Uniforms during the time of Napoleon. 1795 to 1815.
15. Hussar. 1795.
16. Infantry officer. 1806.
17. Grenadier of the guards. 1813.
18. Musketeer. 1806.
19. Foot soldier. 1806.
20. Sapper. 1813.
21. Foot soldier, 1795.

GERMANY (PRUSSIA). *Uniforms. 1730–70.* — 122

Top Group

1. Infantry regiment *Fürst zu Anhalt-Zerbst* (according to an army recruiting pamphlet about 1740).
2. Frederick the Great on horseback (according to D. Chodowiecki).
3. Soldier from the infantry regiment *Fürst zu Anhalt-Zerbst*.

Centre Group

4. Prussian dragoon. 1750. (According to an engraving by J. M. Probst. Augsburg).
5. Cuirassier in billets wearing sleeved waistcoat. Coat and weapons are hung on the wall, cuirass in front of the stool. (According to an engraving by E. Bück. Nuremberg. Germanisches Museum.)
6. Soldier of the giant guard of Frederick William I. (According to a painting formerly in the Charlottenburg Palace.)

Bottom Group

7. Hussar regiment von Kleist, 1758–67 (green uniform).
8. First dragoon regiment.
9. Fifth hussar regiment (black uniform with the emblem of the skull on the helmet: Totenkopfhusaren).
10. Trumpeter of the 12th cuirassier regiment.
11. Grenadier wearing red cap with a tin shield in front.

GERMANY AND FRANCE. LATE ROCOCO, *about 1788* — 123

Women's and men's fashions according to engravings by Riepenhausen from the Göttingen pocket almanac (Göttinger Taschenkalender) 1788. German and French fashions as well as stage costumes are shown in these small almanacs by way of small engravings as early as the seventies of the 18th century, that is to say some time before the appearance of the fashion papers proper (from 1785 on) with their coloured fashion plates.

FRANCE. *Paris Fashions. 1830–35* — 124

1. Evening cape. Paris, February 1834.
2. Evening dress. Paris, February 1833.
3. March 1834.
4. Visite. Paris, April 1834. According to coloured lithographs by Gavarni from the *Journal des gens du monde.* 1833–34.

125 FRANCE AND GERMANY. *Fashion 1850–60. The Time of the Crinoline*

1. Paris fashion, January 1850. Coloured engraving by Compte-Calix from *Modes Parisiennes.*
2. Paris fashion, June 1850. Coloured engraving by Compte-Calix from *Modes Parisiennes.*
3. Berlin fashion, March 1858. Steel engraving from *Hermann Gersons Modezeitung* (Gerson's fashion paper).
4. Berlin fashion, September 1858. Coloured steel engraving from *Herman Gersons Modezeitung* (Gerson's fashion paper).

126 FRANCE AND GERMANY. *Fashion 1870–75. The Time of the Tournure.*

1. Paris evening gown. November 1873. Coloured lithograph by Gustave Janet from *La Mode Artistique.*
2. Paris racing dress, July 1875. Lithograph by Gustave Janet from *La Mode Artistique.*
3. Men's fashion in Germany, July 1872. Coloured lithograph from the *Europäische Modenzeitung* (European Fashion Paper) Leipzig.
4. Women's fashion in Germany, October 1874. Coloured steel engraving from the *Illustrierte Frauenzeitung* (Illustrated Women's Paper) Berlin, Franz Lipperheide.

PLATES

ANCIENT EGYPT

Old Kingdom about 3000 B.

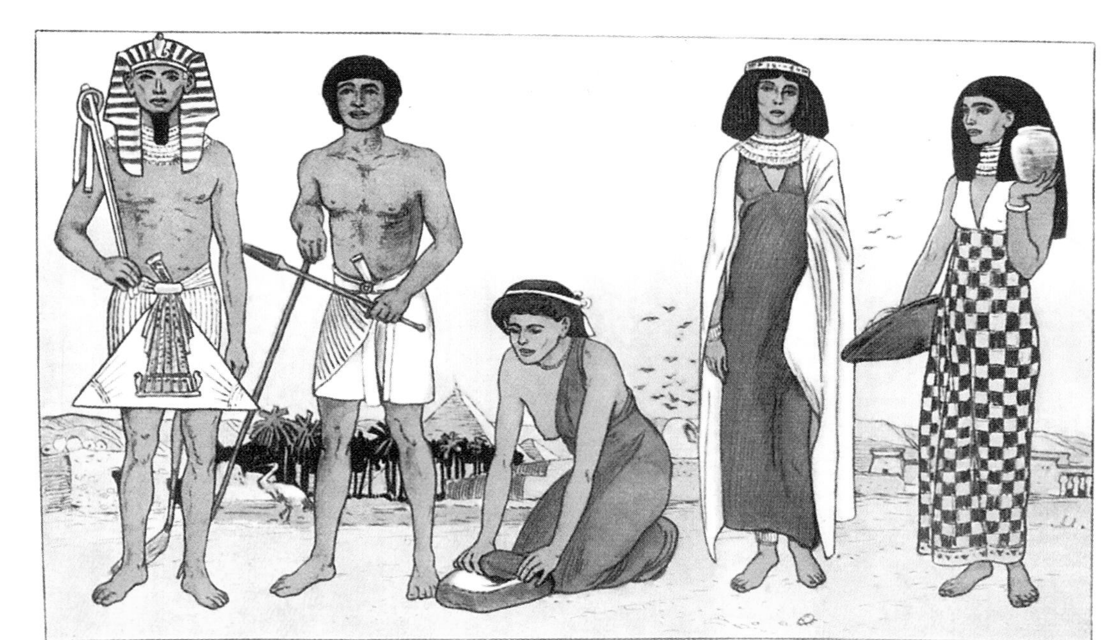

1 2 3 4 5

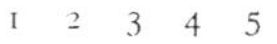

Middle Kingdom about 2100 B. C.

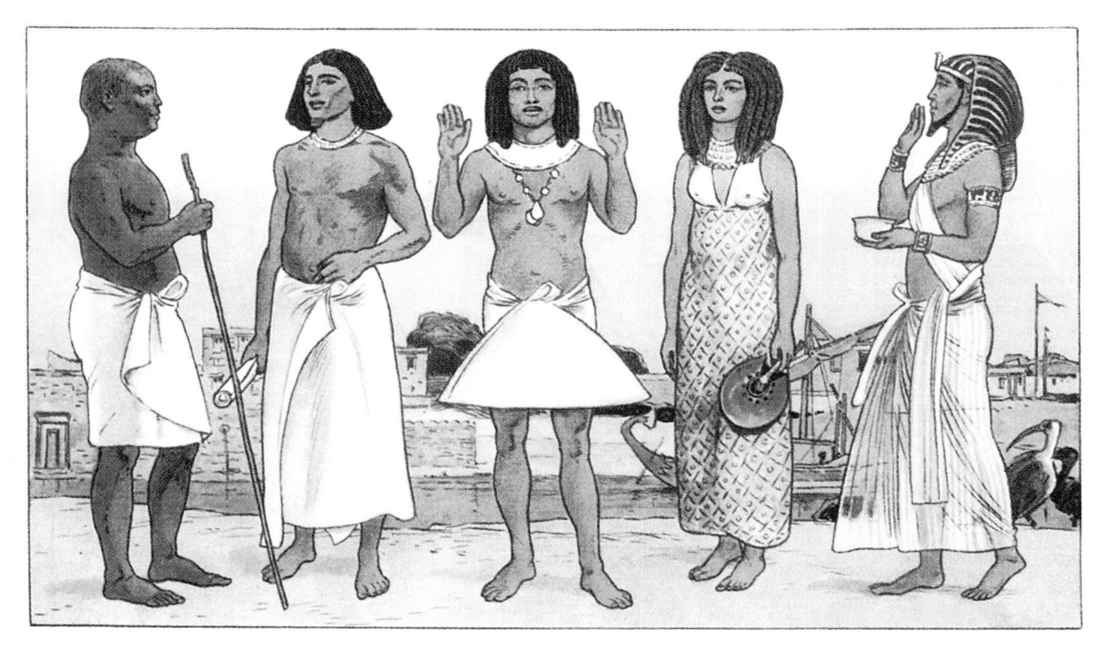

6 7 8 9 10

New Kingdom 1600–1100 B. C.

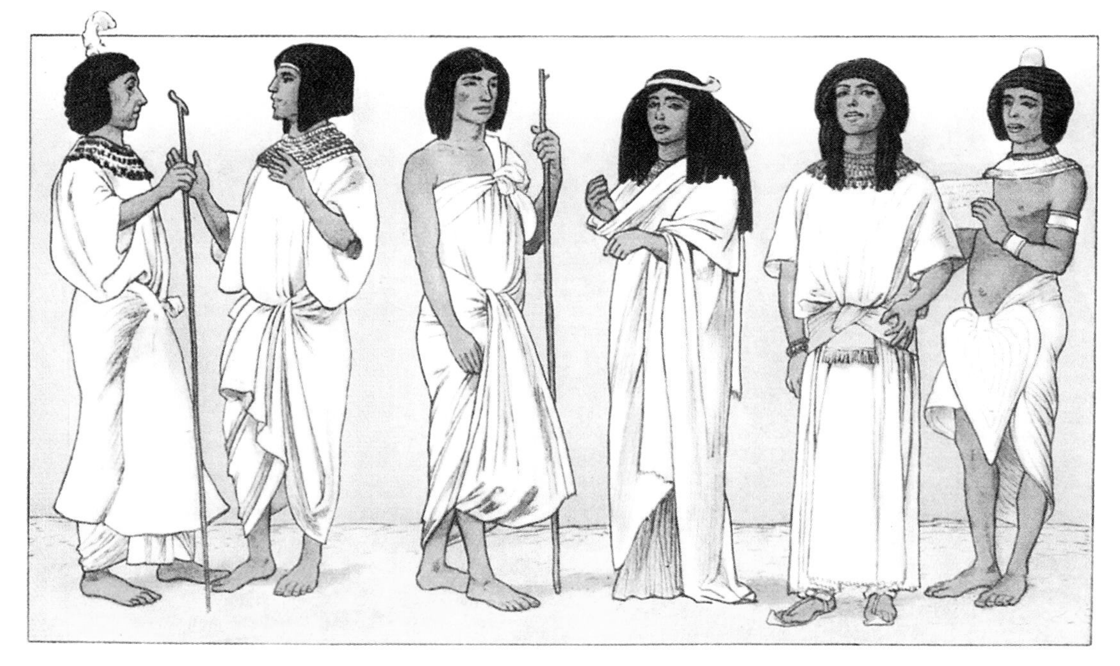

11 12 13 14 15 16

ANCIENT EGYPT

New Kingdom
(Time of Rameses I.
to Rameses III.
1350–1200 B. C.)

Priests, Officials

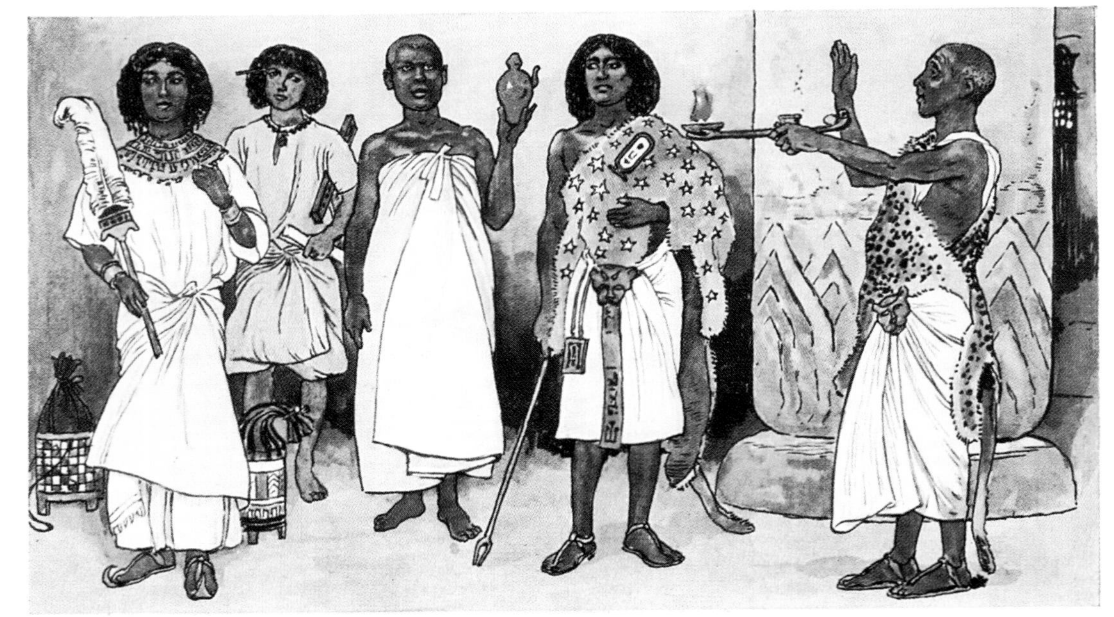

1 2 3 4 5

The King and his Court

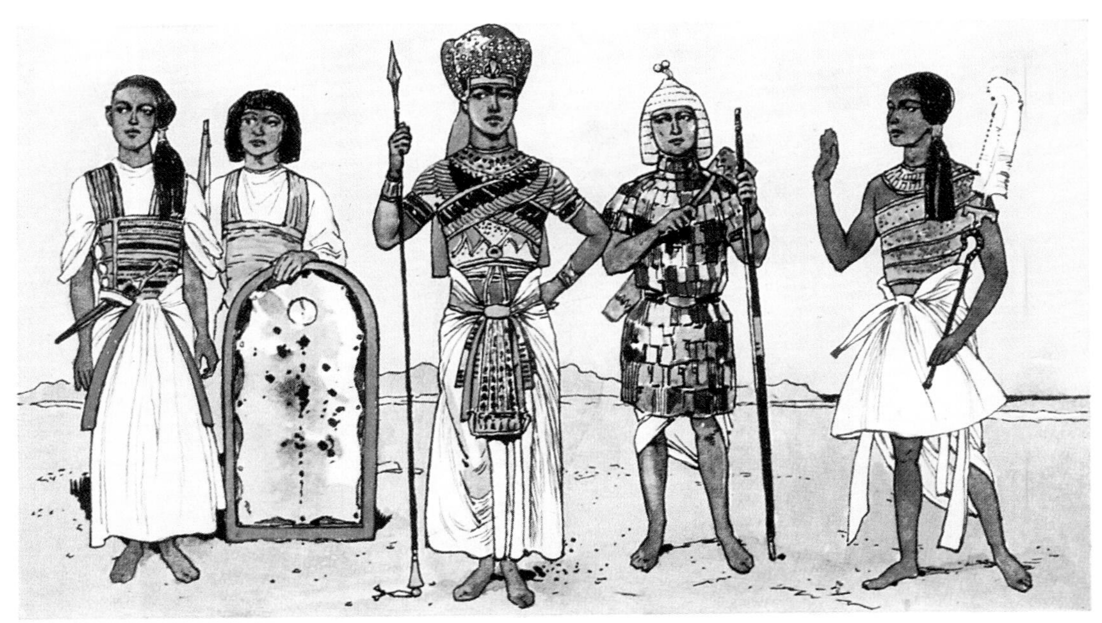

6 7 8 9 10

Soldiers

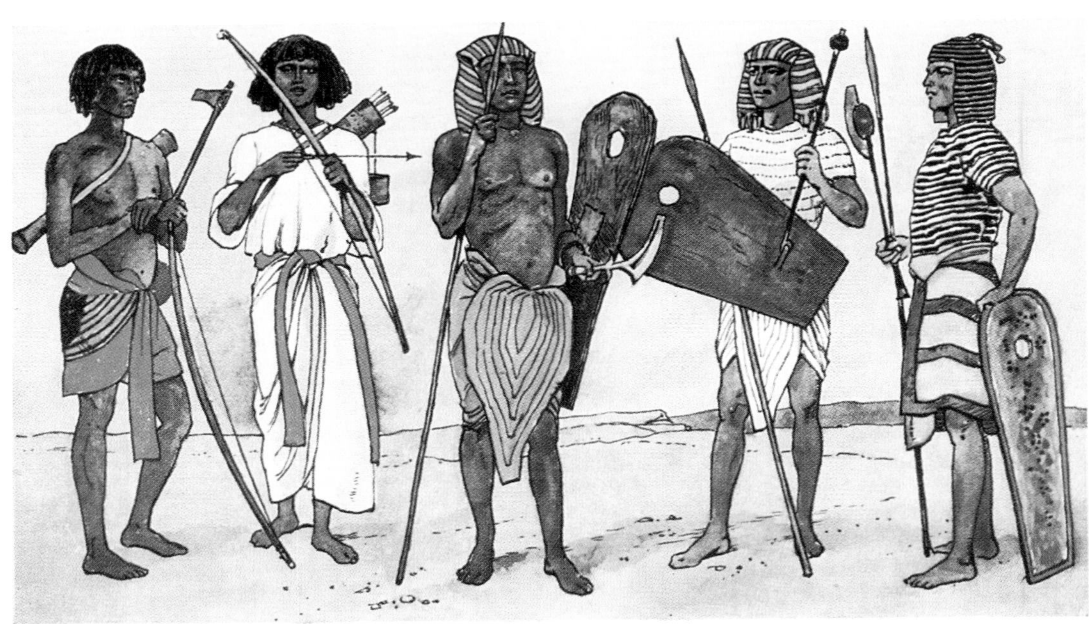

11 12 13 14 15

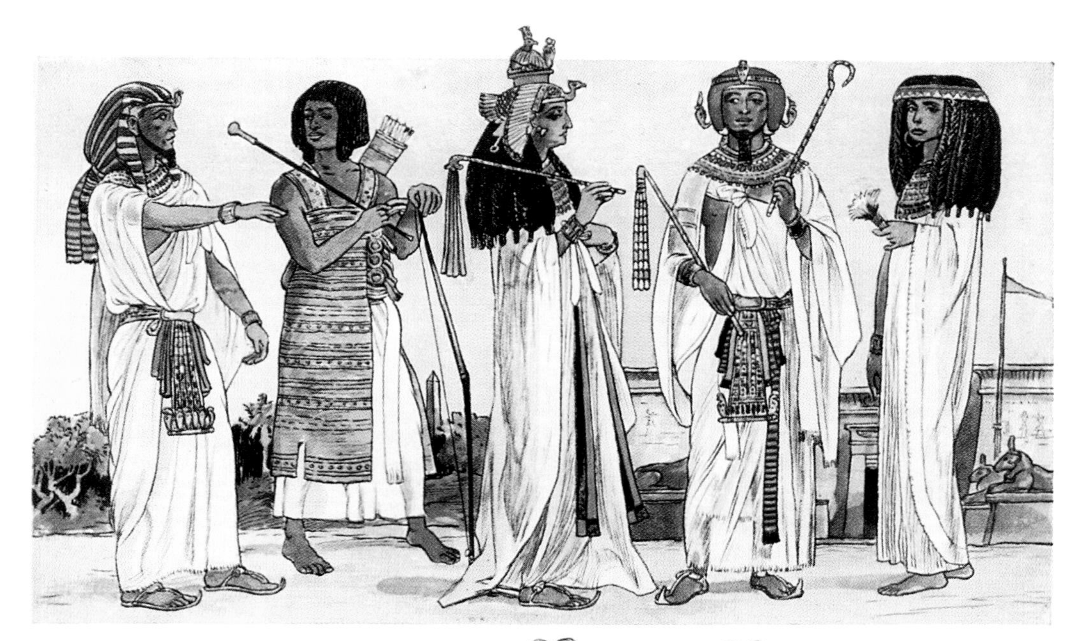

ANCIENT EGYPT

New Kingdom 1600–1100 B. C.
The King and his Court

1 2 3 4 5

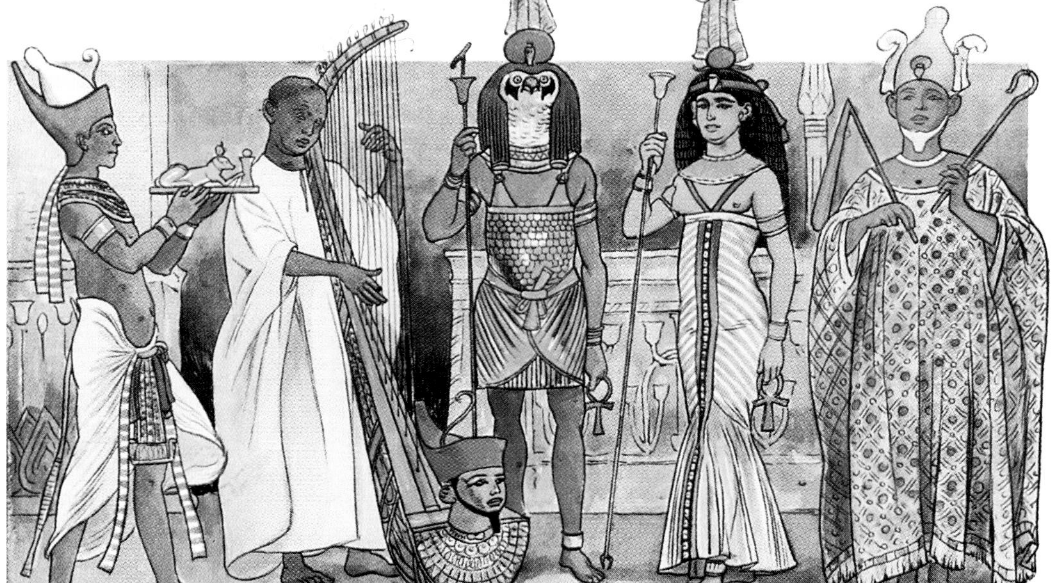

Kings, Priests
and Images of Gods

6 7 8 9 10

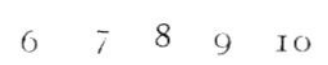

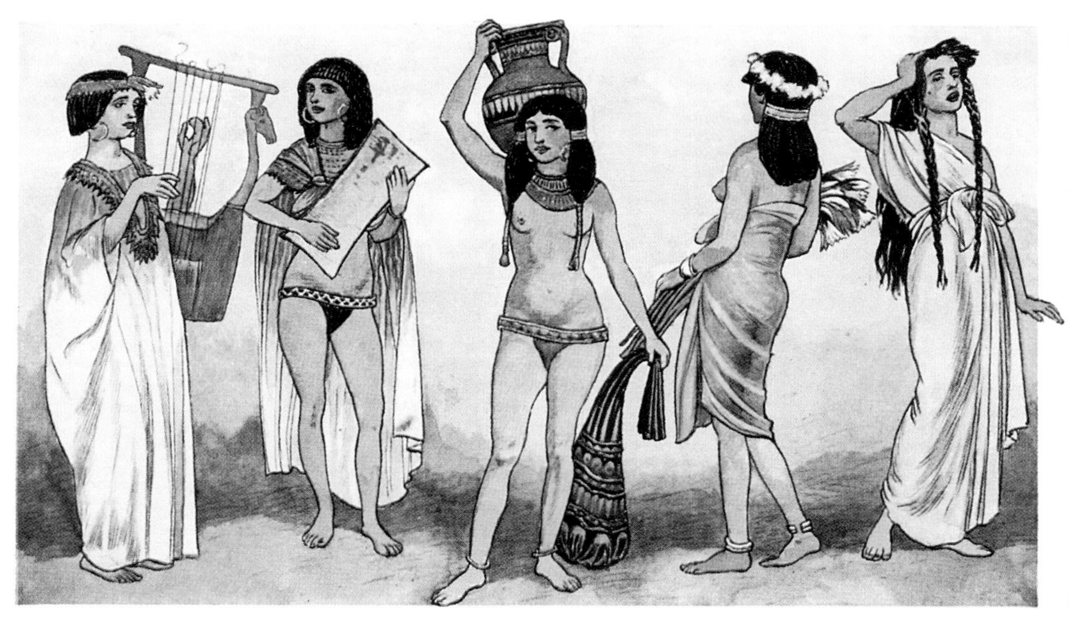

Slave Girls

11 12 13 14 15

ANCIENT EGYPT

New Kingdom
(Late Period: Rameses I. and Successors, 14th and 13th Centuries B. C.)

Kings and their Retinue
Priests, Soldiers, Implements

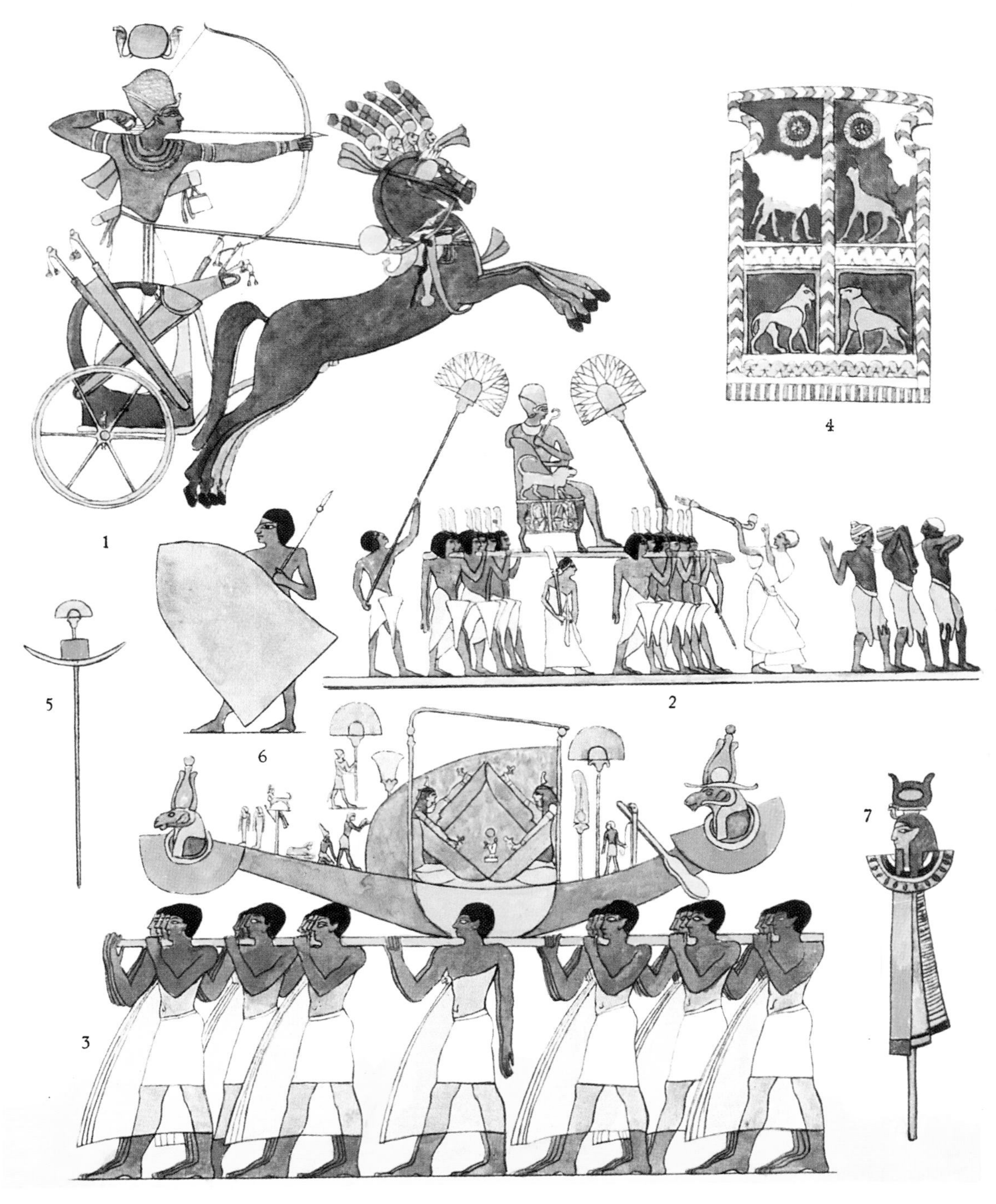

Priestesses, priests, etc.

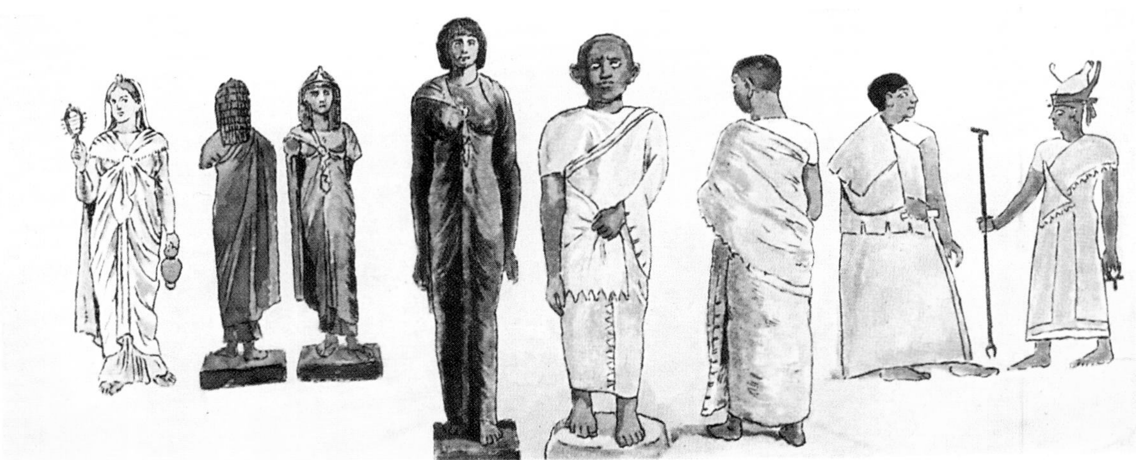

8–15

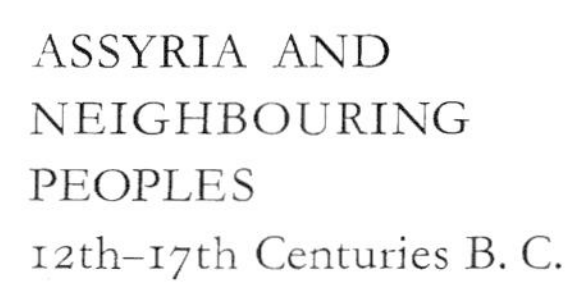

ASSYRIA AND NEIGHBOURING PEOPLES

12th–17th Centuries B. C.

King and Retinue

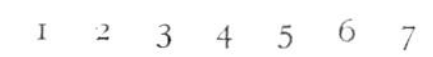

1 2 3 4 5 6 7

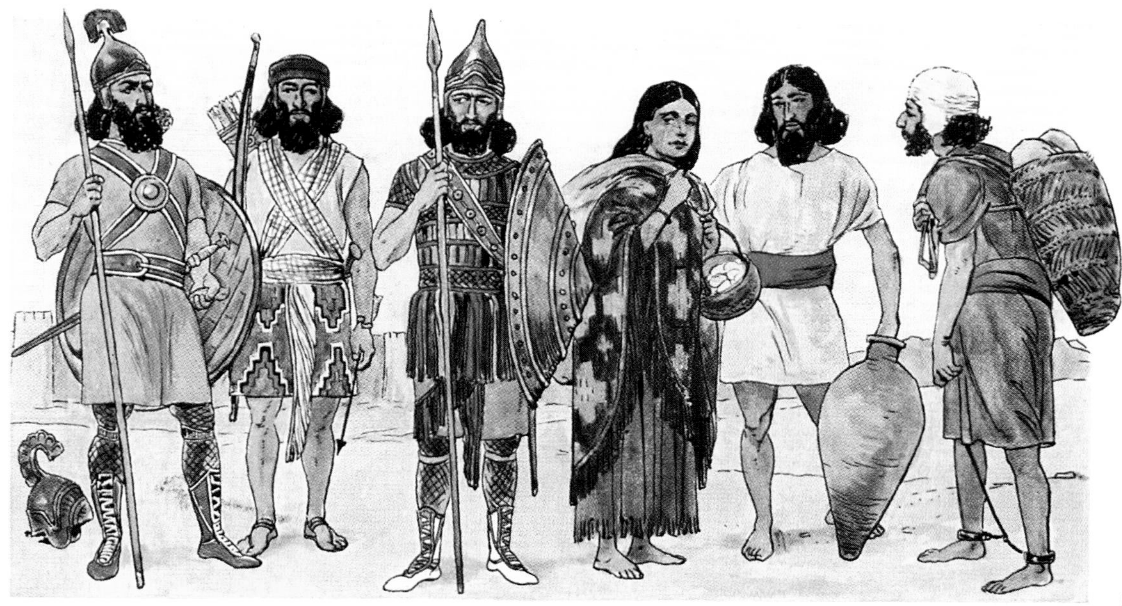

Warriors, etc.

8 9 10 11 12 13

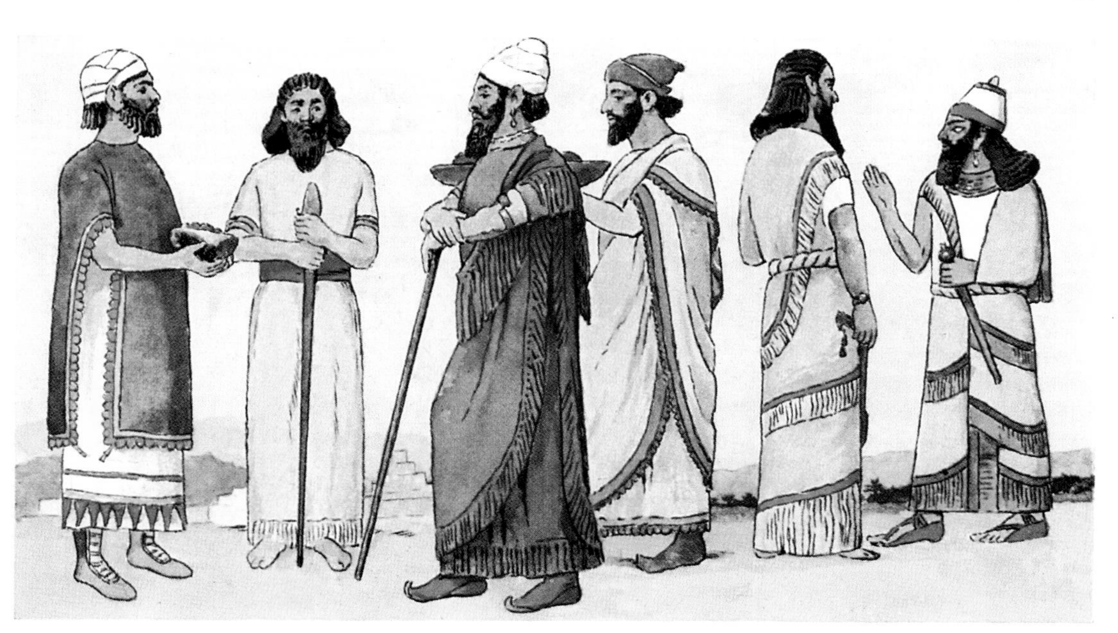

Tribute-bearers
Sacrificial Garments

14 15 16 17 18 19

BABYLONIA AND ASSYRIA (2800–700 B.C.)

Babylonia

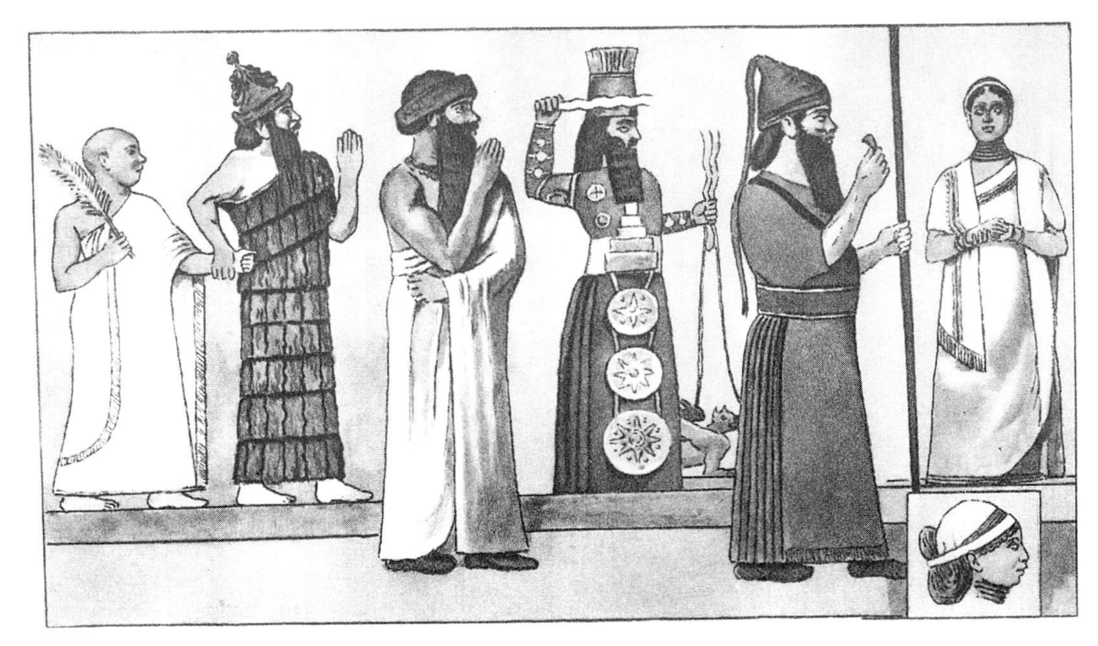

1 2 3 4 5 6

Assyria, King and his Court

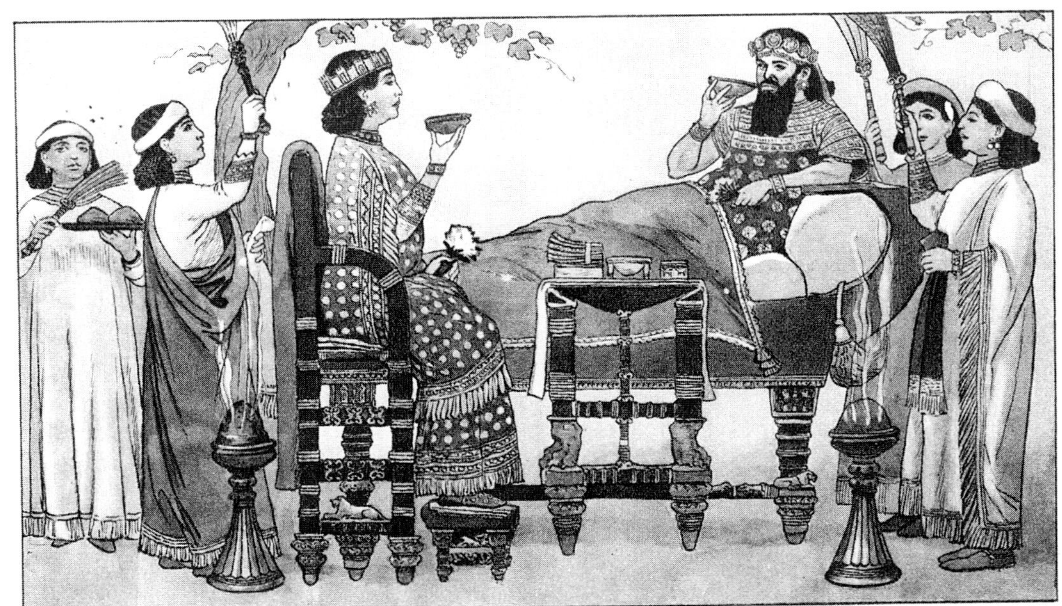

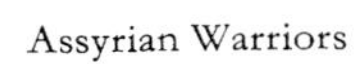

7 8 9 10 11 12

Assyrian Warriors

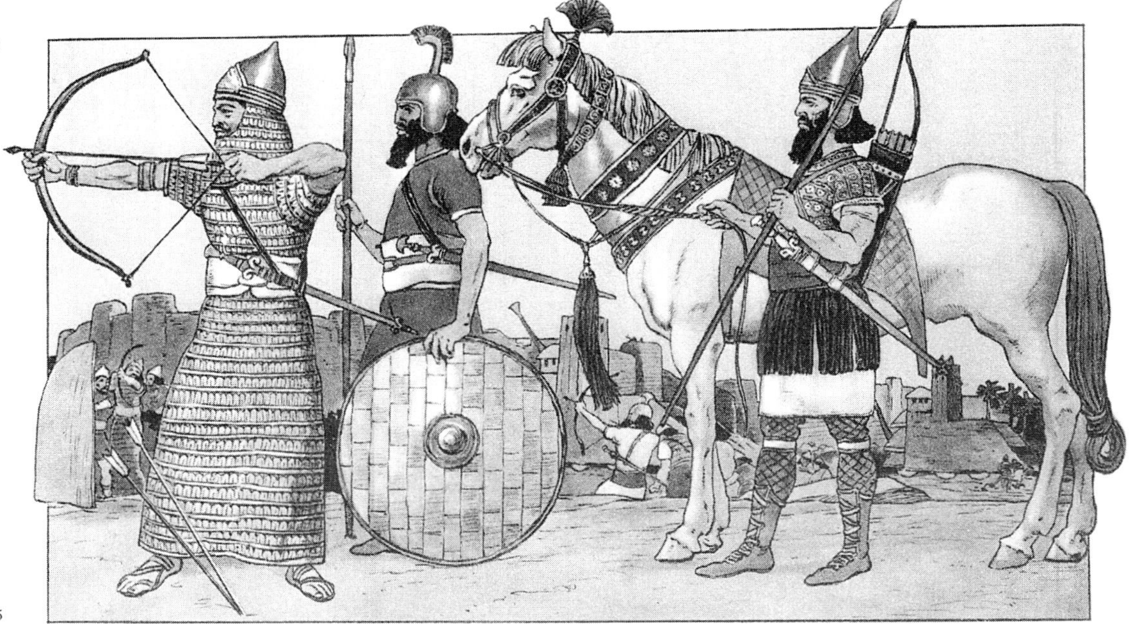

13 14 15

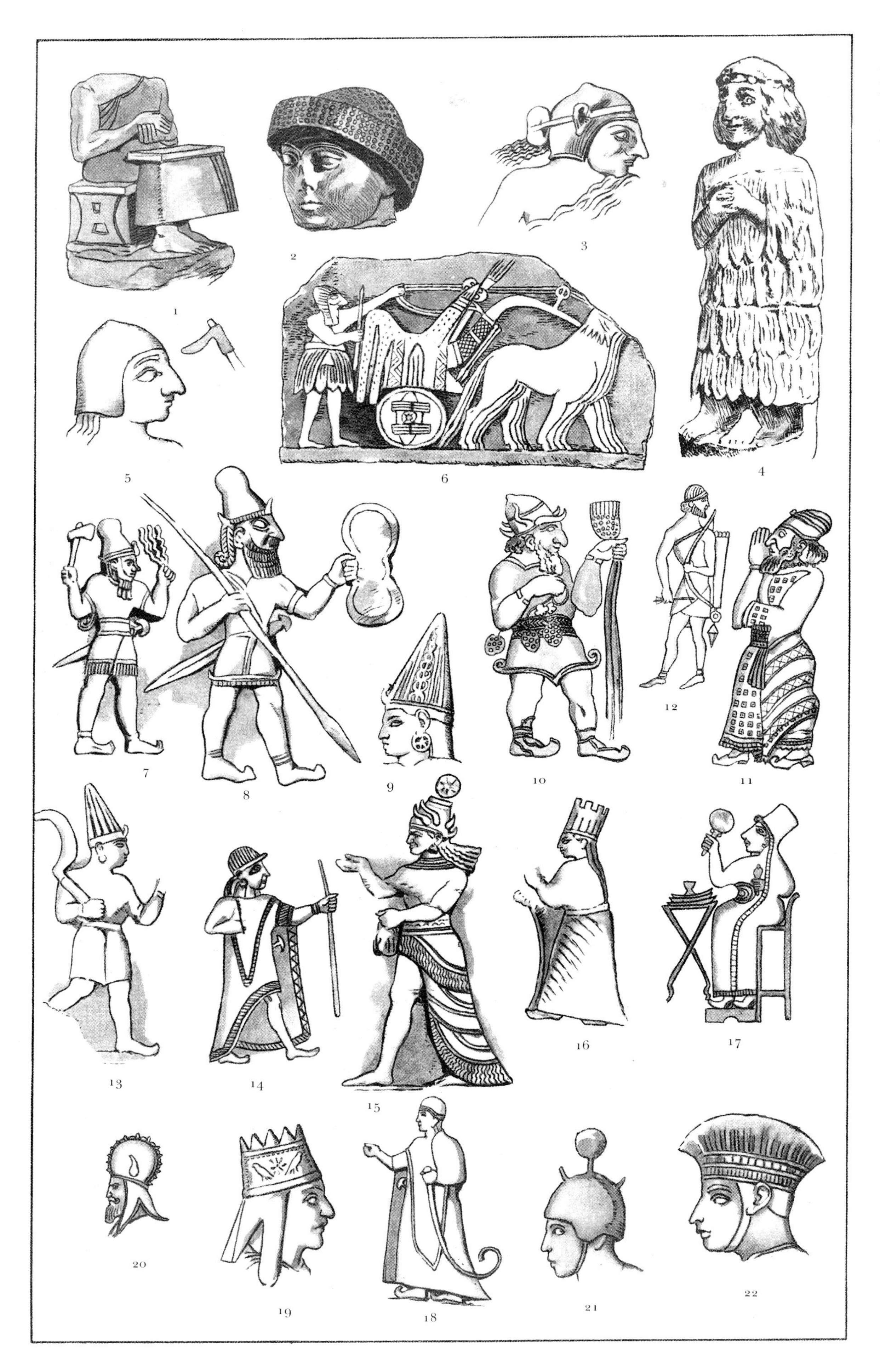

ARMENIANS, PARTHIANS, PHILISTINES, SUMERIANS, HITTITES, ARABS

WESTERN ASIA IN ANTIQUITY

Crete, Palestine, Syria

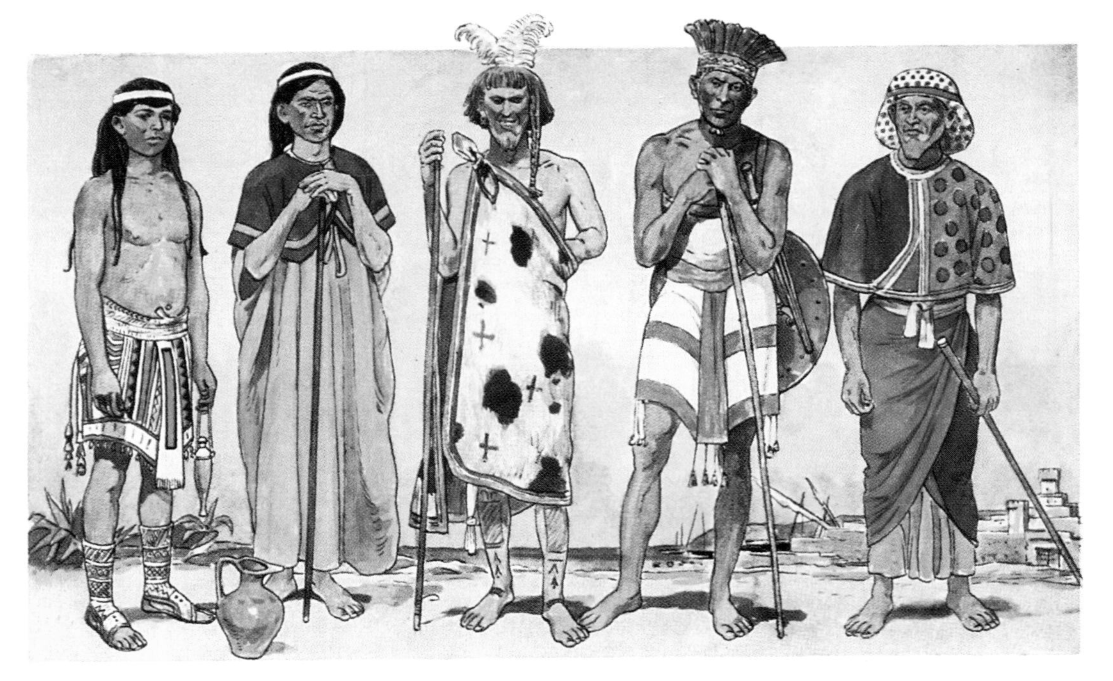

1 2 3 4 5

Bedouins, Syria, Palestine

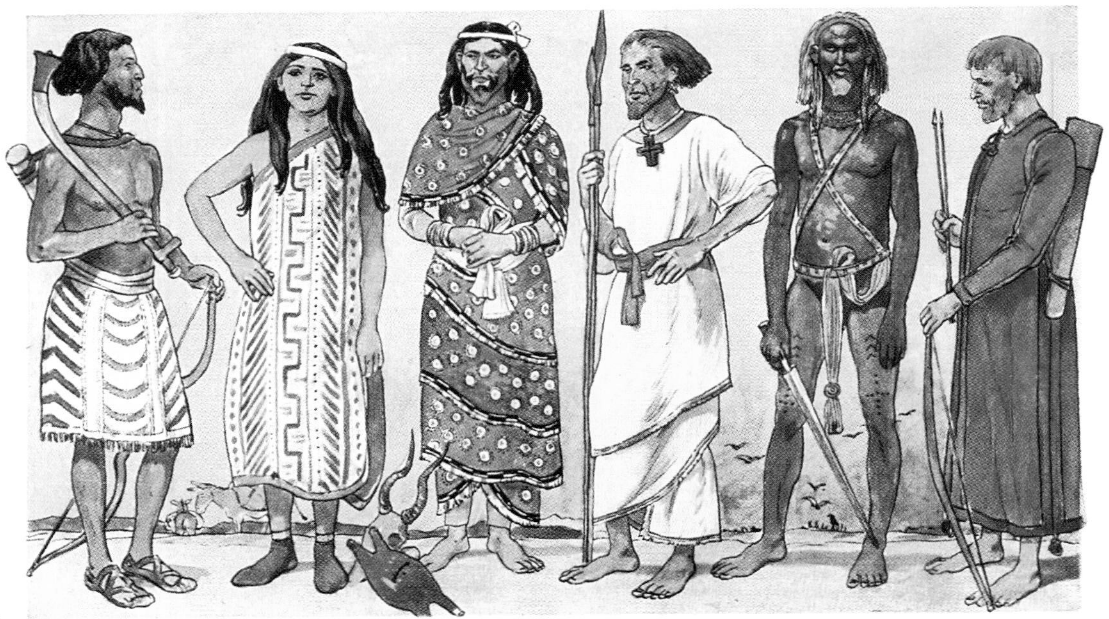

6 7 8 9 10 11

Hebrews

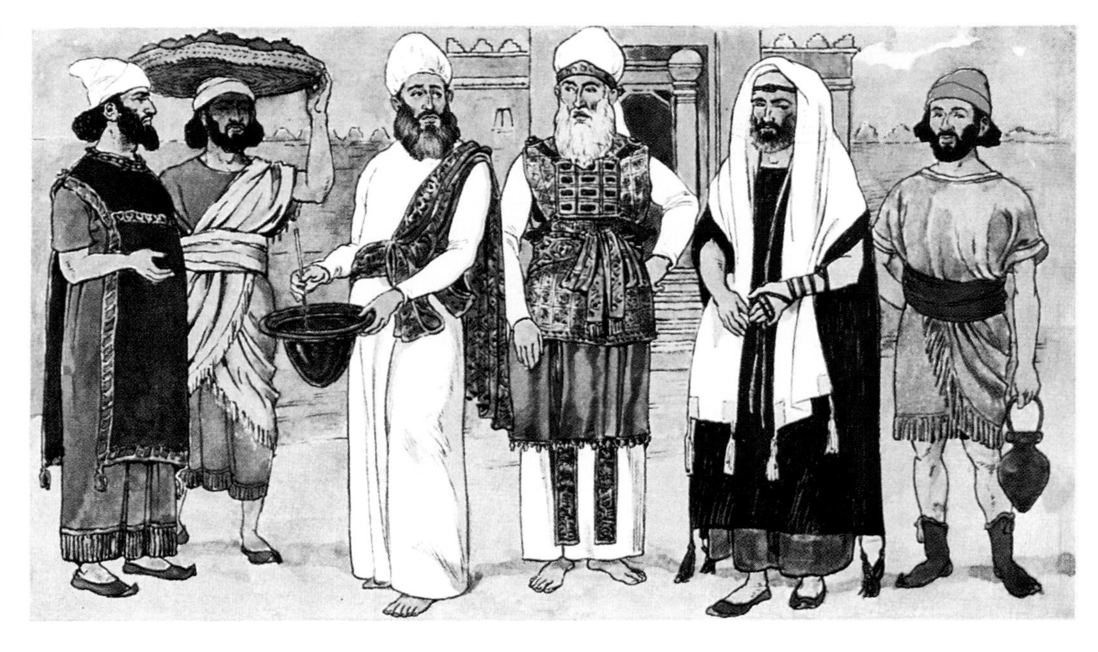

12 13 14 15 16 17

MYCENAE, CRETE, CYPRUS

(Aegean and Phoenician Cultures) 2000–500 B.C.

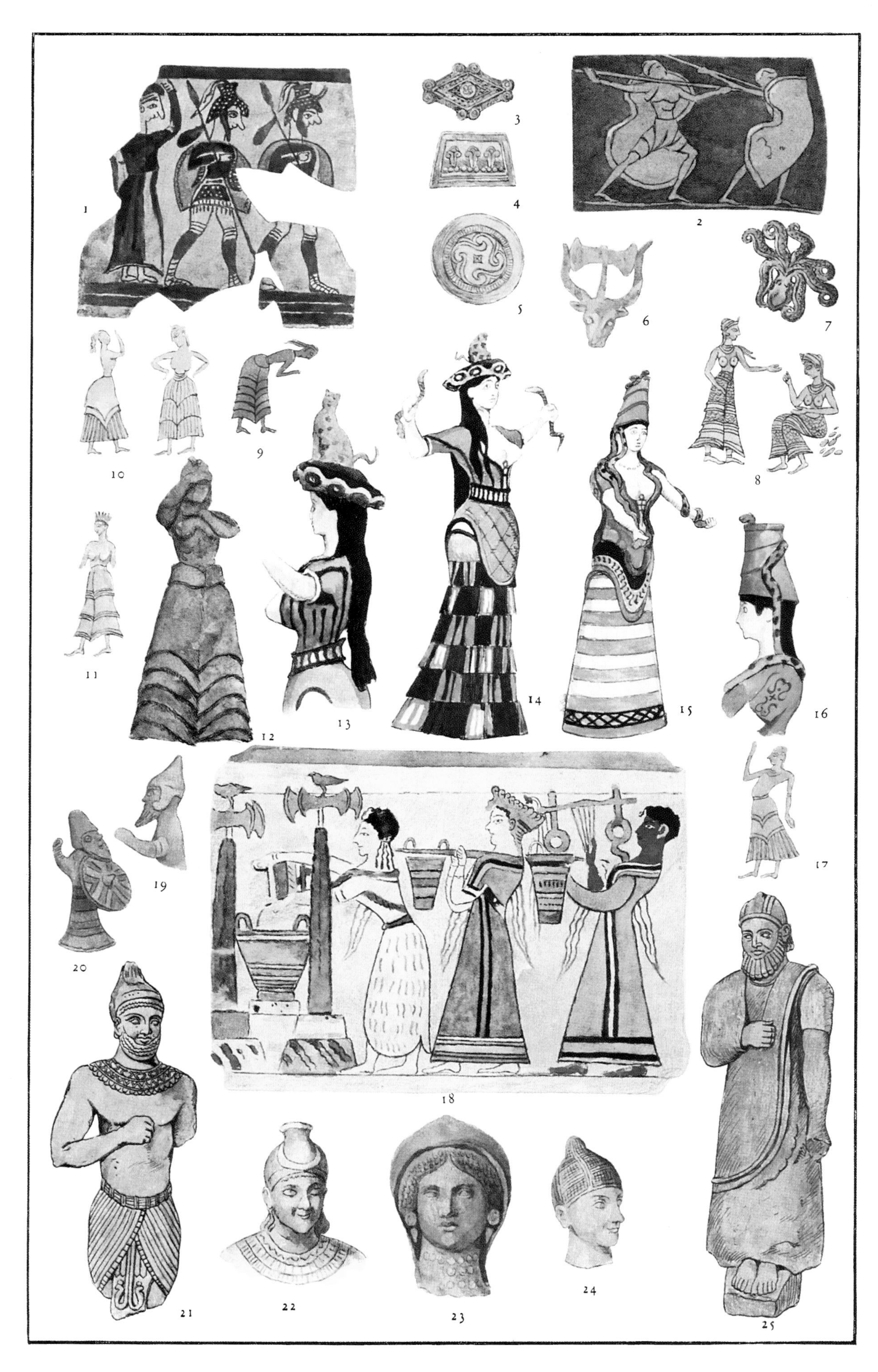

Mycenae
1–11

Crete
12–18

Cyprus
19–25

PERSIA
Antiquity and Early Middle Ages

Ancient Persia
6th–5th Centuries B.C.

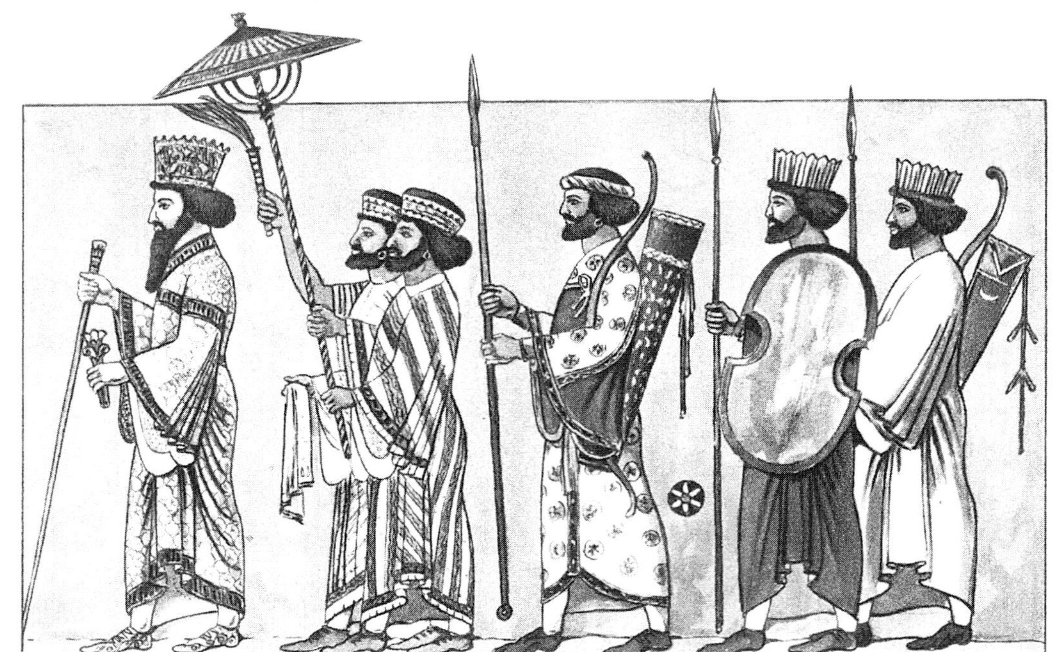

1 2 3 4 5 6

Ancient Persia
6th–5th Centuries B.C.

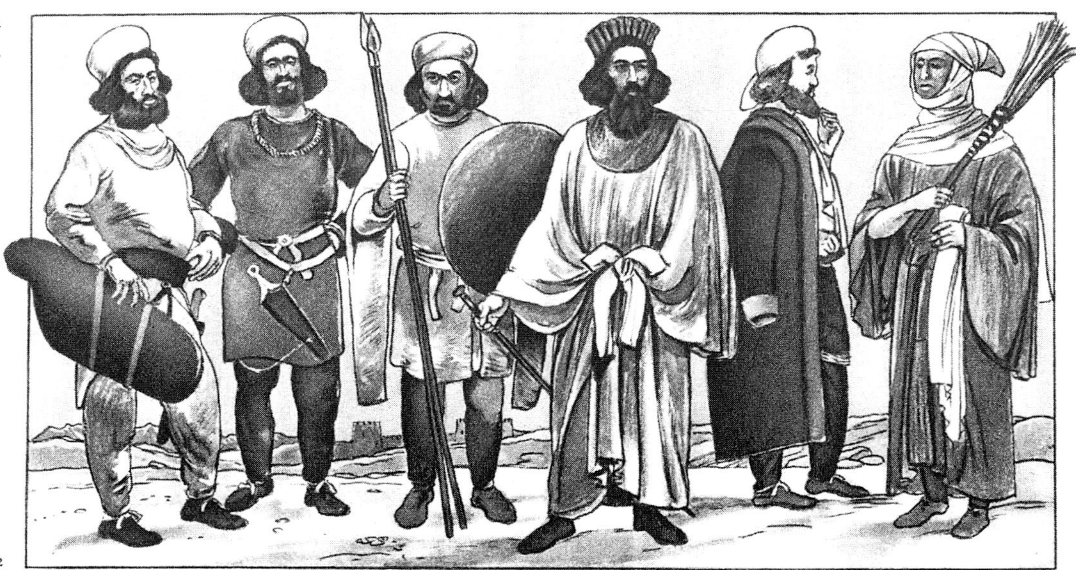

7 8 9 10 11 12

Persia about 600 A.D.

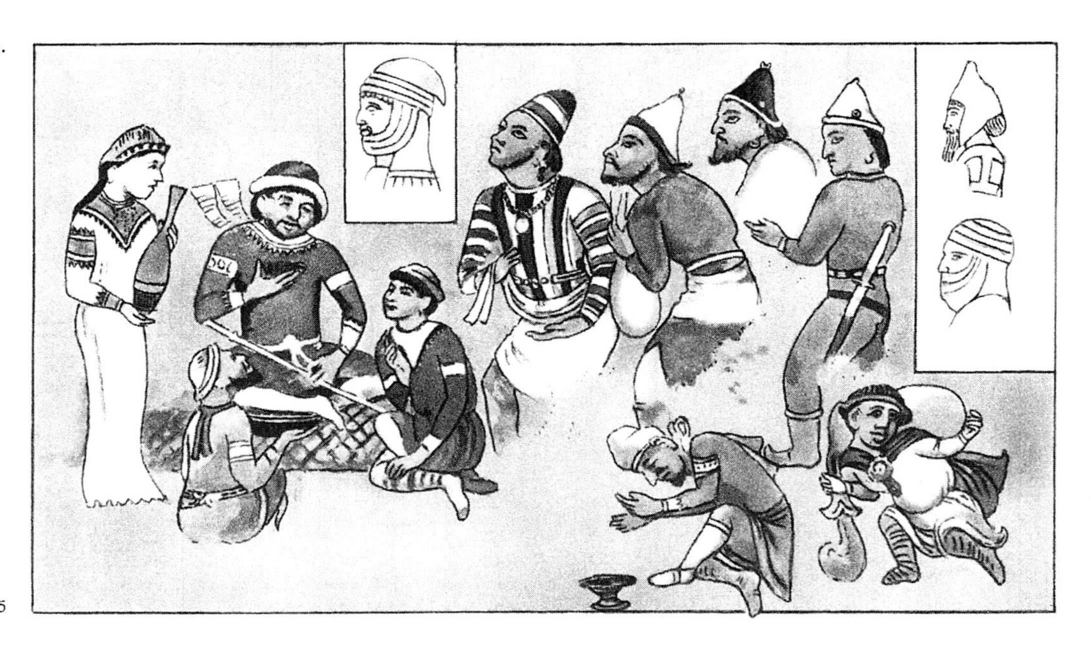

13–25

SCYTHIANS AND INHABITANTS OF ASIA MINOR
8th and 7th Centuries B. C.

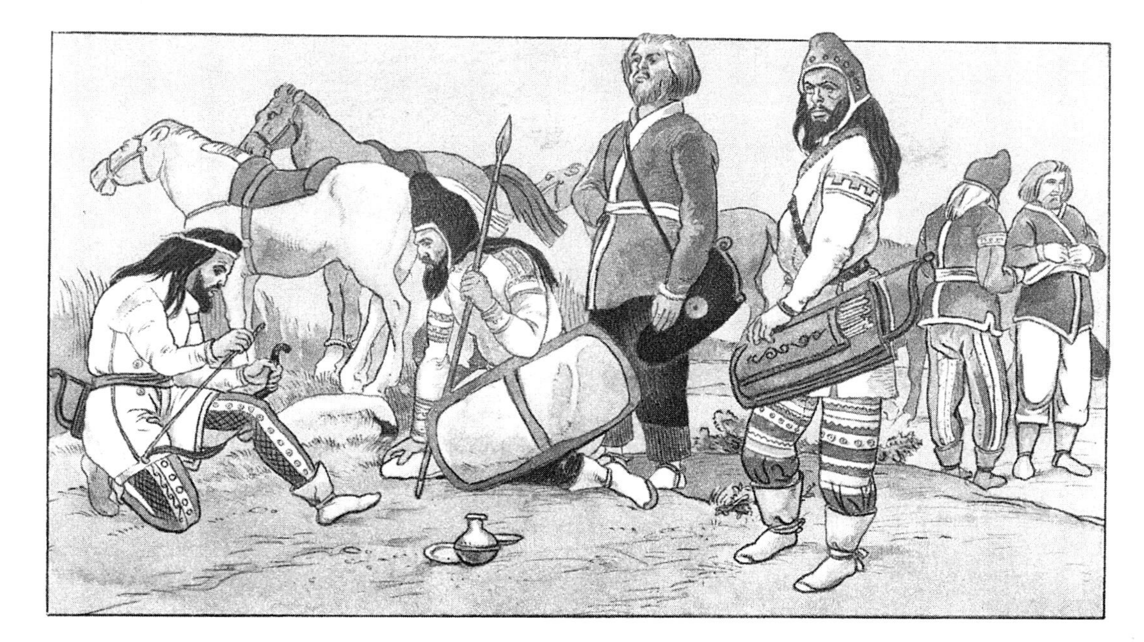

Scythians

1 2 3 4 5 6

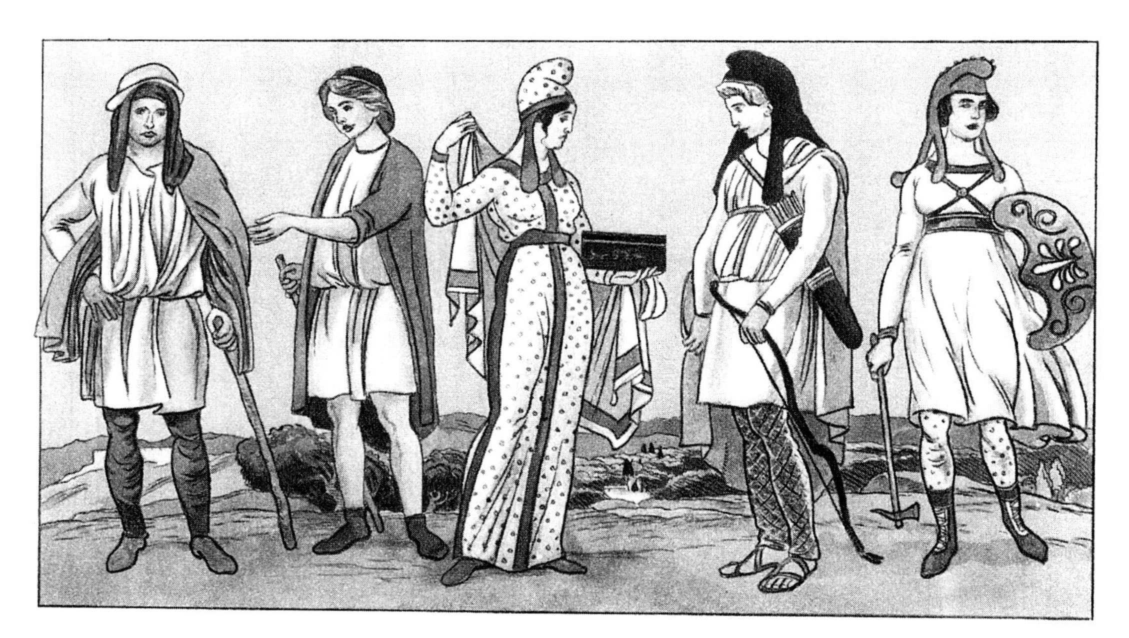

Phrygians

7 8 9 10 11

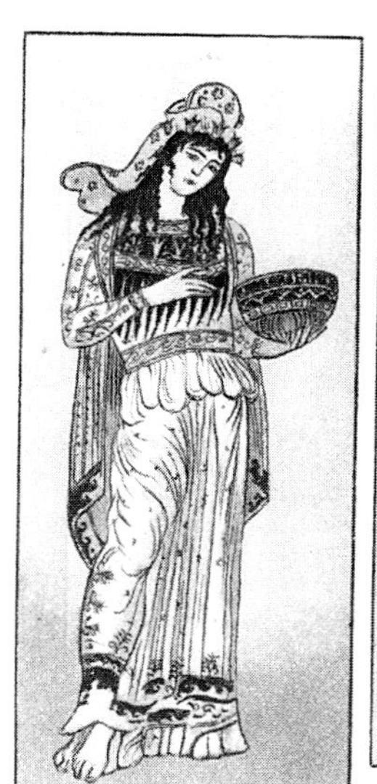

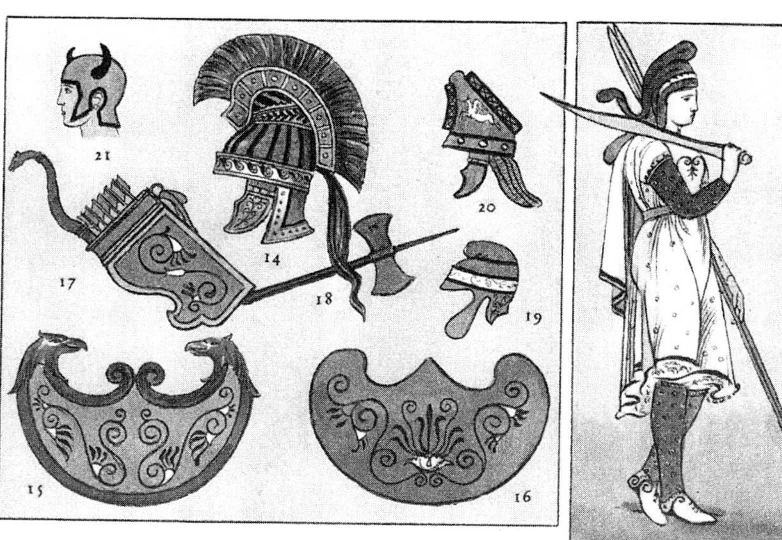

Other Inhabitants of Asia Minor

12 13 14–21

GREECE

6th and 5th Centuries B. C.

1st Half of 6th Century

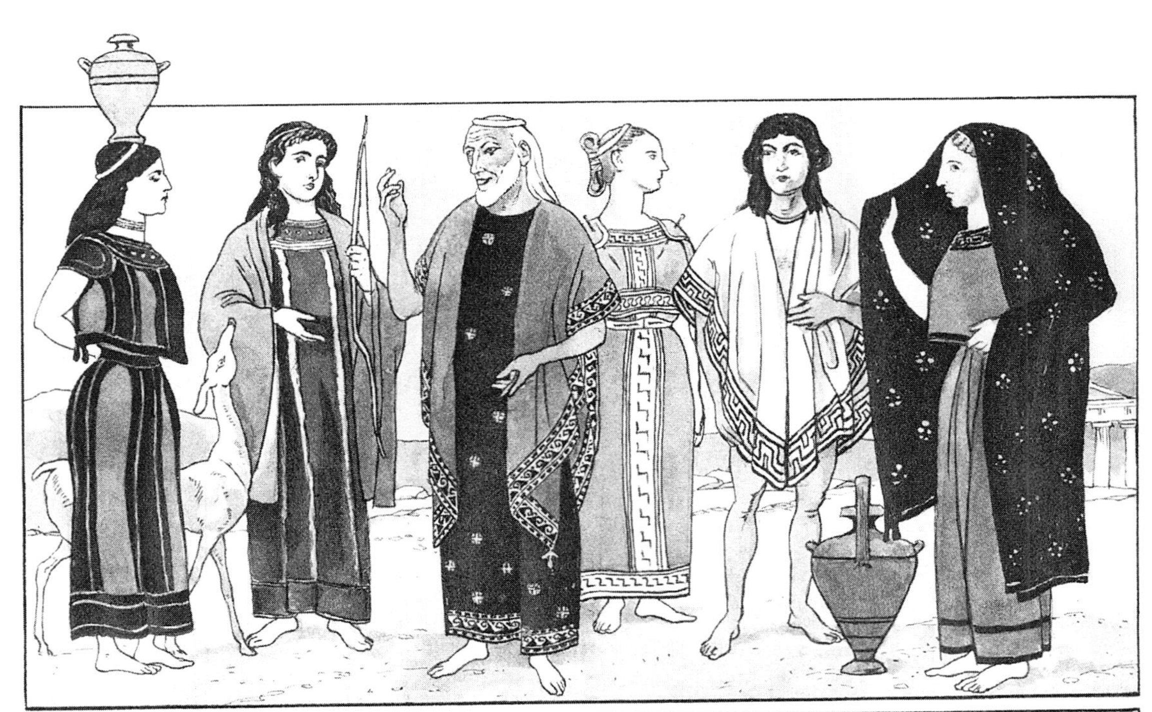

1 2 3 4 5 6

6th and 5th Centuries

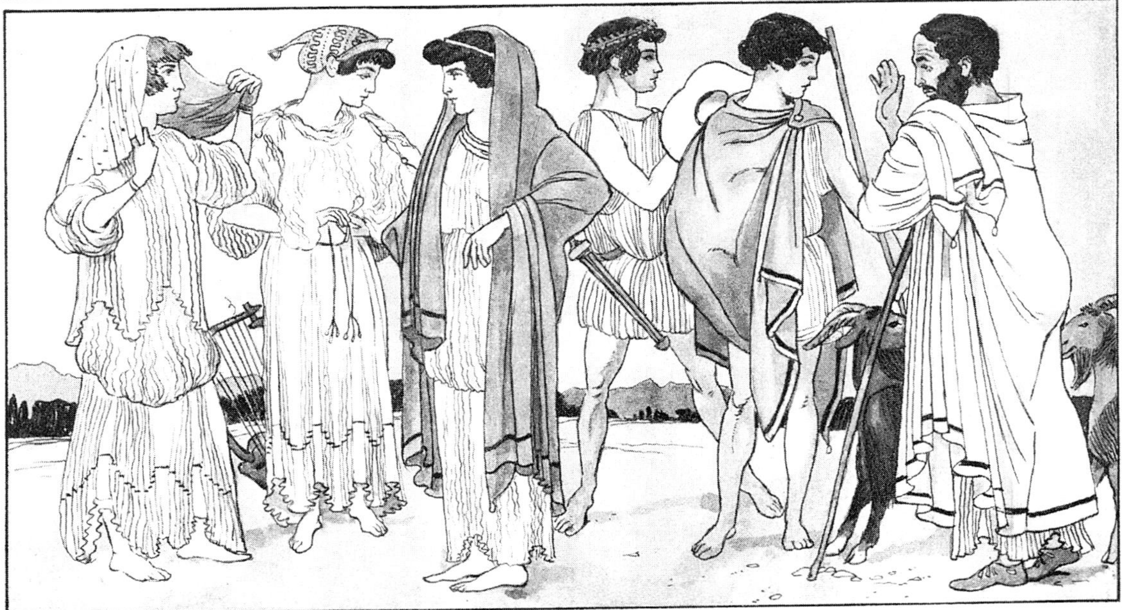

7 8 9 10 11 12

5th Century

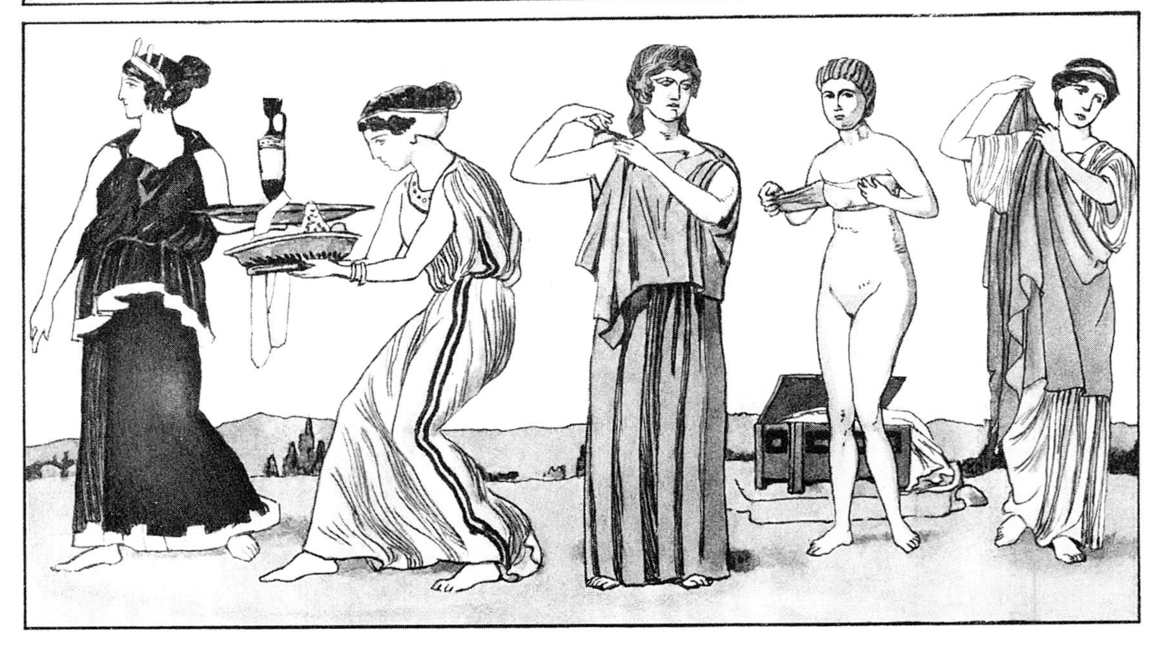

13 14 15 16 17

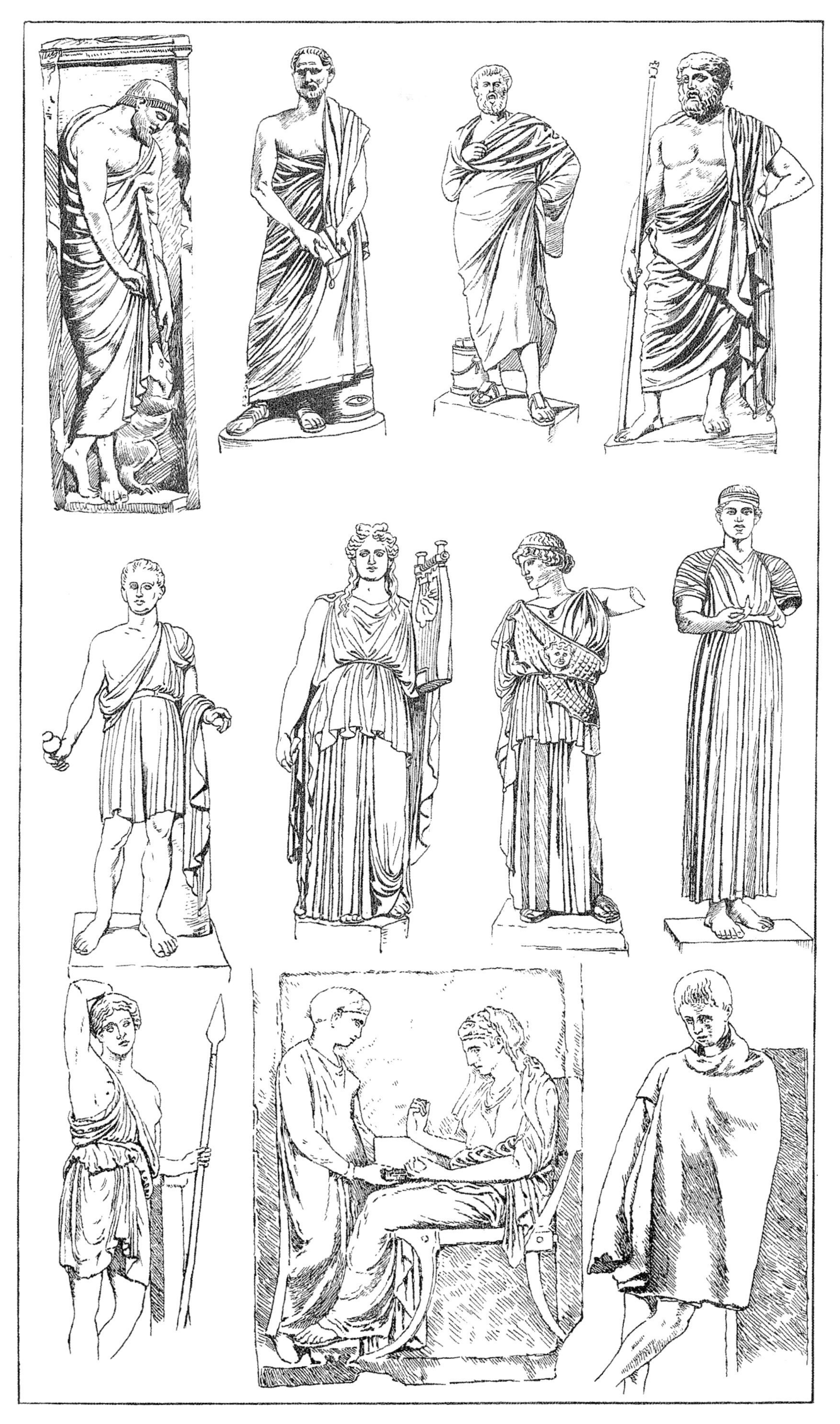

GREECE
5th–4th Centuries

Himation

1 2 3 4

Chiton and Peplos

5 6 7 8

Chiton, Chlamys

9 10 11 12

GREECE

Armour, Banqueting, Games, Music

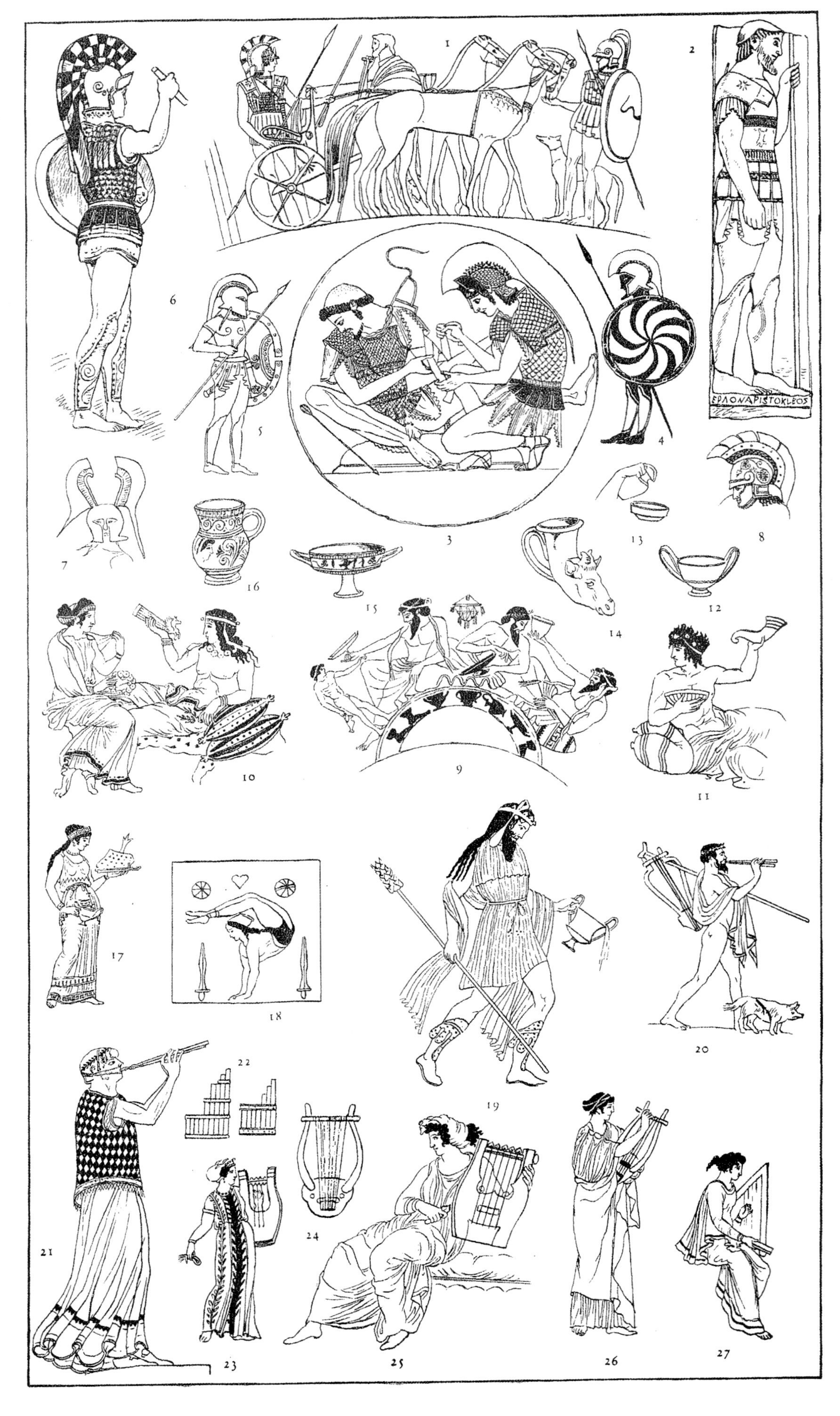

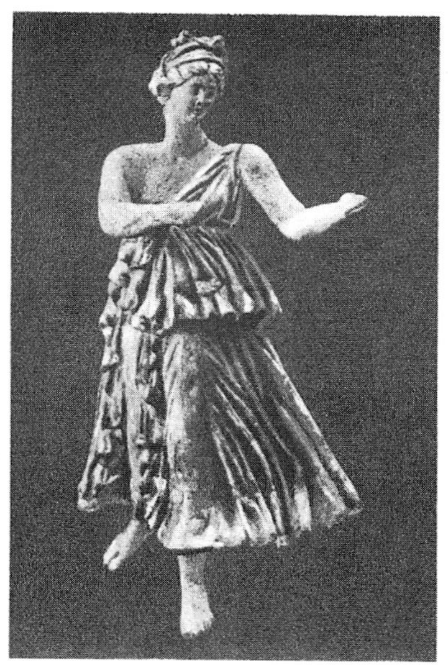
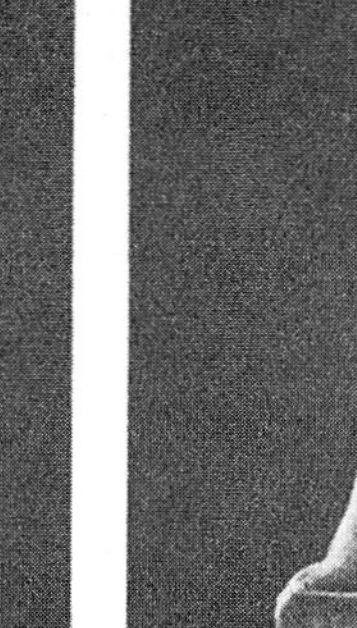
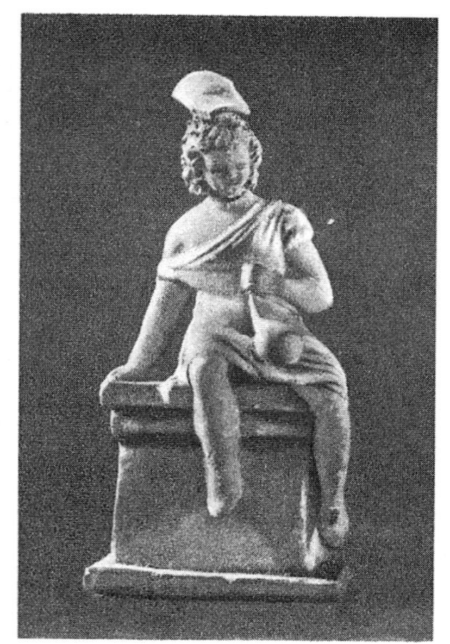
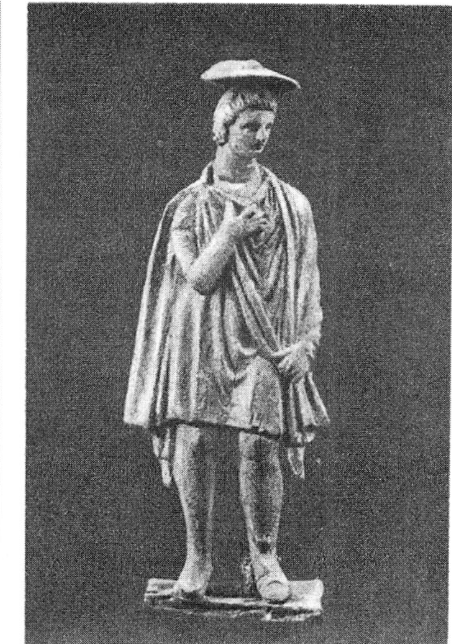
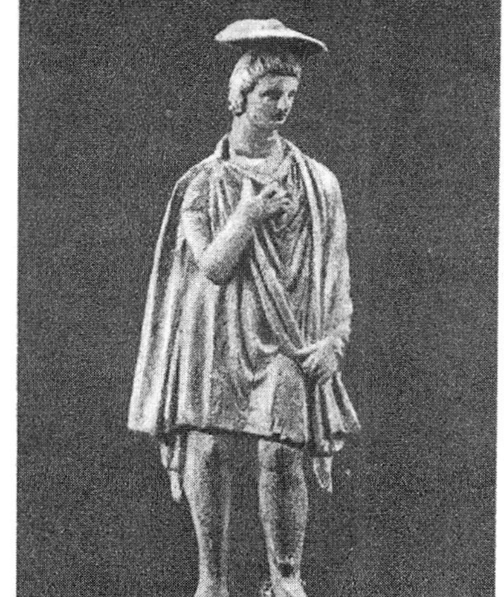

GREECE
Late Period
4th Century B.C.

Late Greek Town Costume

Painted Terra-cotta
Figures from
Tanagra, Boeotia

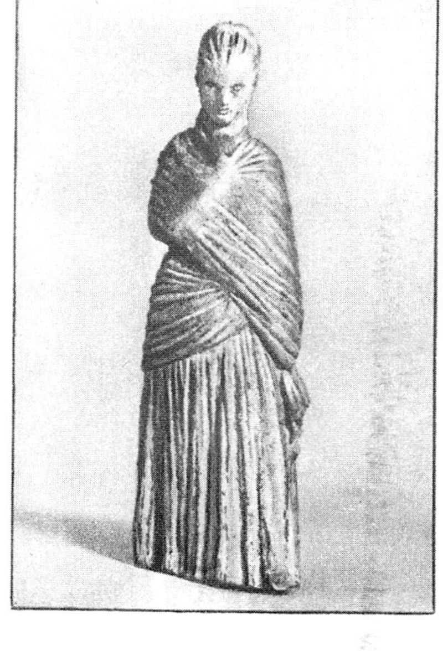
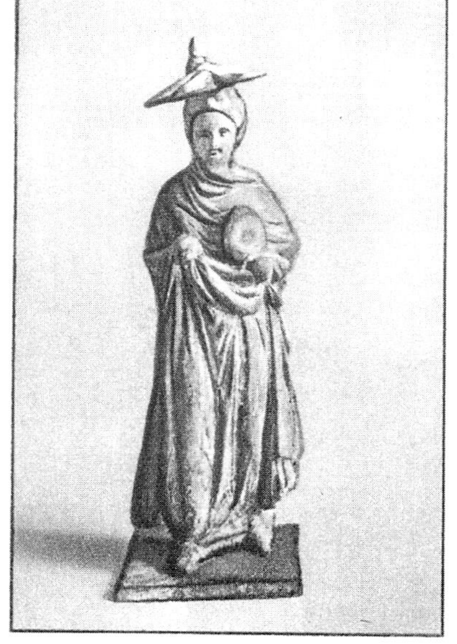
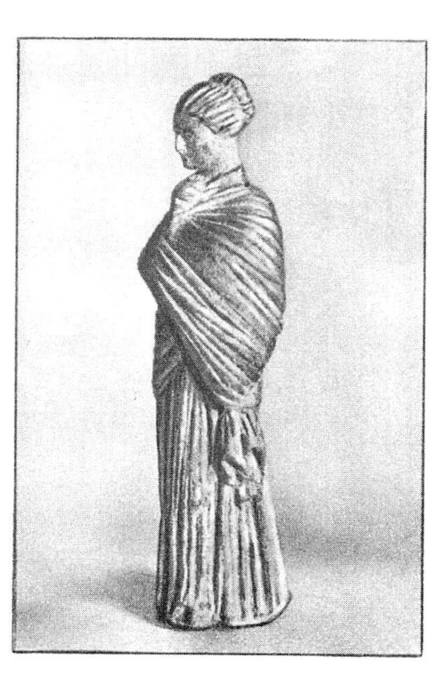

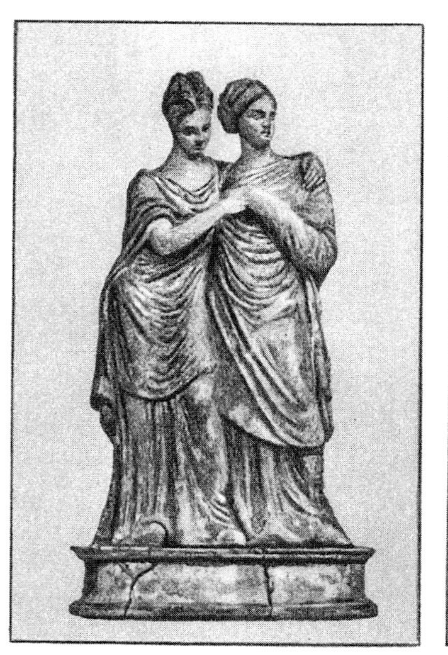
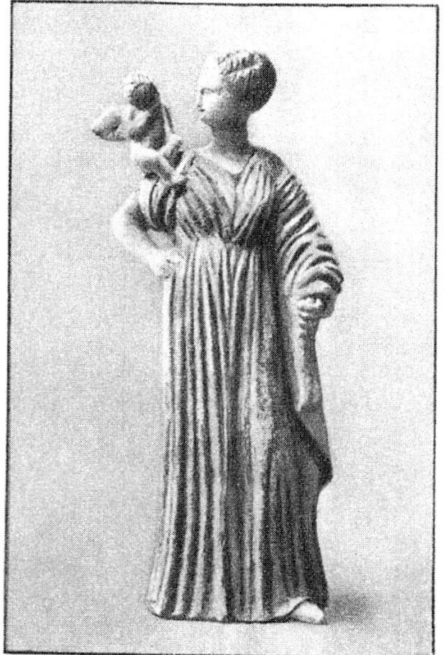

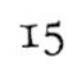

ETRUSCANS
About 750 B. C.

Costume
1–18

Warriors

19 20 21 22 23 24

Banquet, Dance, Music

25–35

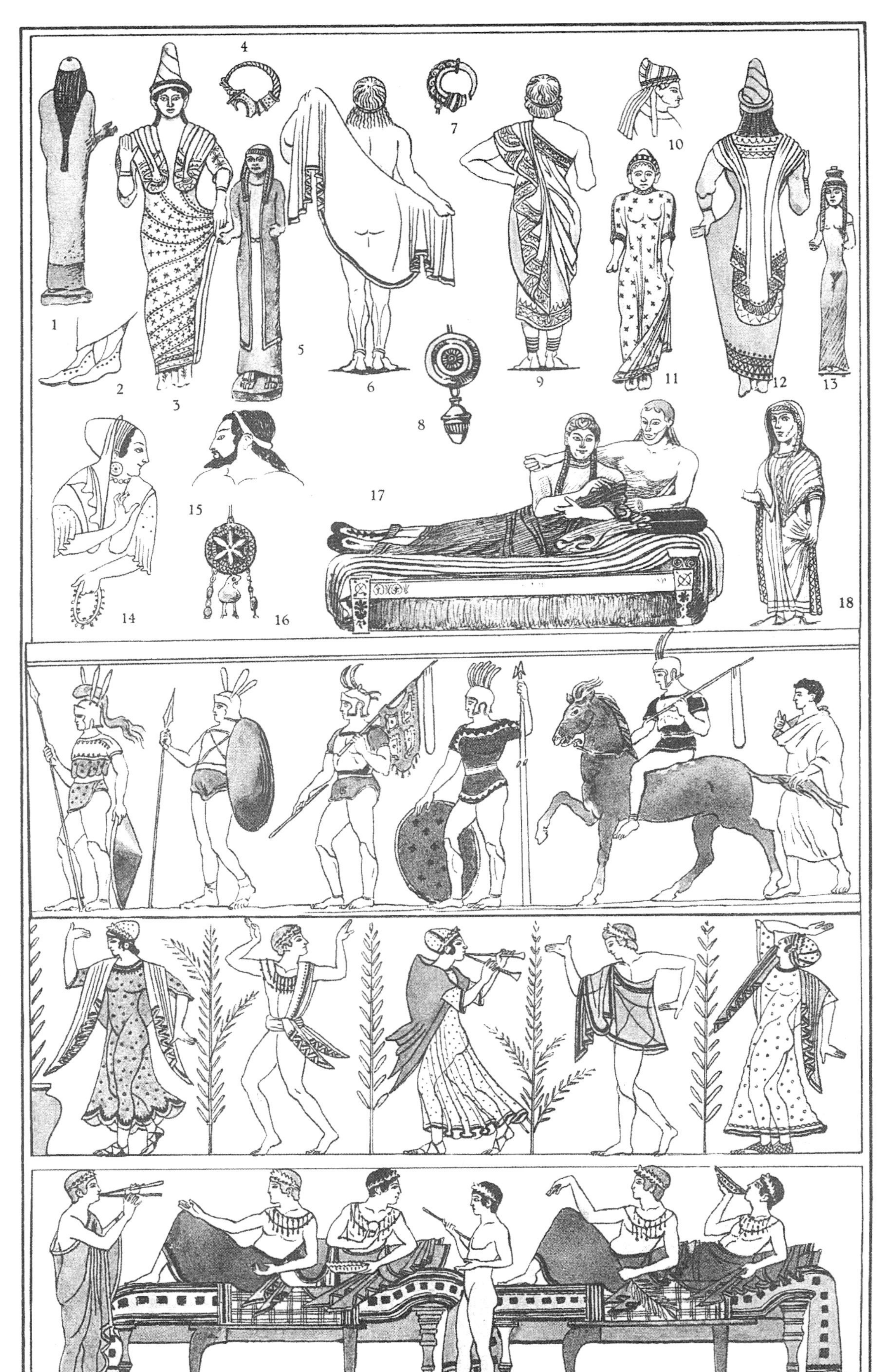

ROME

Men's Costume

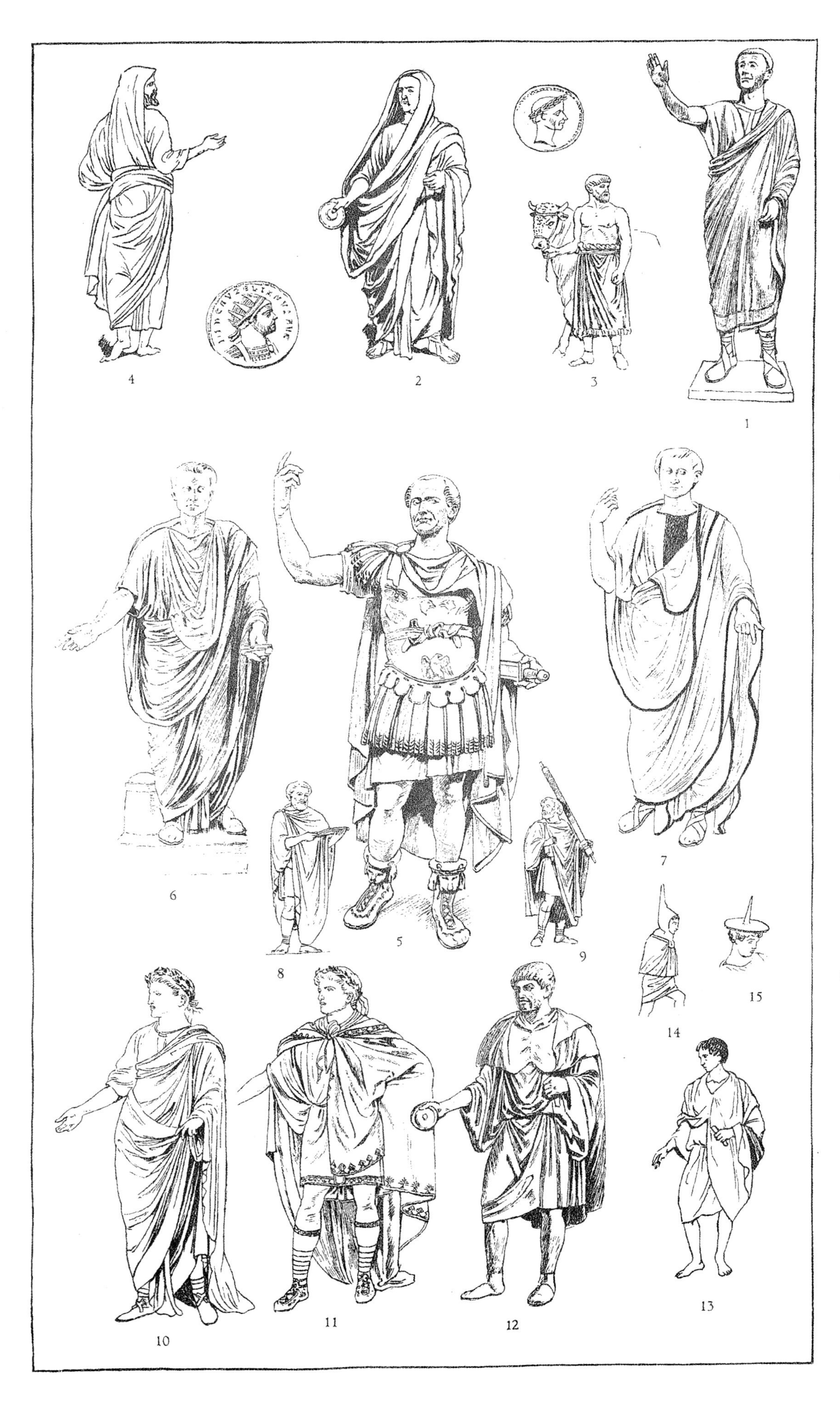

Toga, Paludamentum, Sagum

Toga, Toga, Paenula

Cucullus, etc.

ROME
Ordinary People, Women, Priestesses

Ordinary People
1 2 3 4 5

Women, Priestesses
6–14

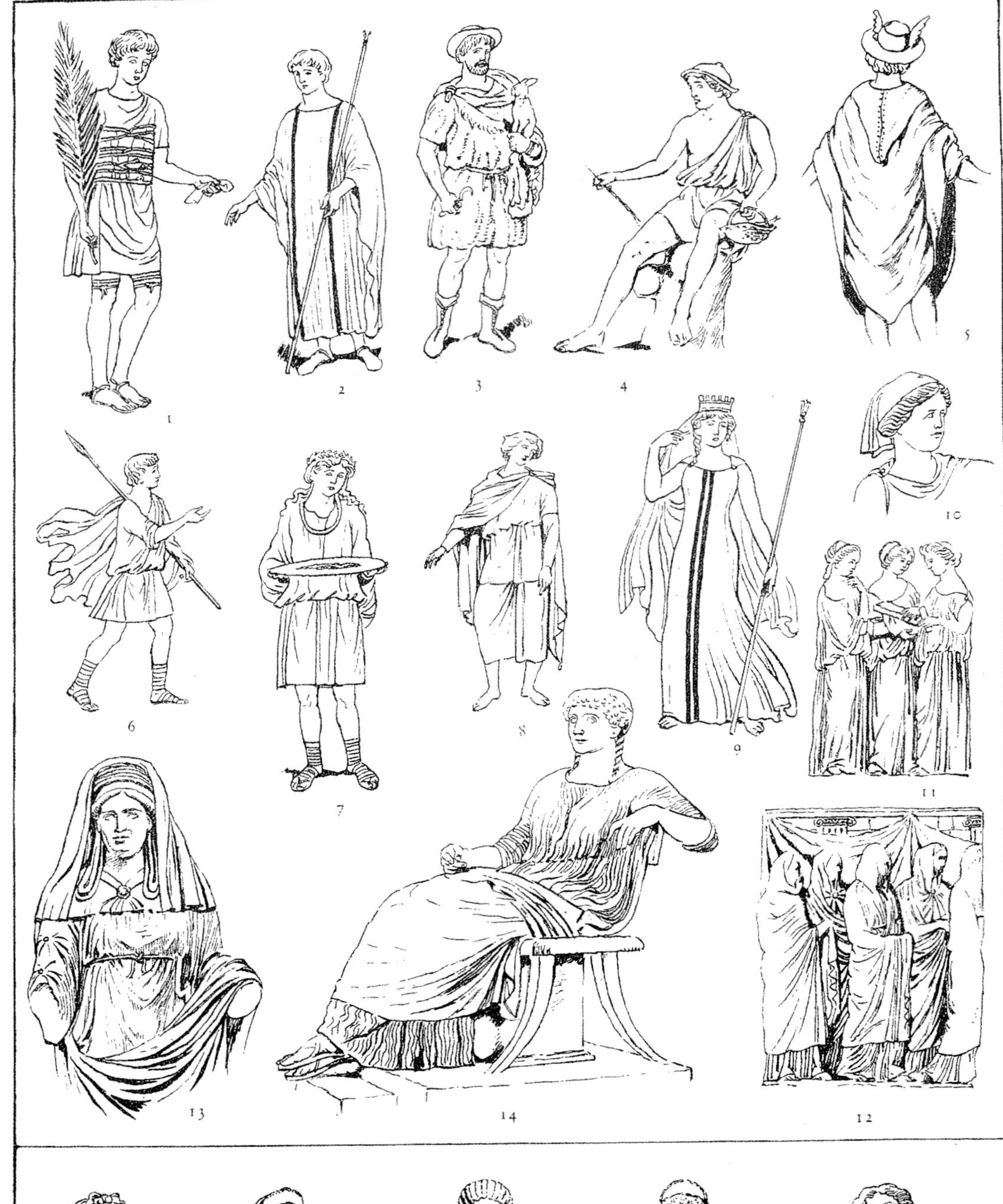

Women dressed in the Palla

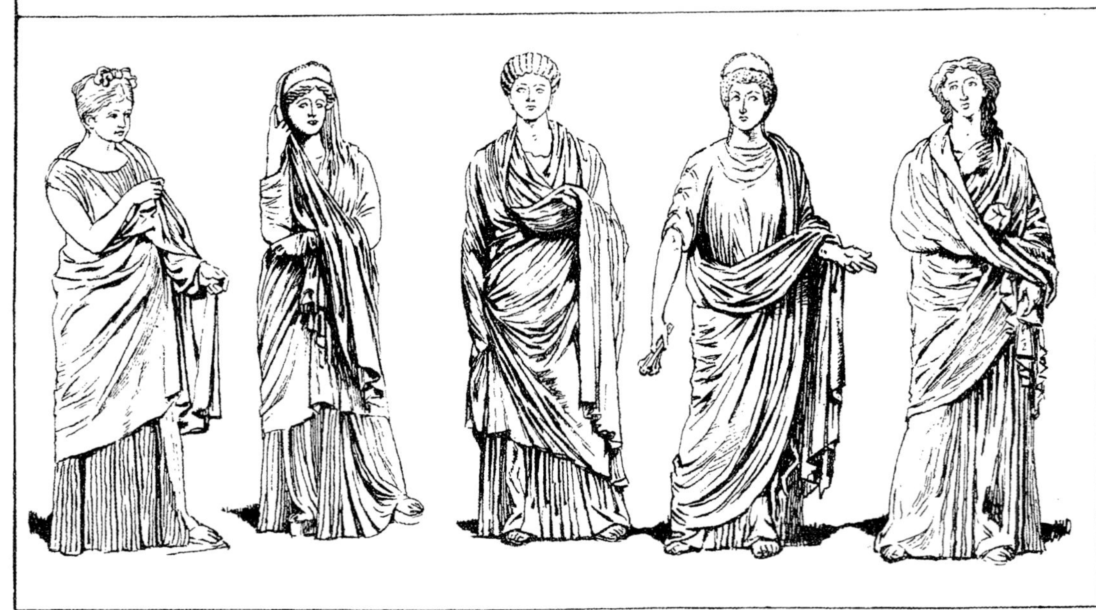

15 16 17 18 19

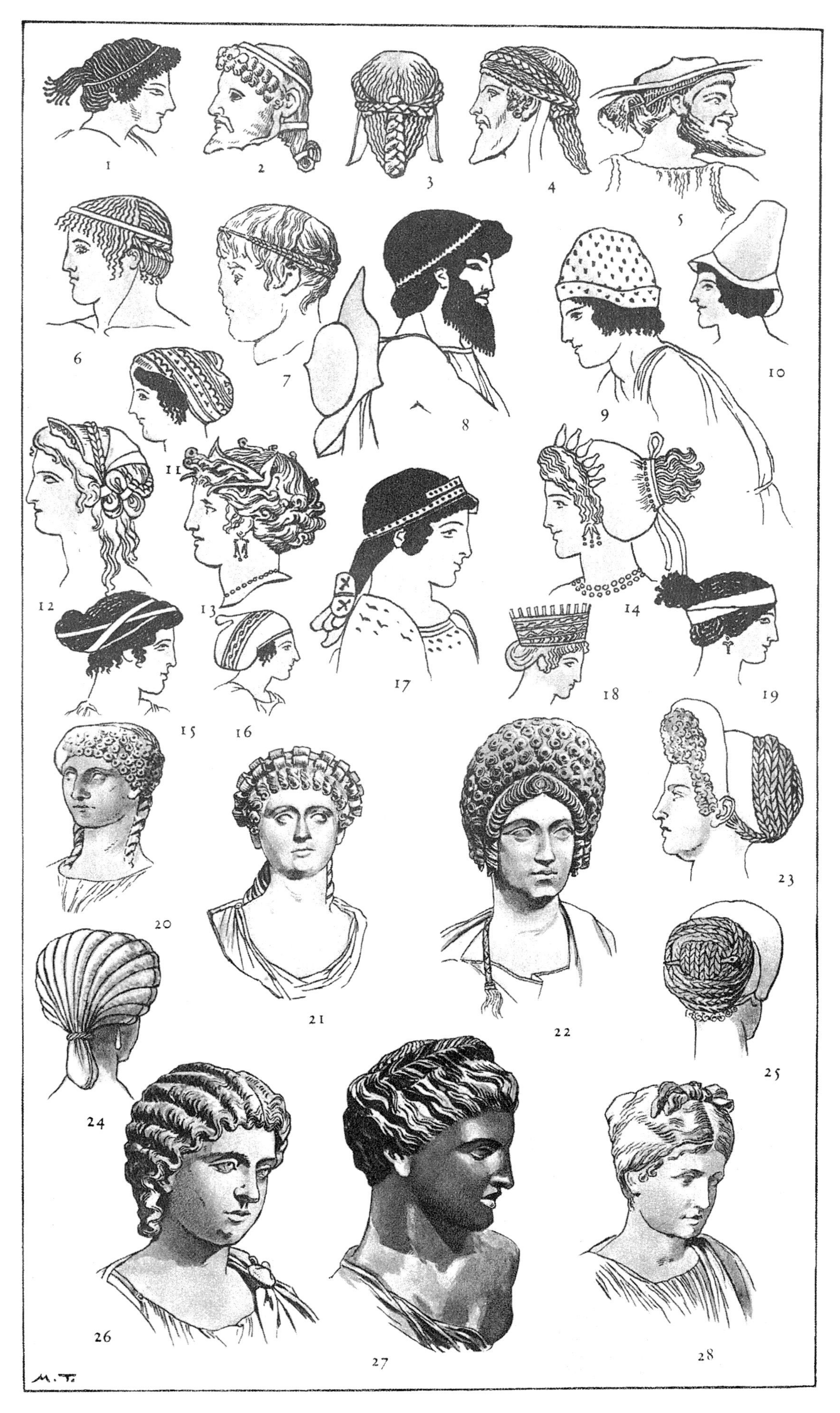

GREECE AND ROME

Ancient Hair Styles and Head-dresses

Greek Hair Styles

1 - 19

Roman Hair Styles

20 - 28

GREECE AND ROME
Footwear (Greek, Roman, Coptic)

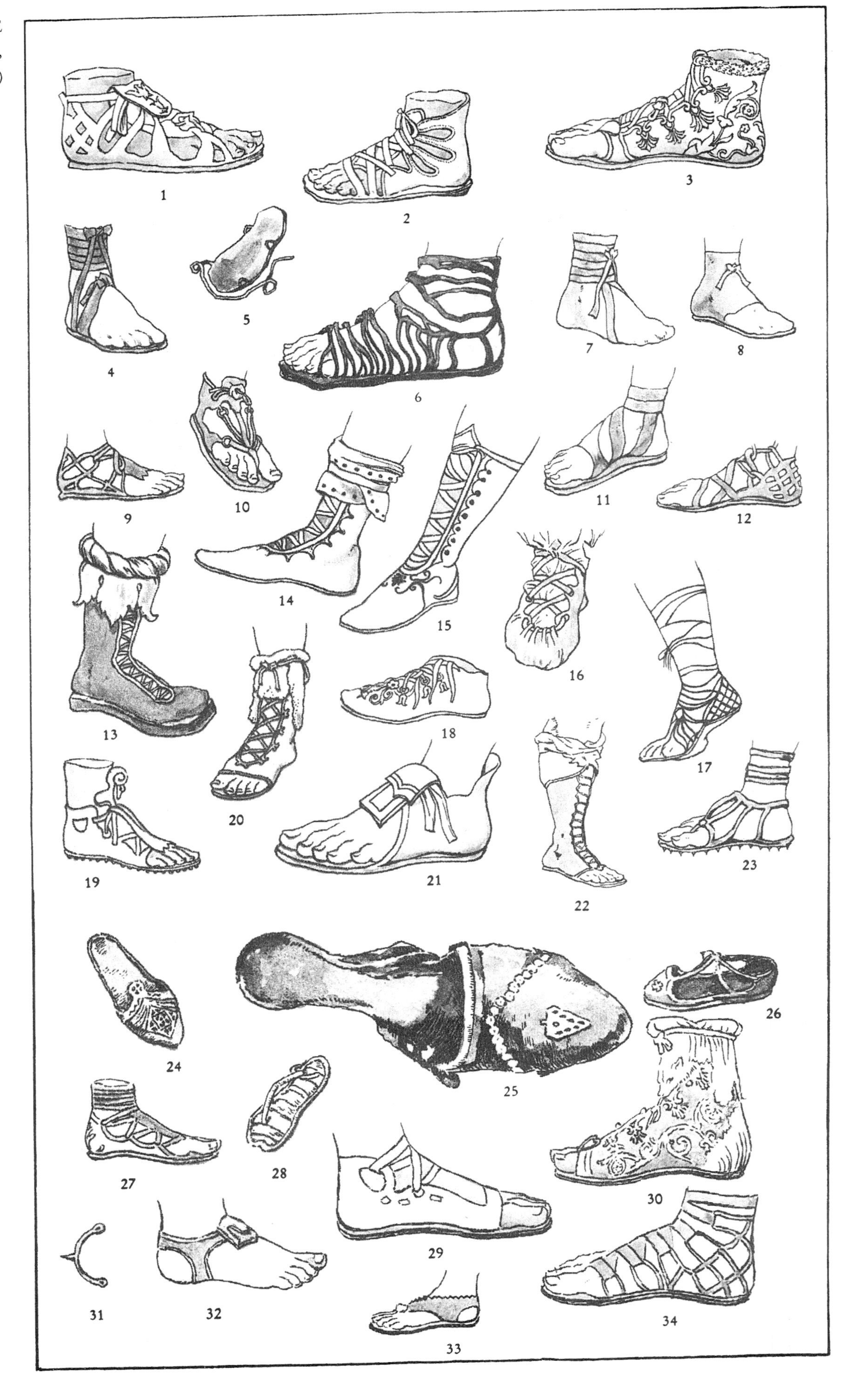

TEUTONS
Prehistoric to Roman Times

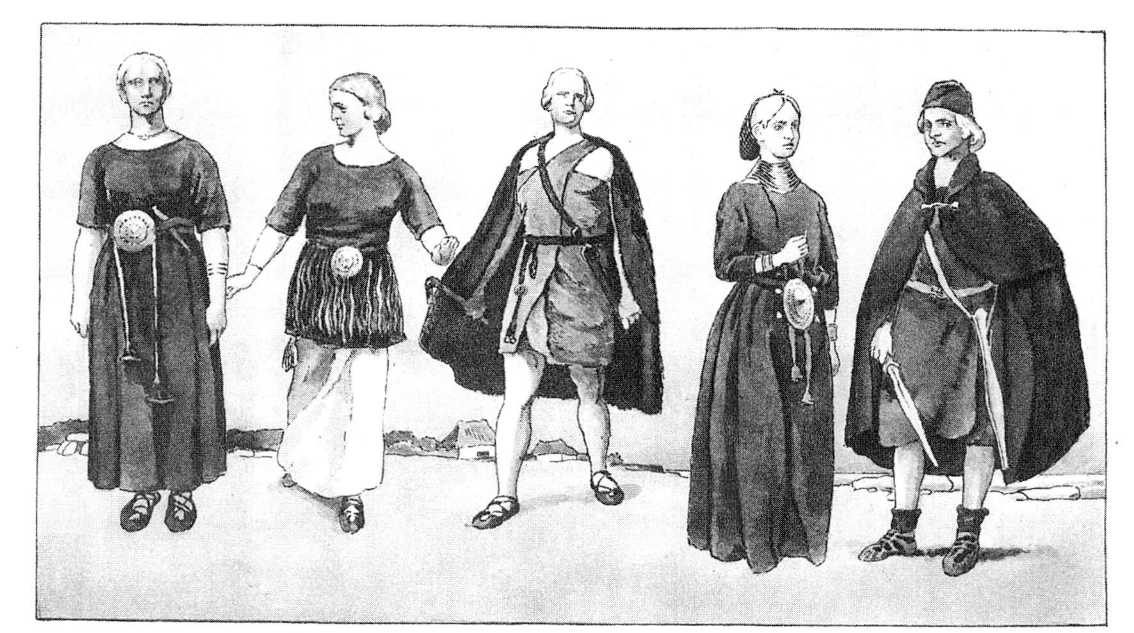

Teutons in Jutland
(Bronze Age 2000–800 B. C.)

1 2 3 4 5

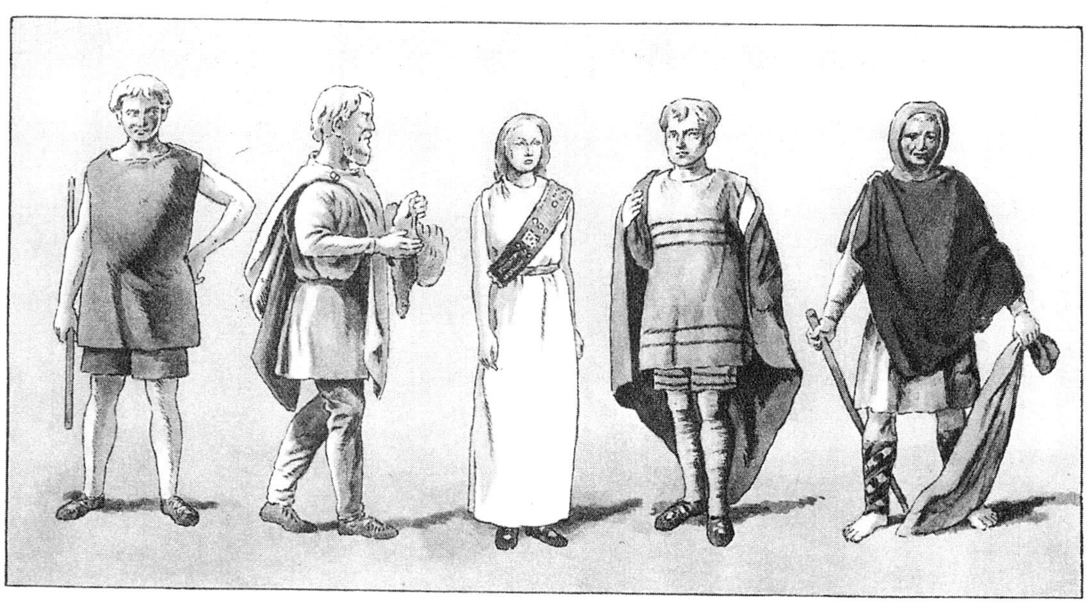

Teutons in North Germany
(Bronze Age 2000–800 B. C.)

6 7 8 9 10

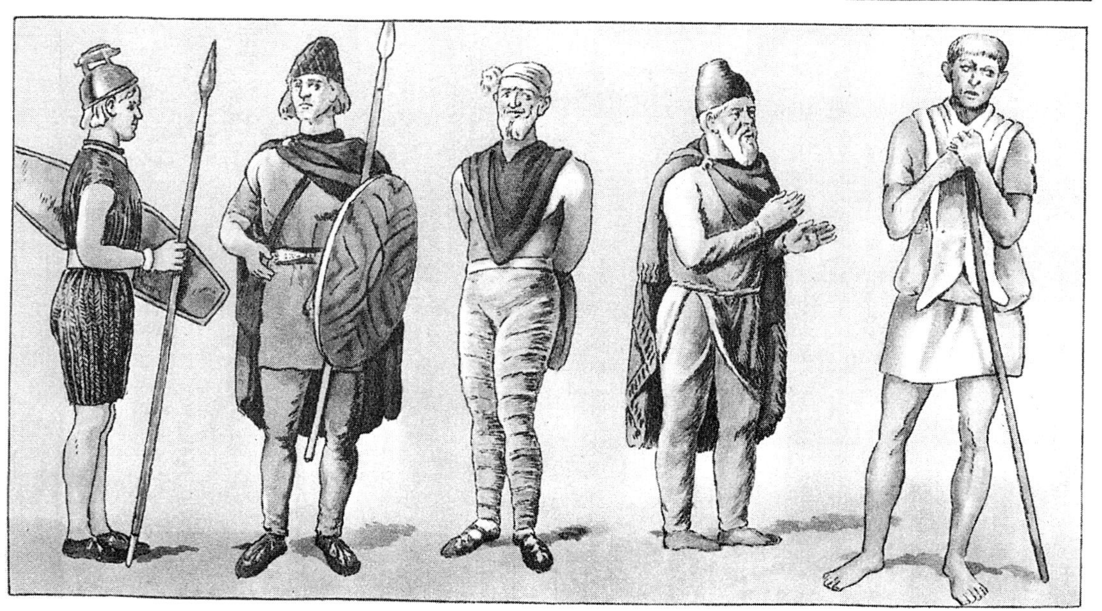

East Teutons (Roman Period)

11 12 13 14 15

TEUTONS
Prehistoric
and Roman Times

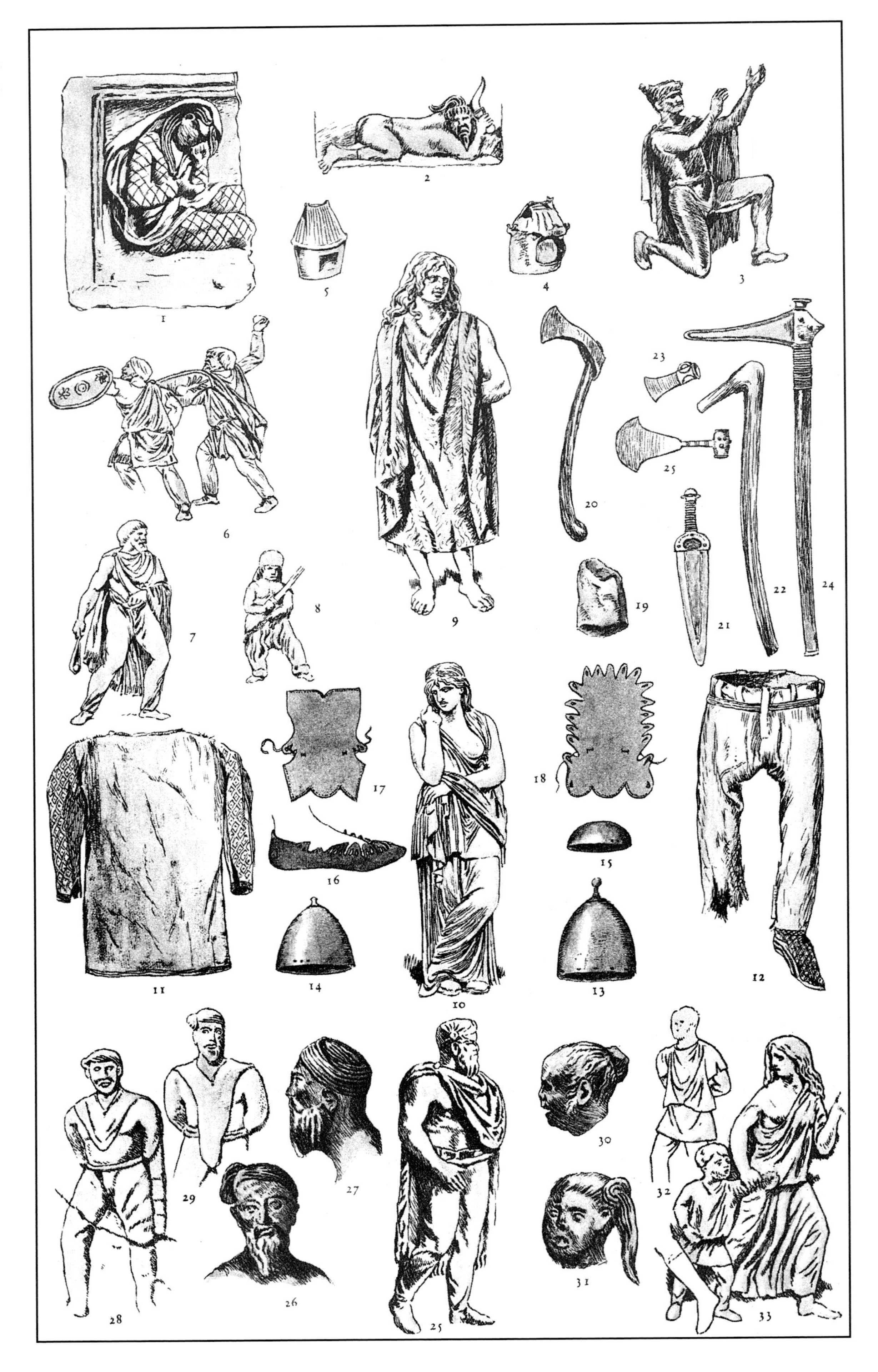

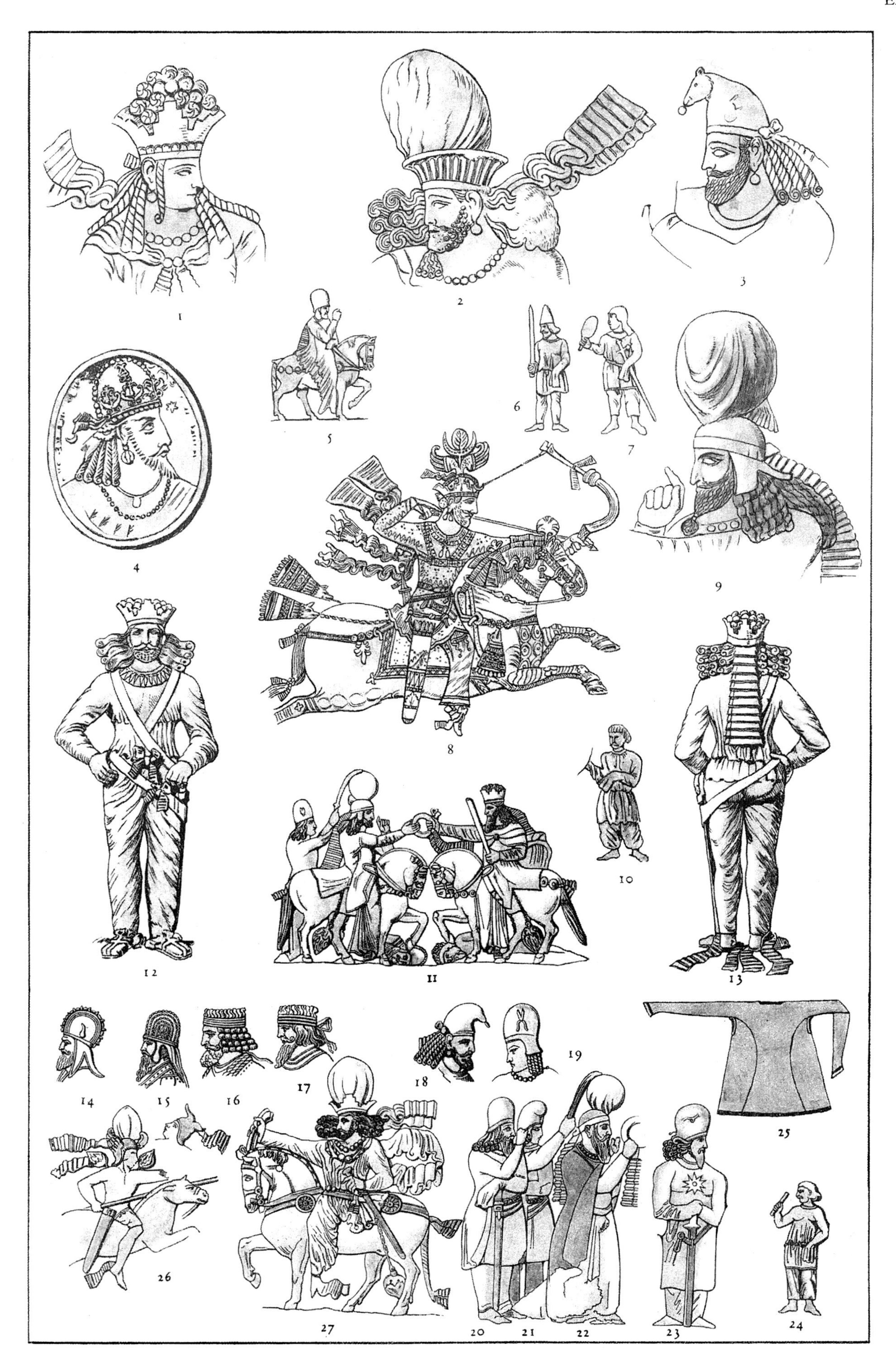

PERSIA
227–651 A.D.
Sassanian Period

Gods, Kings, Parthians, Huntsmen, Horsemen

GAULS, VIKINGS AND NORSEMEN

Gauls

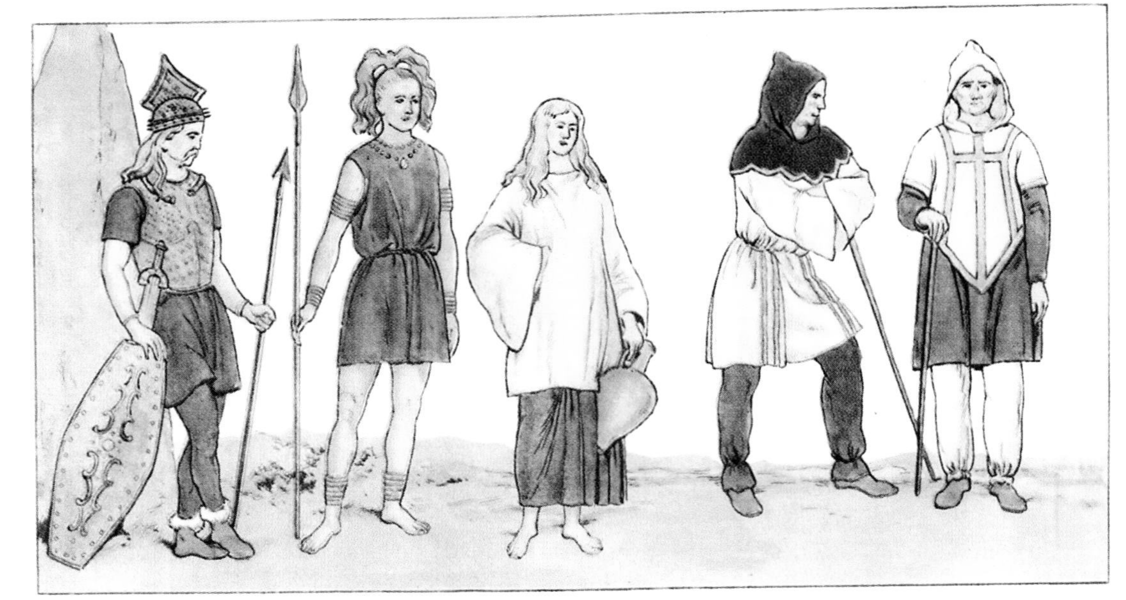

1 2 3 4 5

Gauls

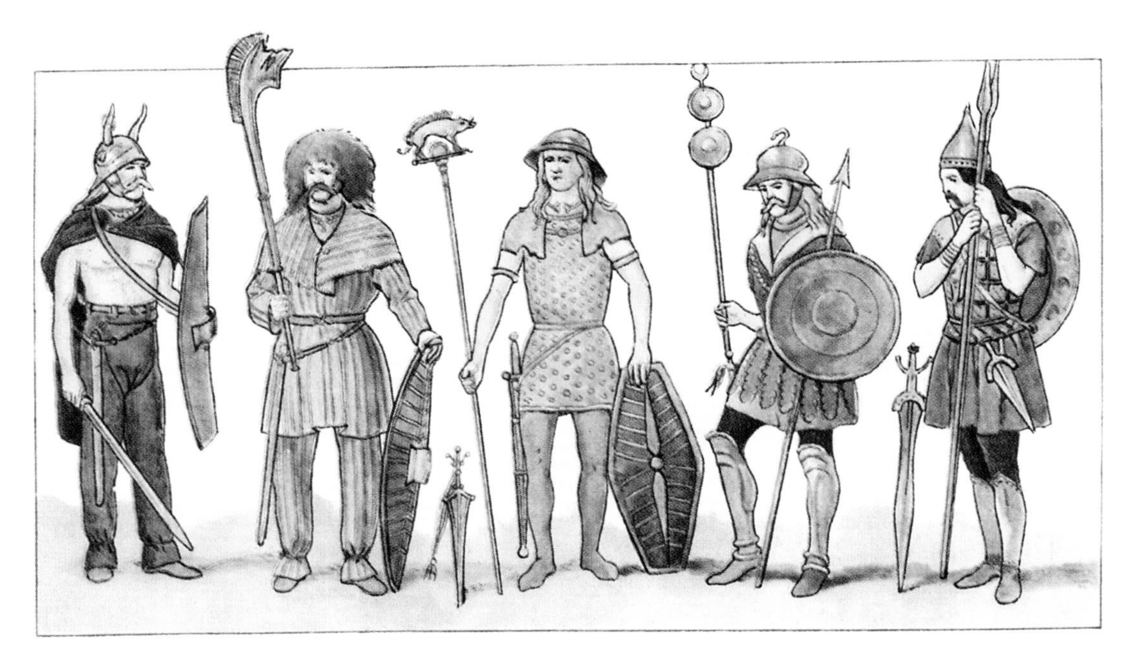

6 7 8 9 10

Vikings and Norsemen

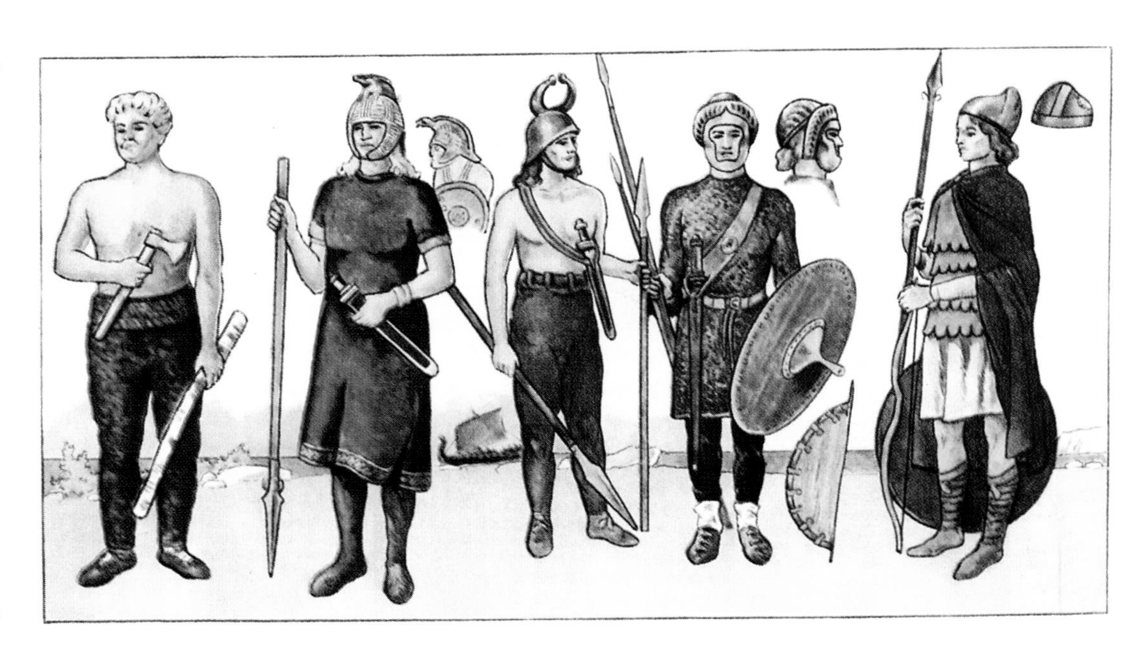

11 12 13 14 15

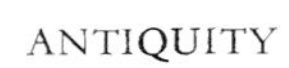

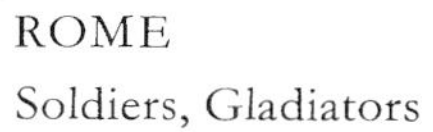

ROME
Soldiers, Gladiators

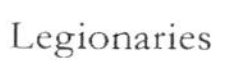

Legionaries

1 2 3 4

Officers, Horsemen, Auxiliary Troops

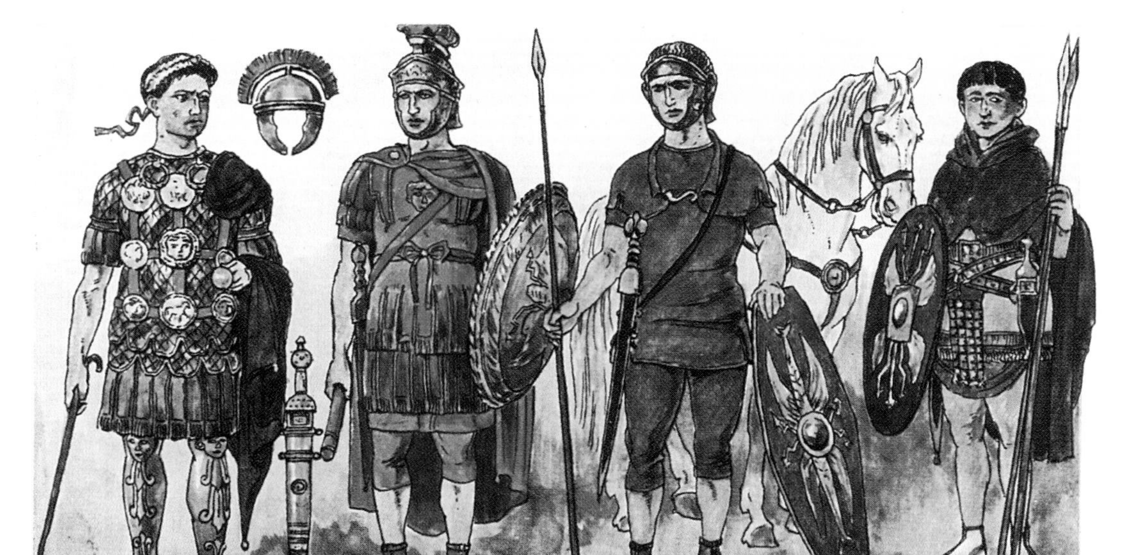

5 6 7 8

Gladiators

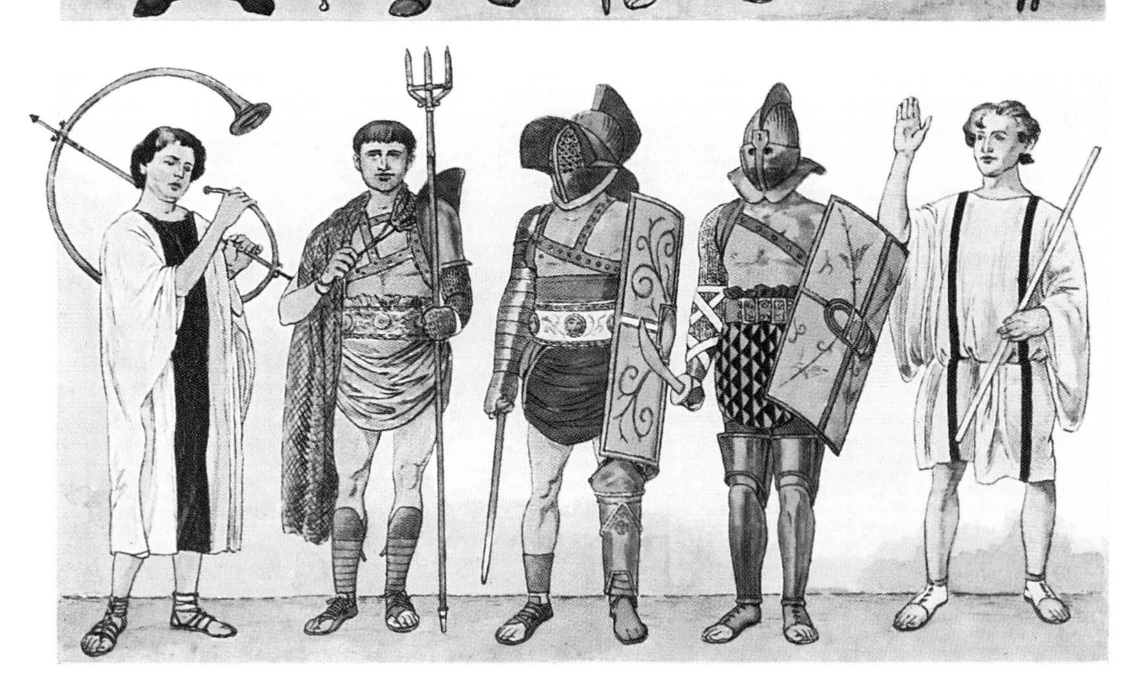

9 10 11 12 13

EARLY CHRISTIAN PERIOD
300–600 A.D.

Dalmatic, Tunic

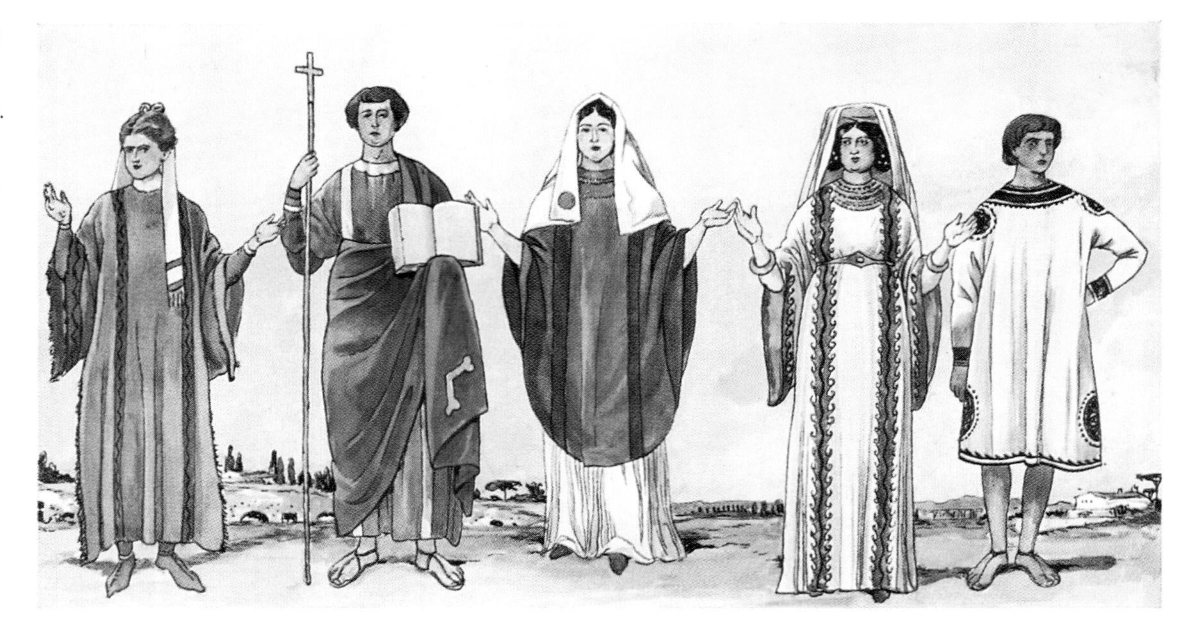

1 2 3 4 5

Dalmatic, Tunic

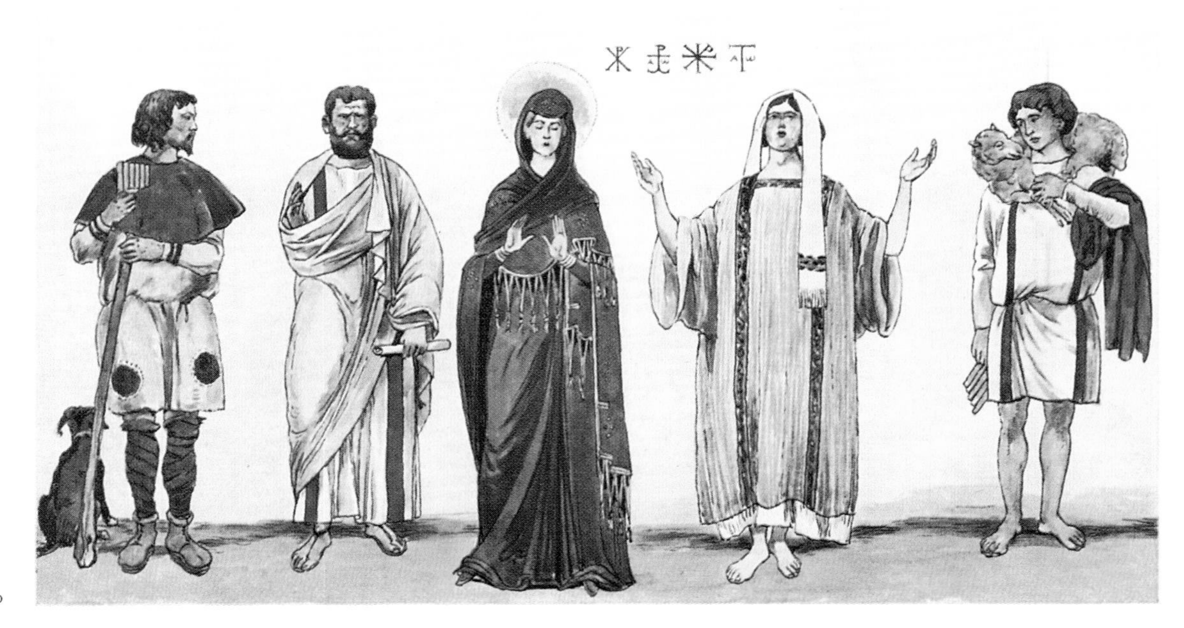

6 7 8 9 10

Various Forms of Tunic and Toga

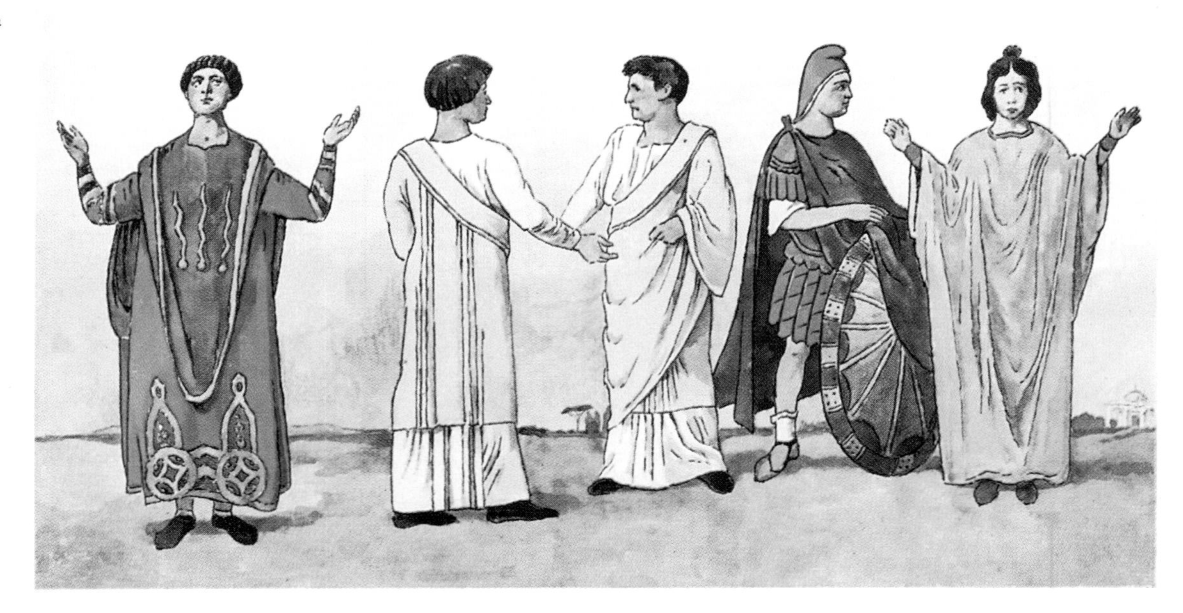

11 12 13 14 15

BYZANTINE EMPIRE
4th–11th Centuries

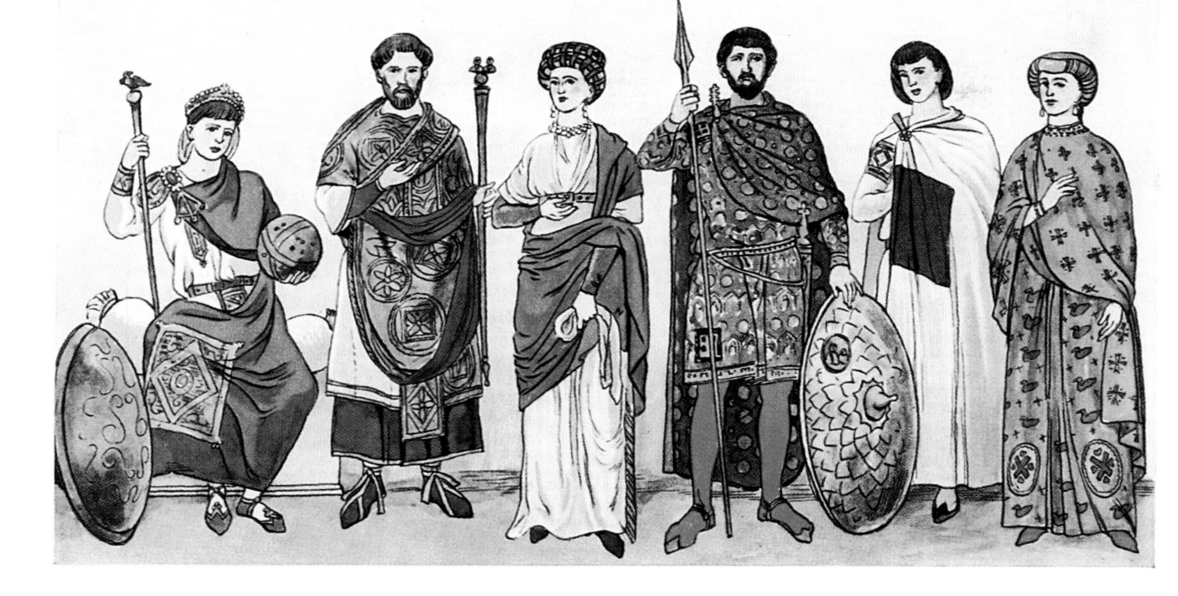

Emperor's Court
4th–5th Centuries

1 2 3 4 5 6

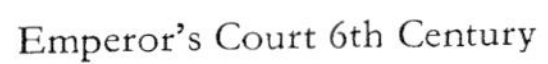

Emperor's Court 6th Century

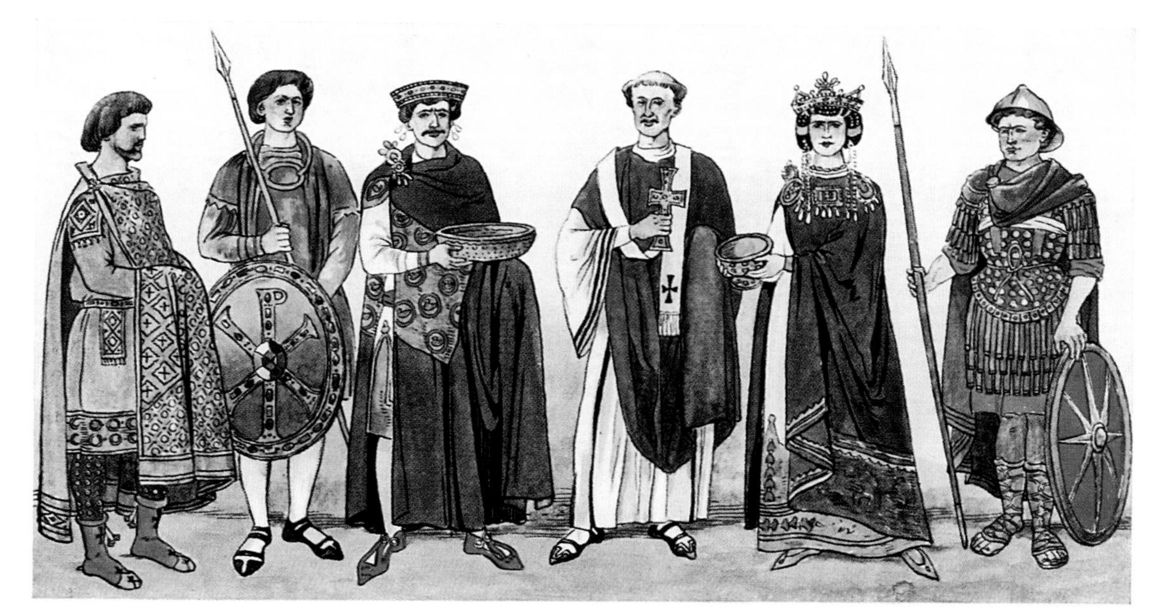

7 8 9 10 11 12

Emperor's Court
10th–11th Centuries

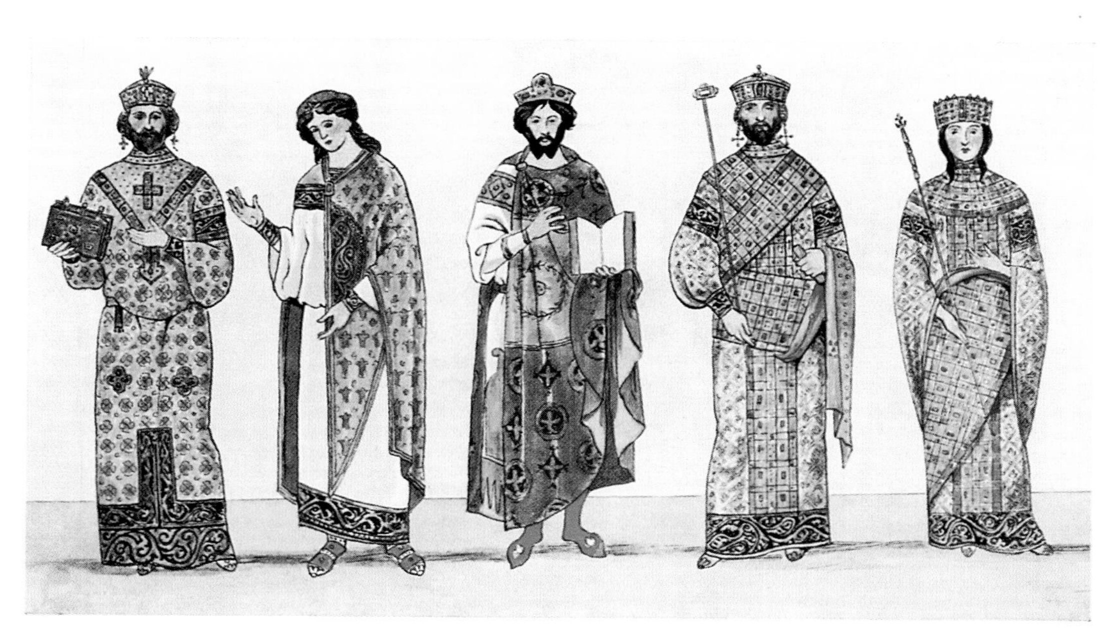

13 14 15 16 17

MONASTIC ORDERS AND ORDERS OF KNIGHTS

Orders of Knights

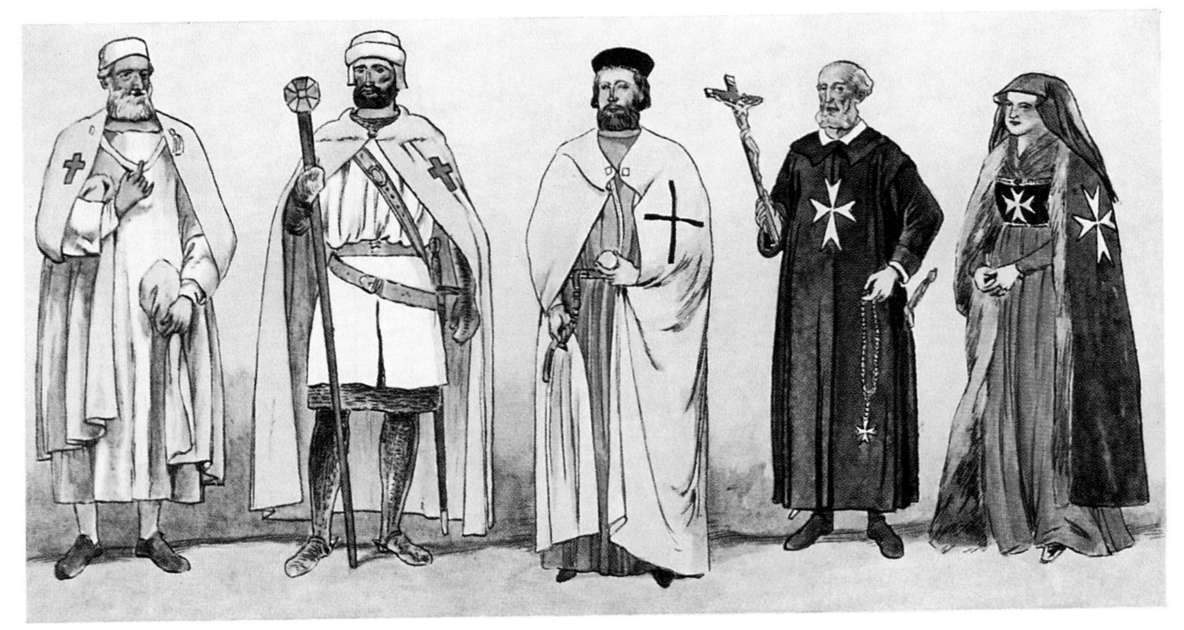

1 2 3 4 5

Monastic Orders

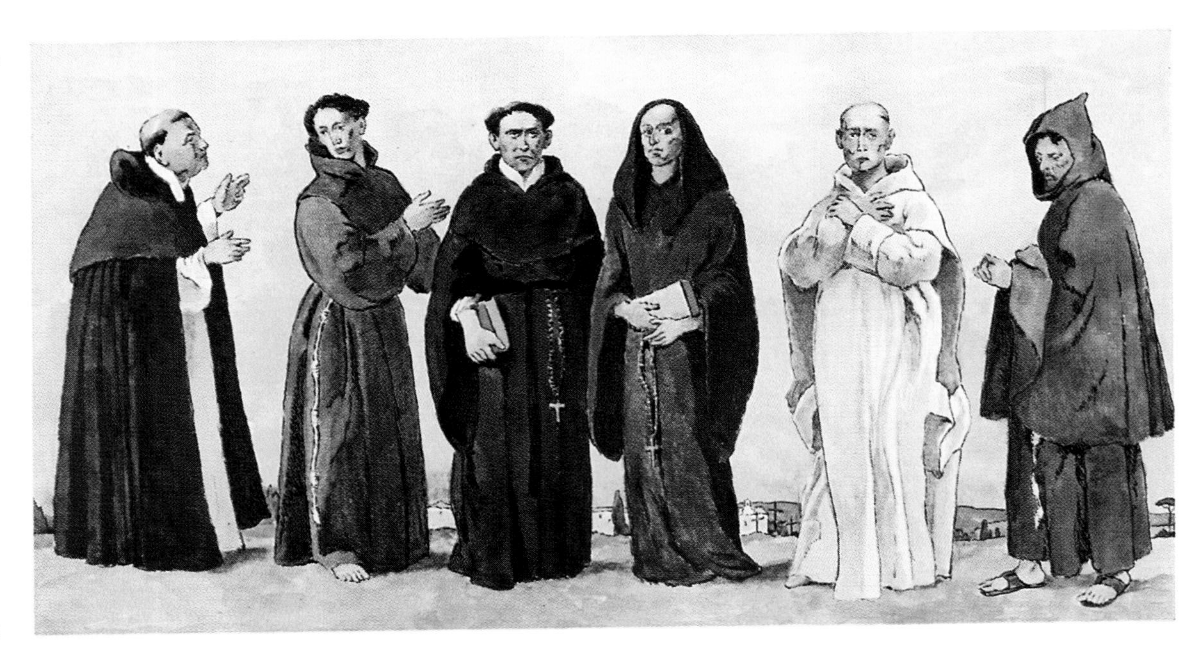

6 7 8 9 10 11

Monks and Nuns

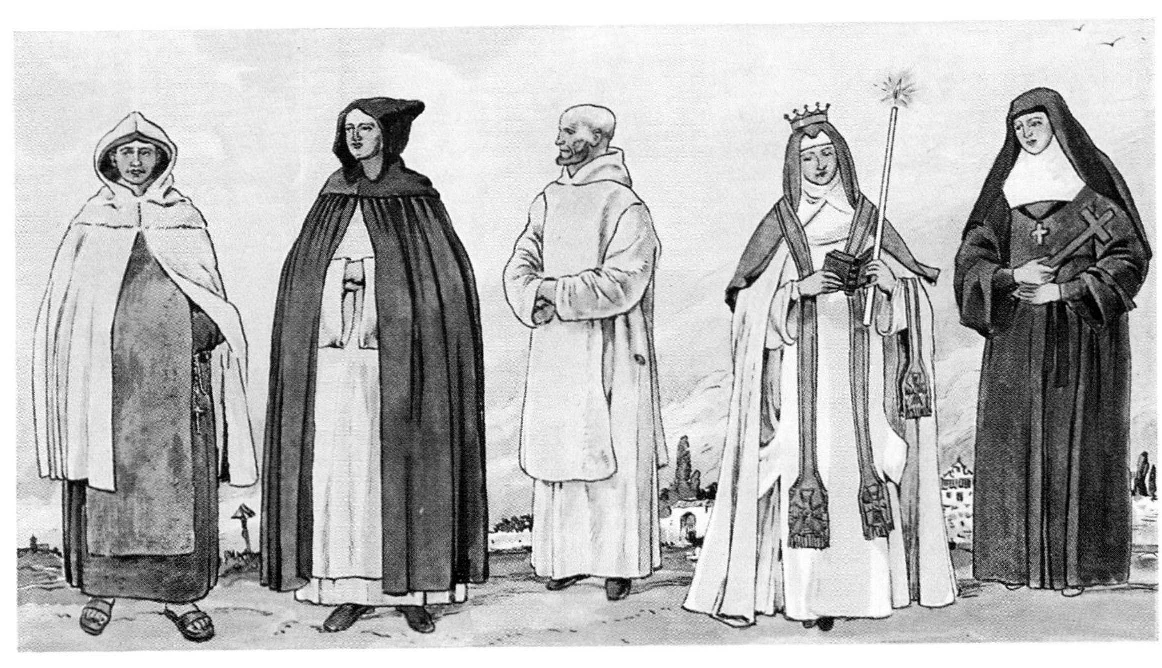

12 13 14 15 16

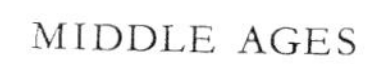

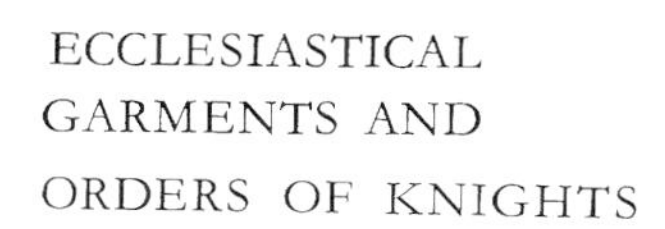

ECCLESIASTICAL GARMENTS AND ORDERS OF KNIGHTS

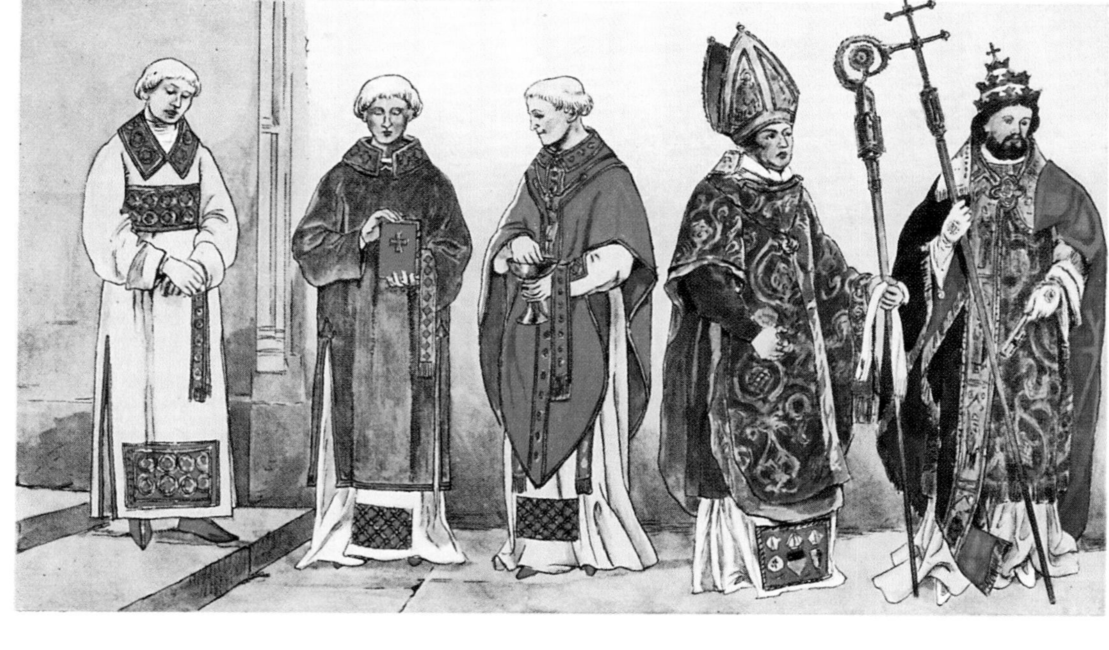

Priests, Bishops, Popes

1 2 3 4 5

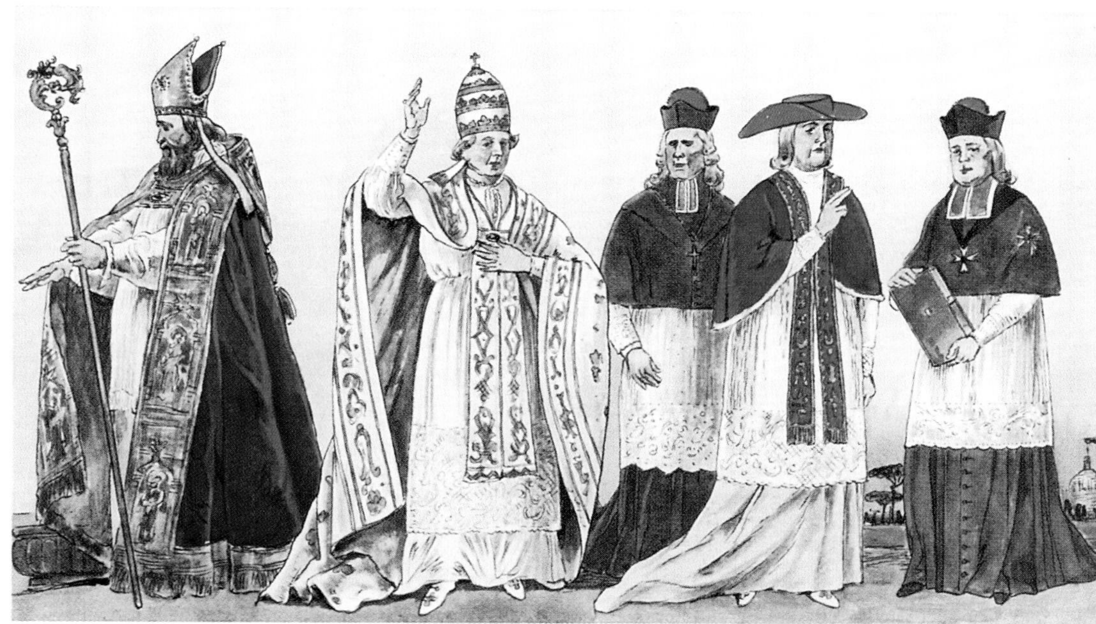

Bishops, Popes

6 7 8 9 10

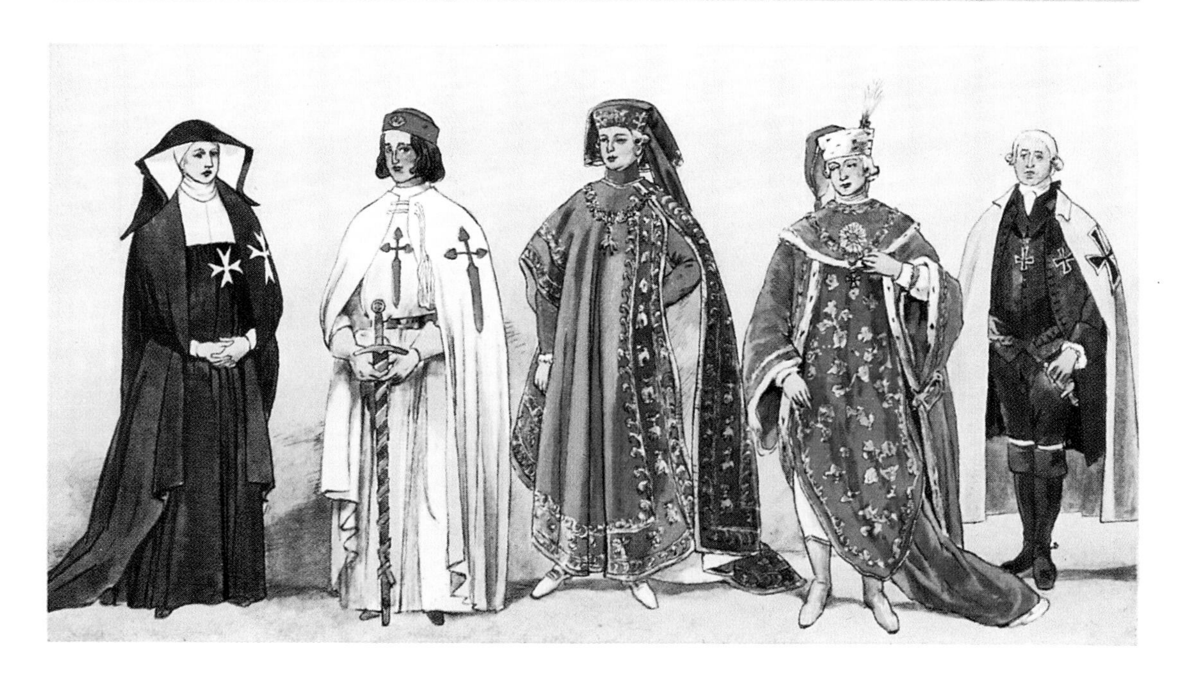

Costumes of Orders of Knights
15th–18th Centuries

11 12 13 14 15

GERMANY
500–1200 A.D.

Frankish Kingdom
(Merovingian and
Carlovingian Periods)
7th–9th Centuries

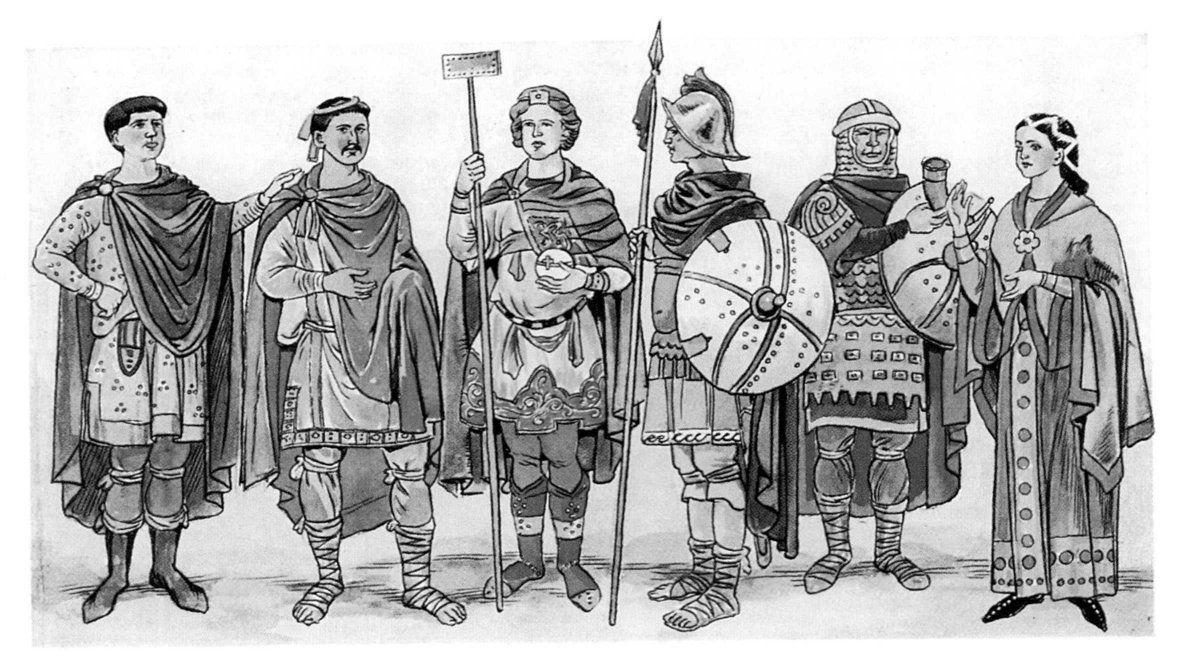

1 2 3 4 5 6

Frankish Men and Women
(9th–11th Centuries)

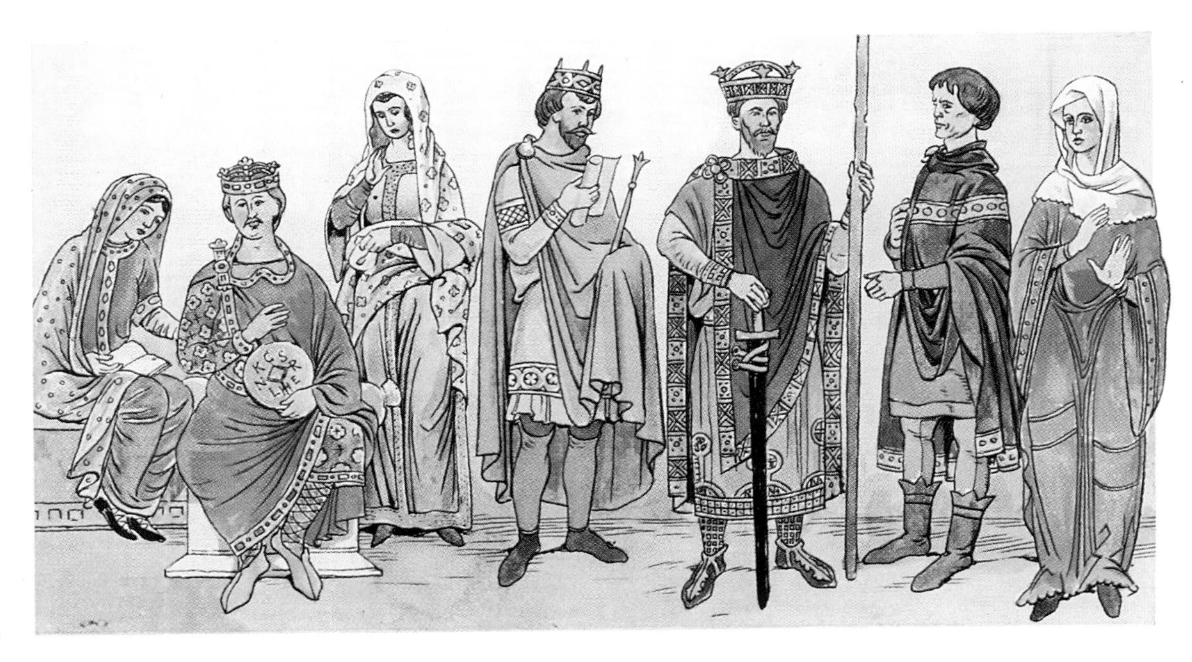

7 8 9 10 11 12 13

Men and Women
(11th–12th Centuries)

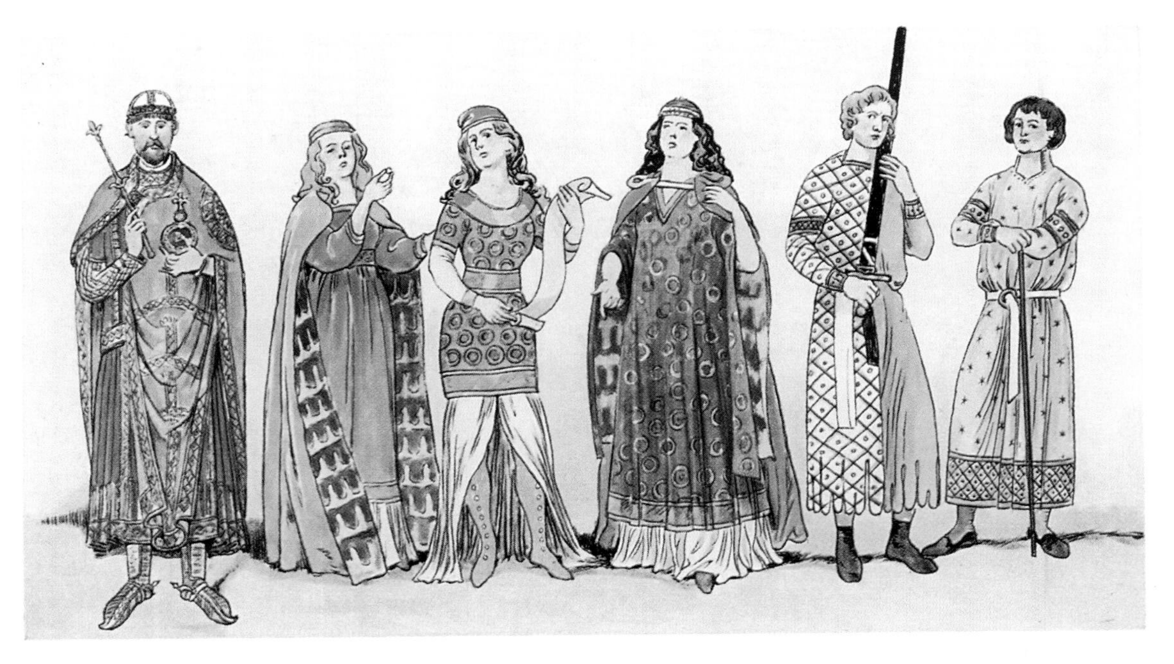

14 15 16 17 18 19

EARLY

MIDDLE AGES AND BYZANTINE EMPIRE

(300–1000 A.D.)

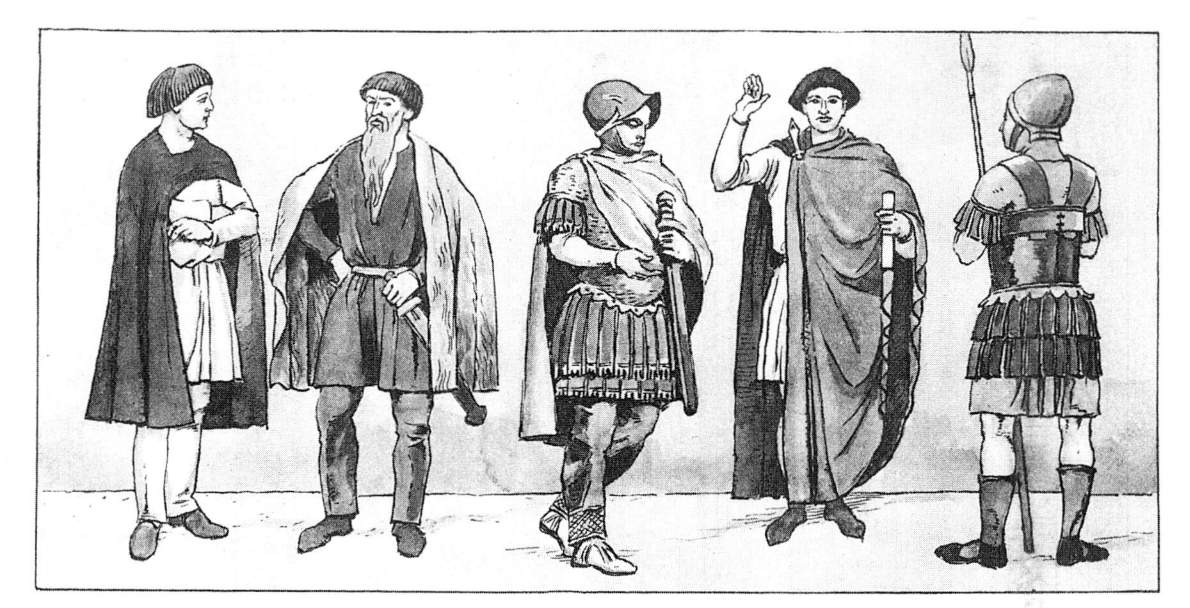

Men, Warriors

1 2 3 4 5

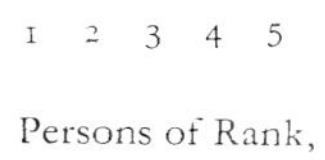

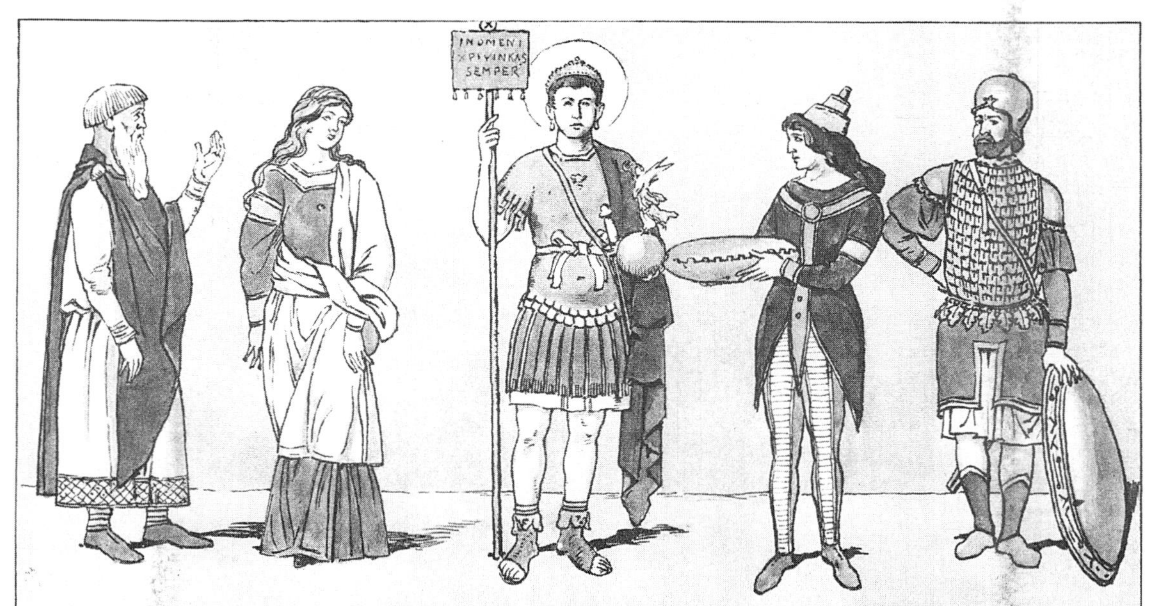

Persons of Rank, Emperor, Warriors

6 7 8 9 10

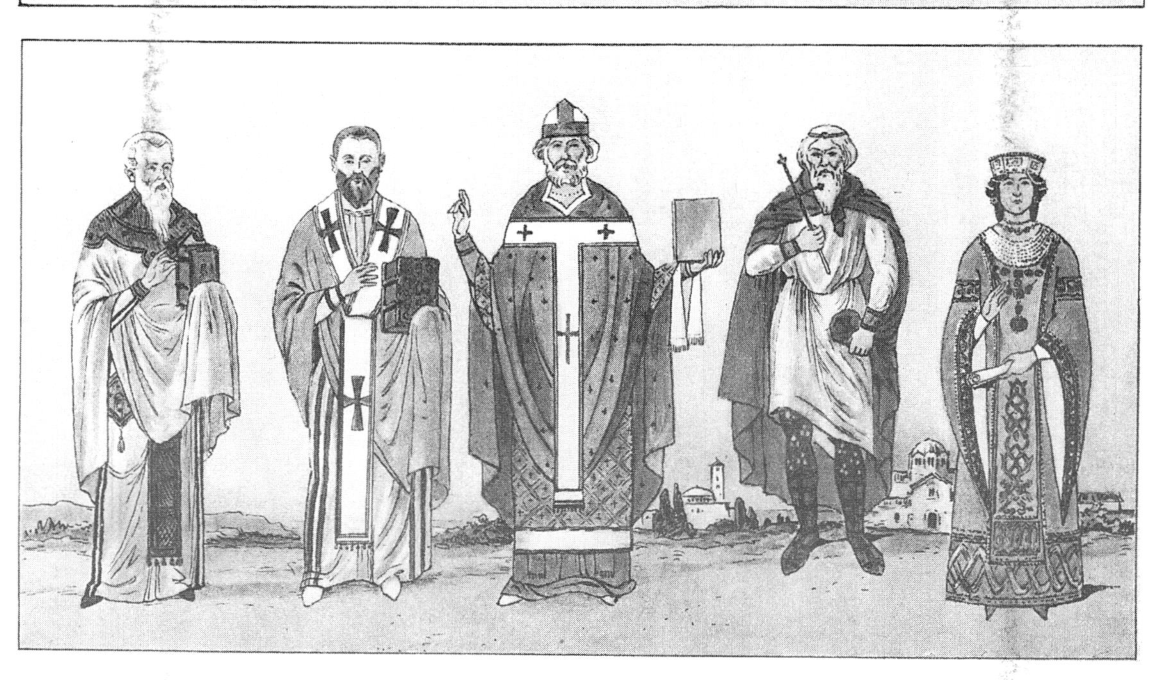

Ecclesiastics, etc.

11 12 13 14 15

GERMANY

Time of the Minnesingers and Crusades 12th–13th Centuries

People of High and Low Ranks

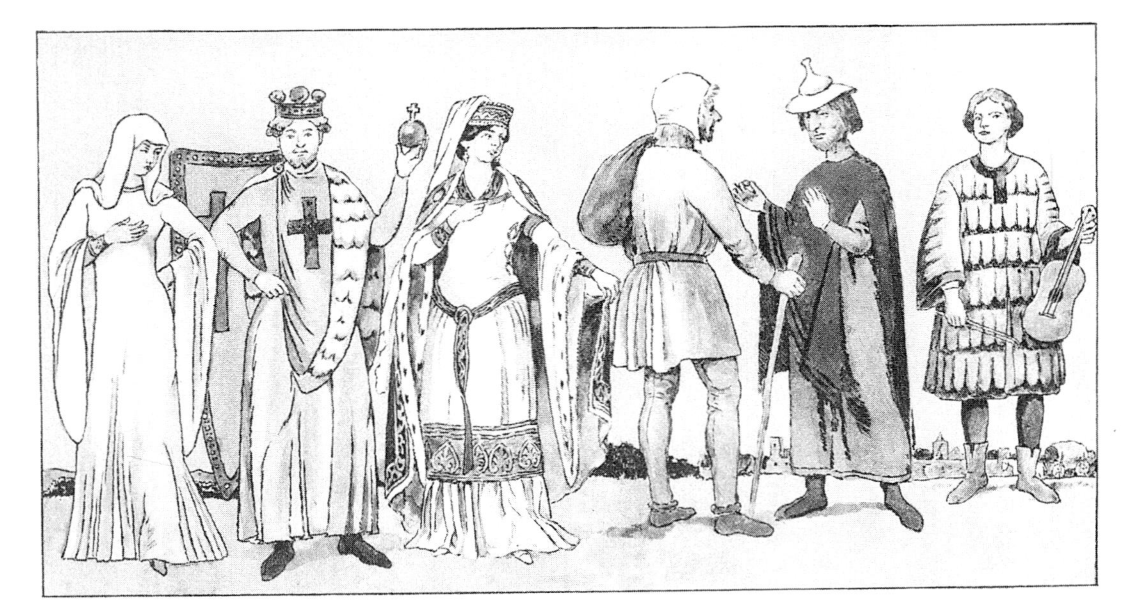

1 2 3 4 5 6

Minnesingers and Courtiers

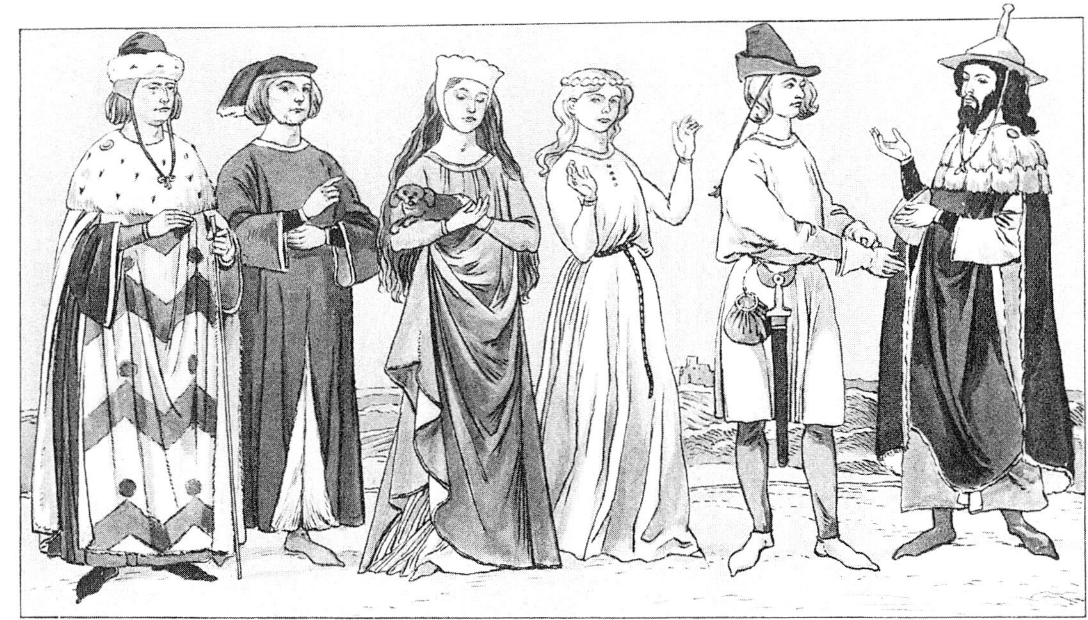

7 8 9 10 11 12

Singers and Minstrels

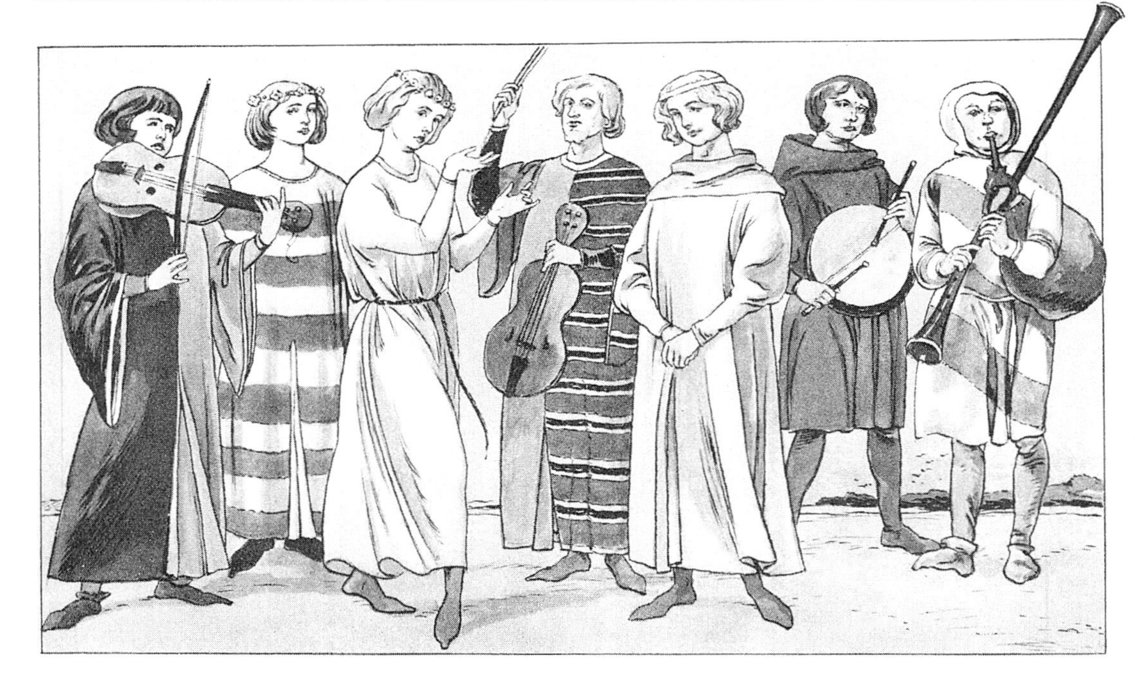

13 14 15 16 17 18 19

FRANCE
900–1400

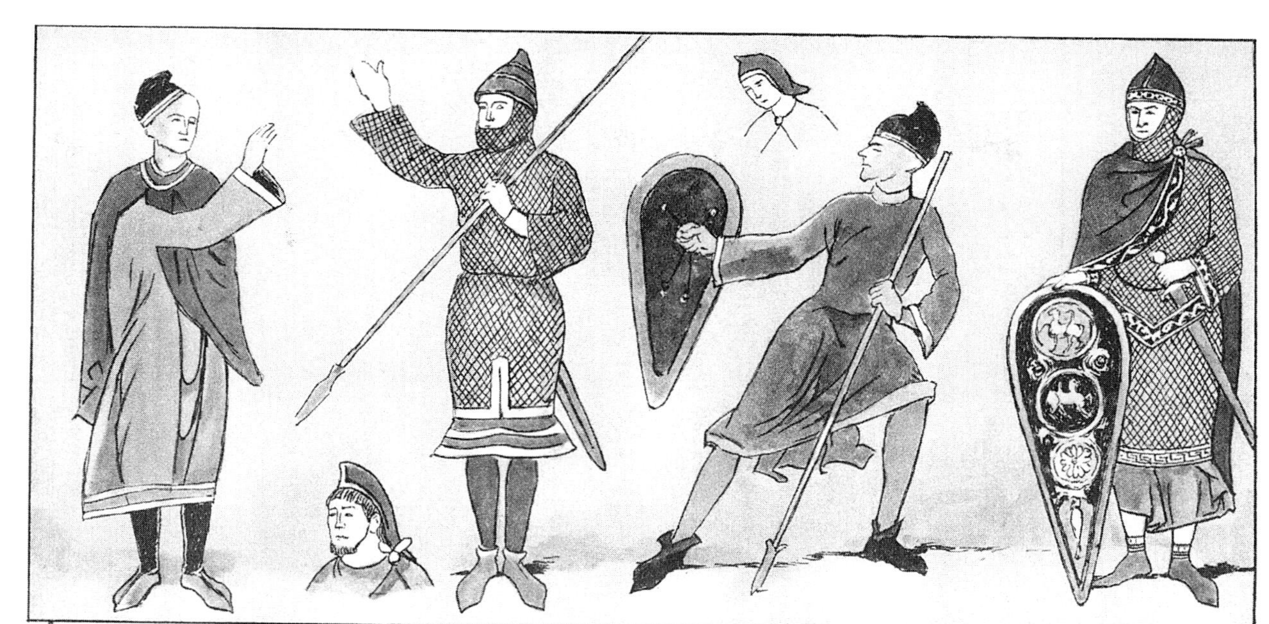

Warriors

1 2 3 4 5 6

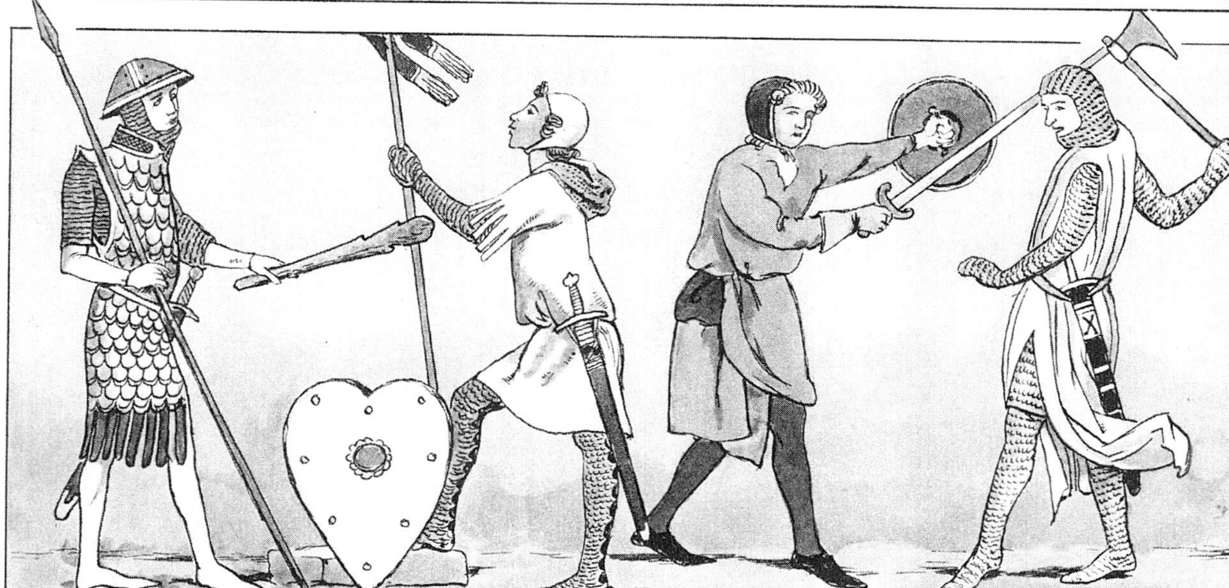

Knights and Squires

7 8 9 10

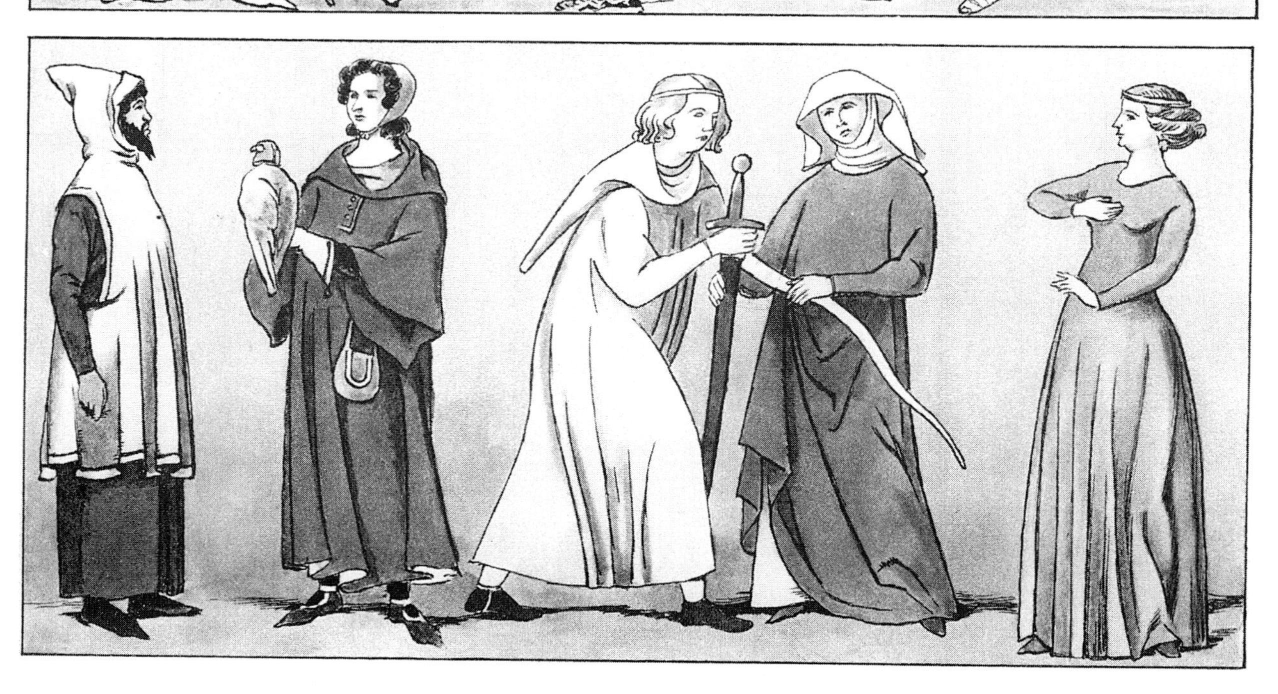

Men and Women

11 12 13 14 15

NORMANS AND ANGLO-SAXONS
11th–14th Centuries

Warriors

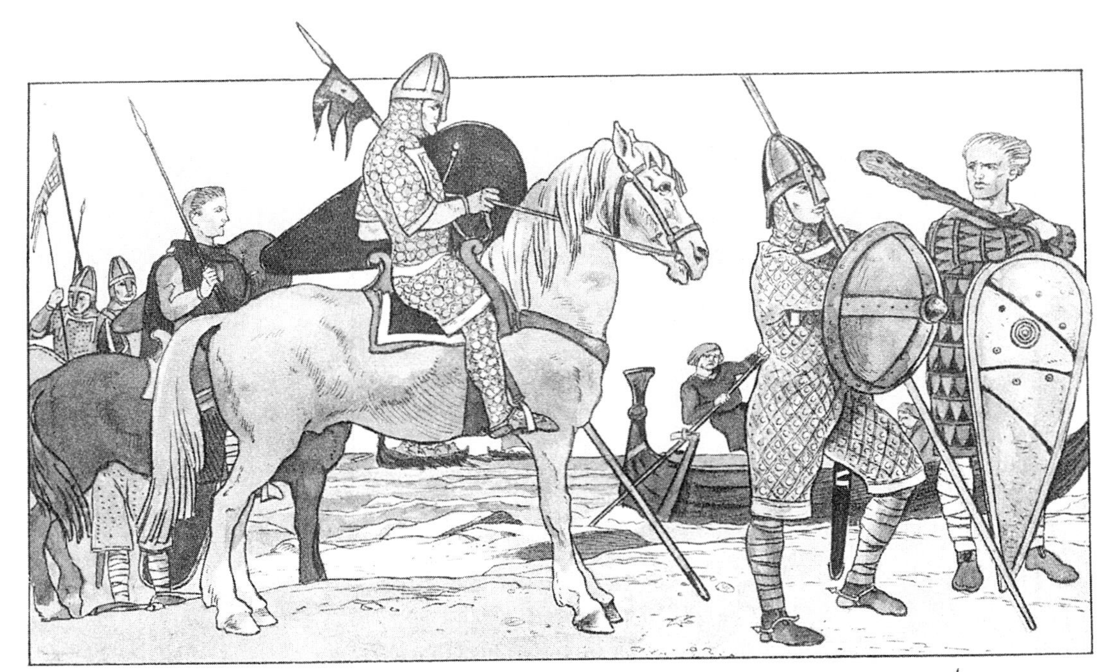

1 2 3 4

Warriors

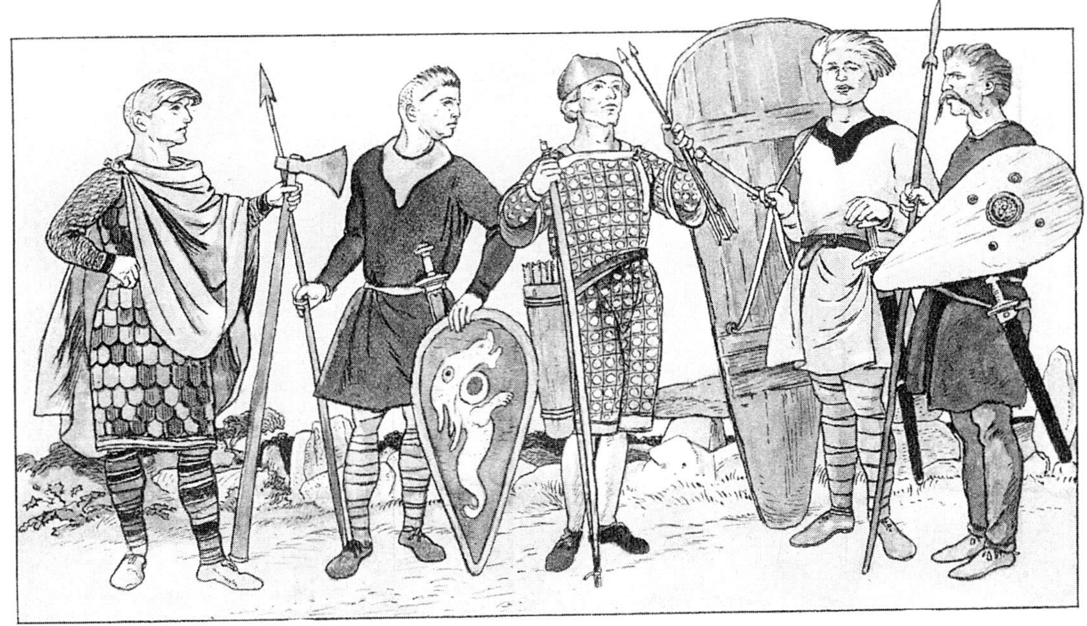

5 6 7 8 9

Peasants and Travellers

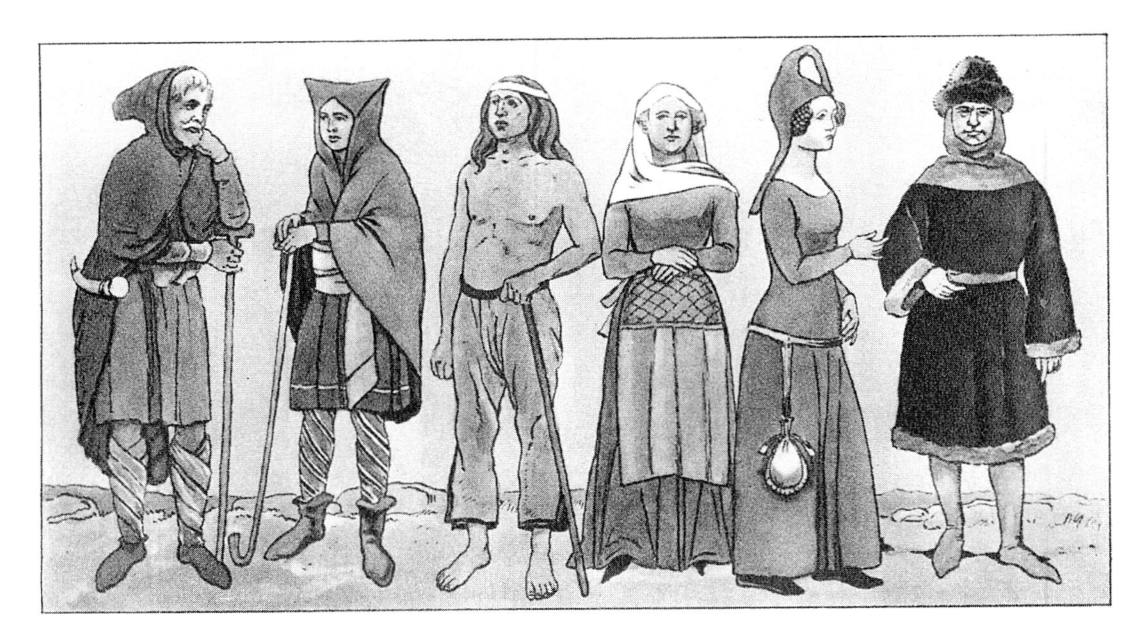

10 11 12 13 14 15

ARMOURED KNIGHTS
800–1300

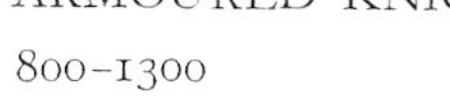

Knights

1 2 3 4 5

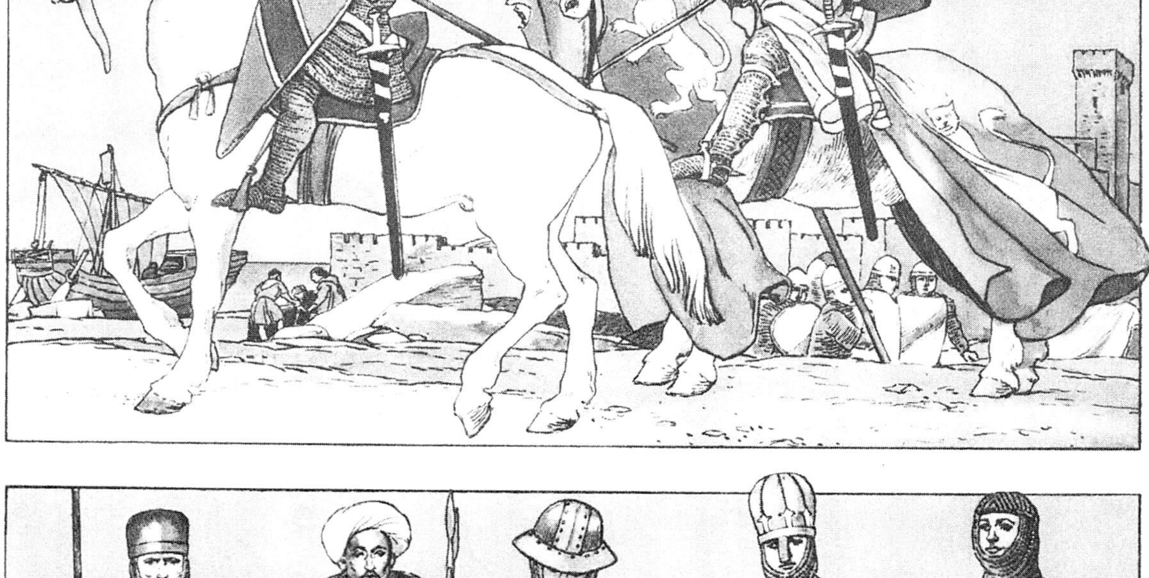

Crusaders on Horseback

6 7

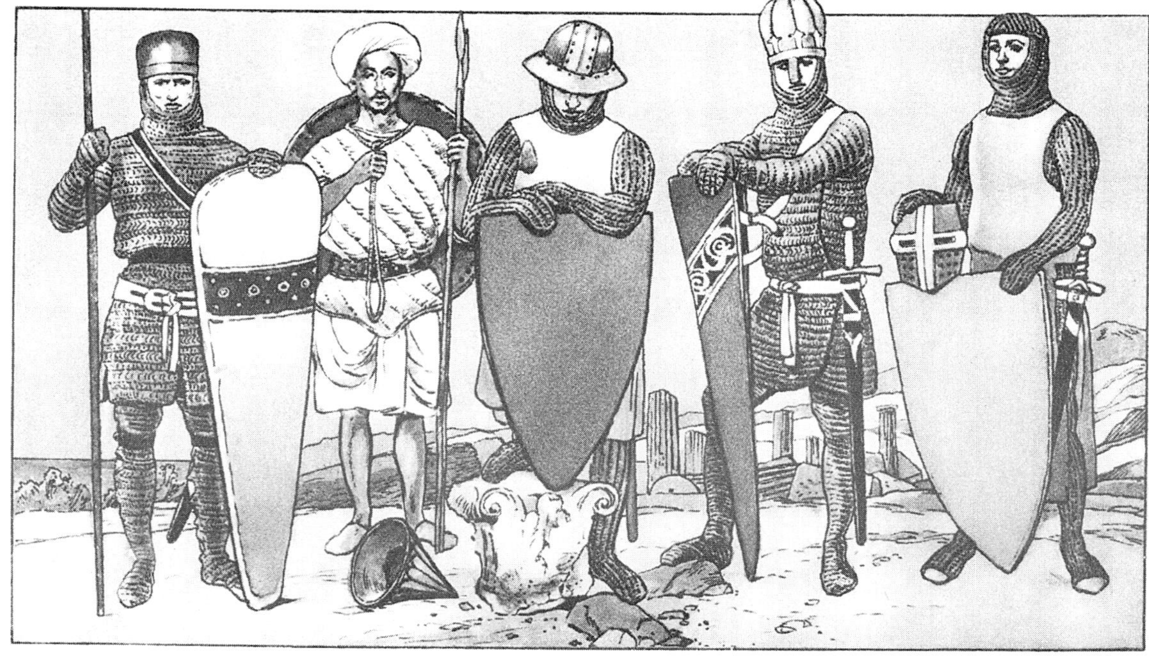

Knights in various types of Armour

8 9 10 11 12

ARMOURED KNIGHTS

14th–15th Centuries

Burgundy, England, France

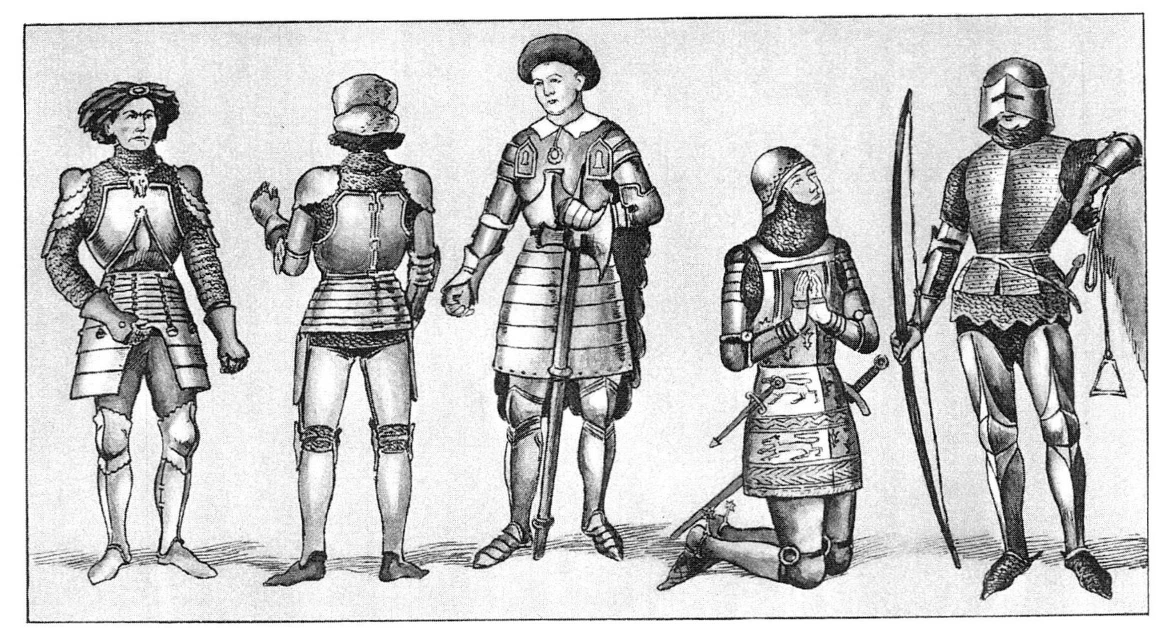

1 2 3 4 5

Burgundy, Poland, France

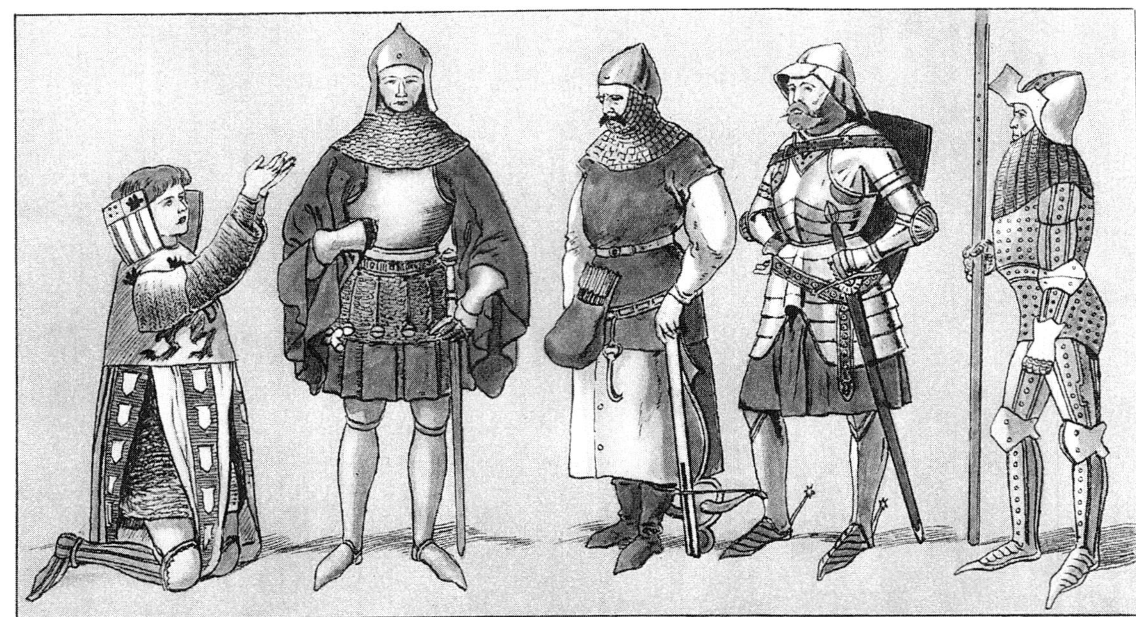

6 7 8 9 10

Italy

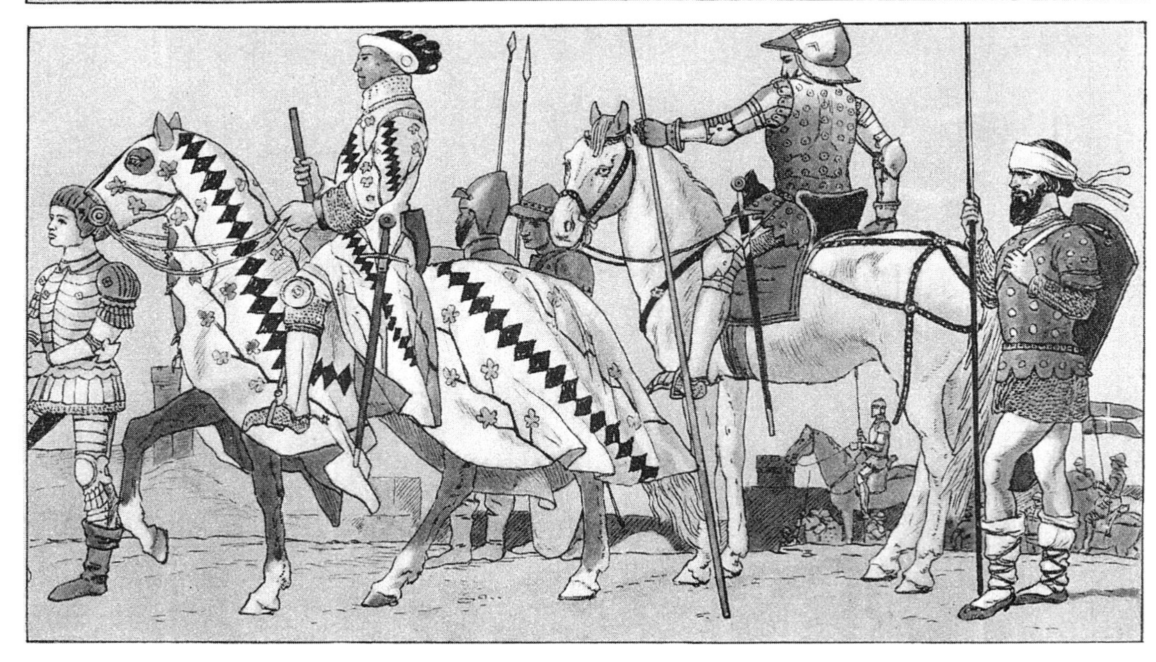

11 12 13 14 15 16 17

ENGLAND
10th–15th Centuries

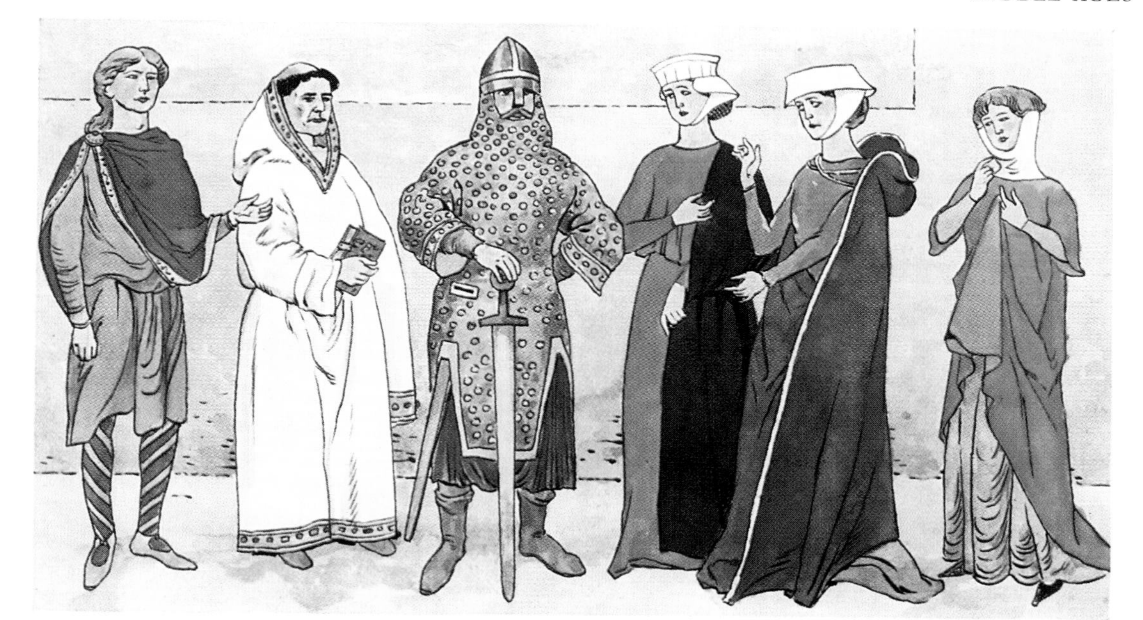

10th–13th Centuries

1 2 3 4 5 6

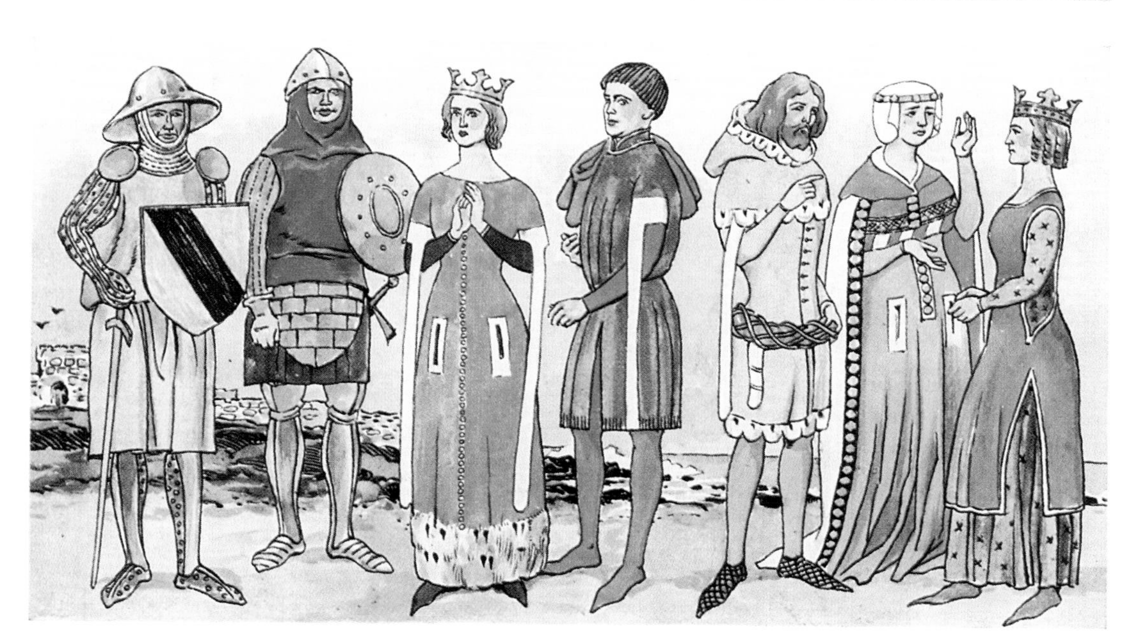

14th Century

7 8 9 10 11 12 13

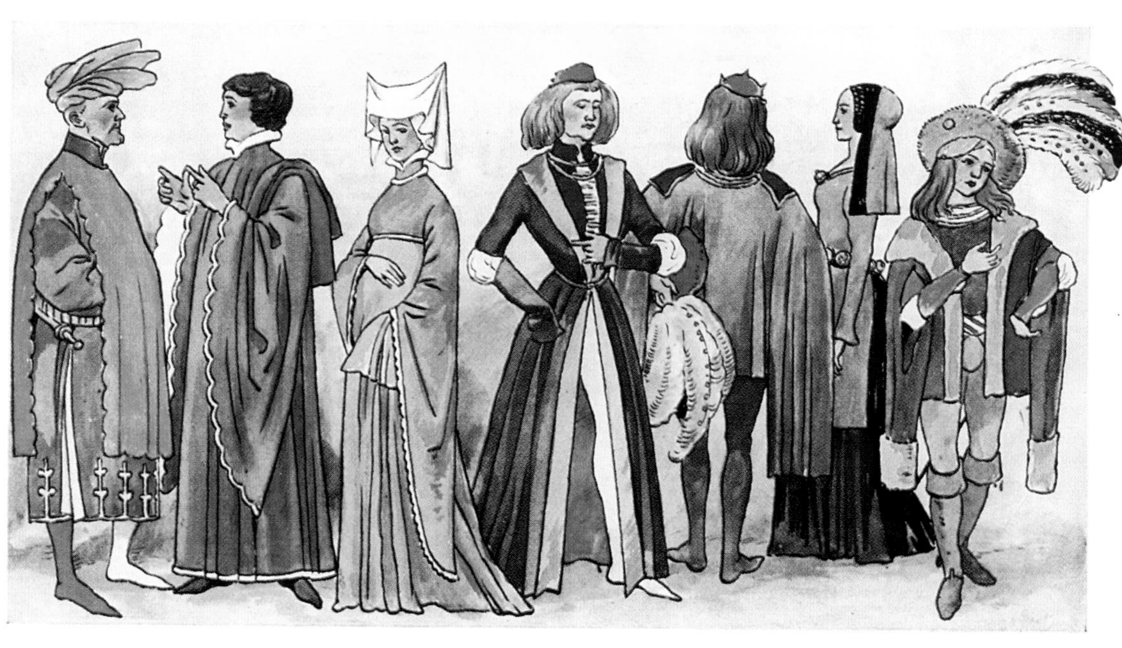

15th Century

14 15 16 17 18 19 20

ARMOURED KNIGHTS

France and Germany
15th Century

French Knights

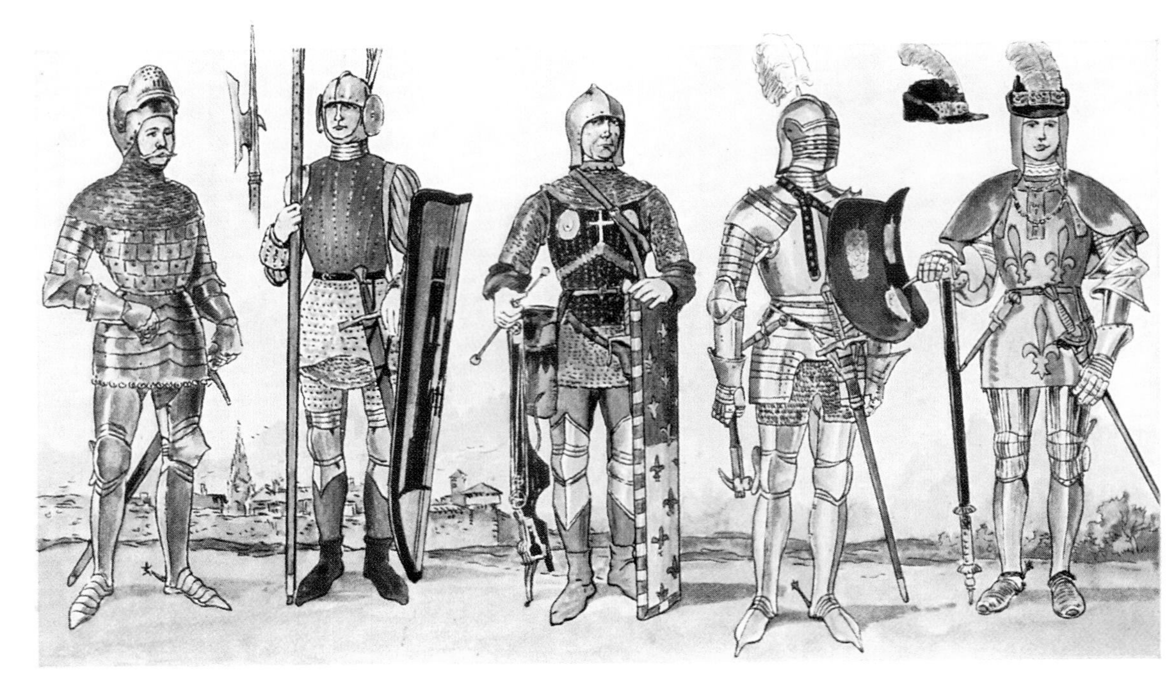

1 2 3 4 5

German Knights

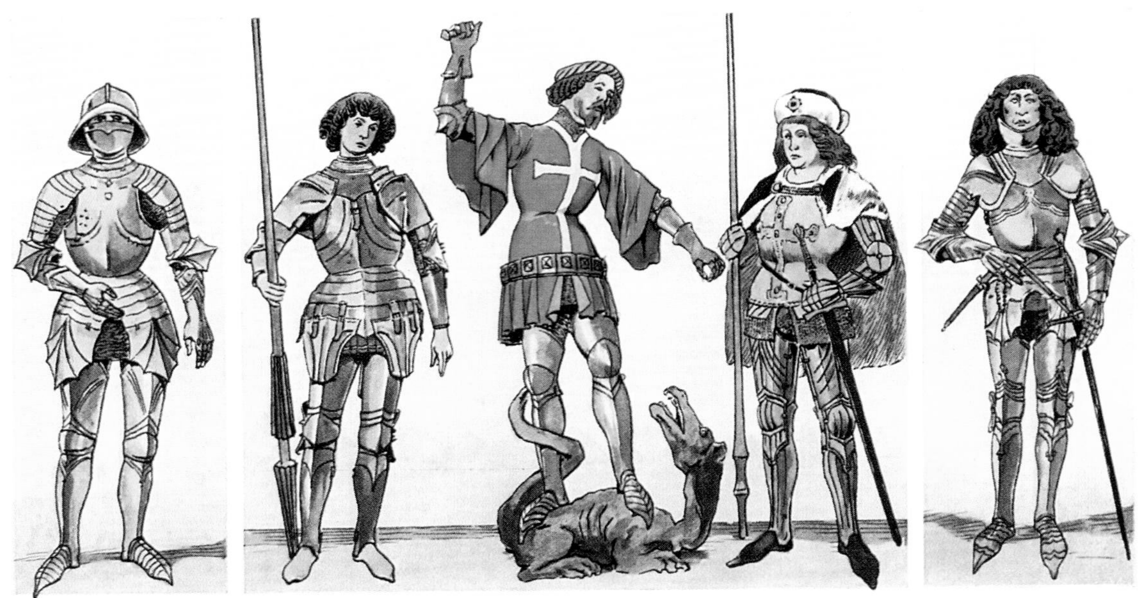

6 7 8 9 10

German Knights

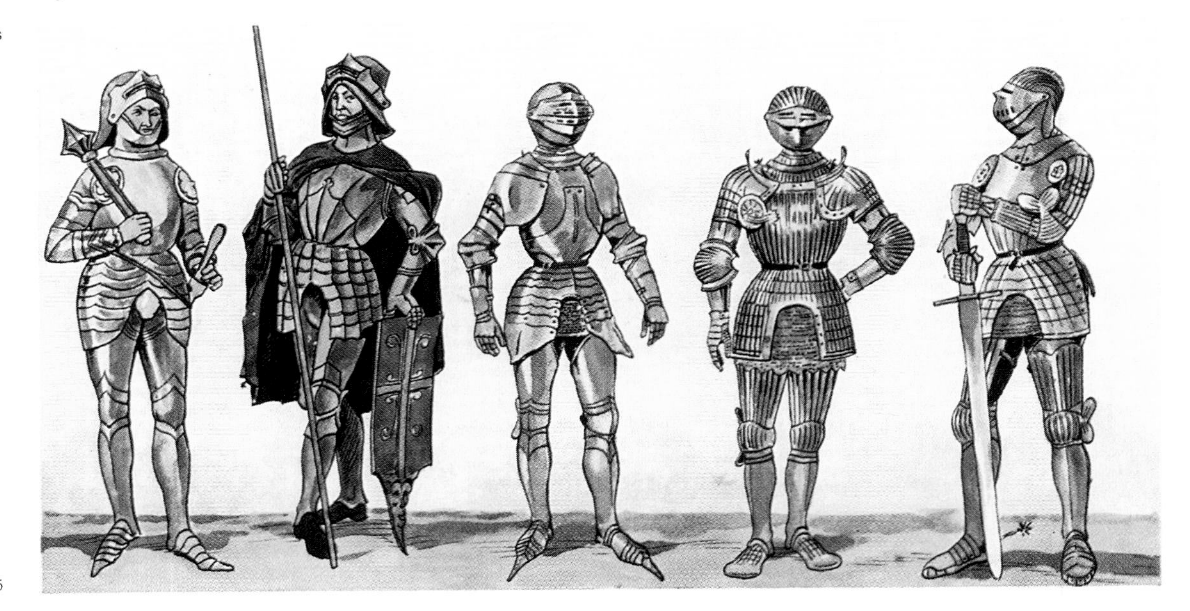

11 12 13 14 15

ARMOURED KNIGHTS

Italy 13th–15th Centuries

Verona
Florence
Genoa

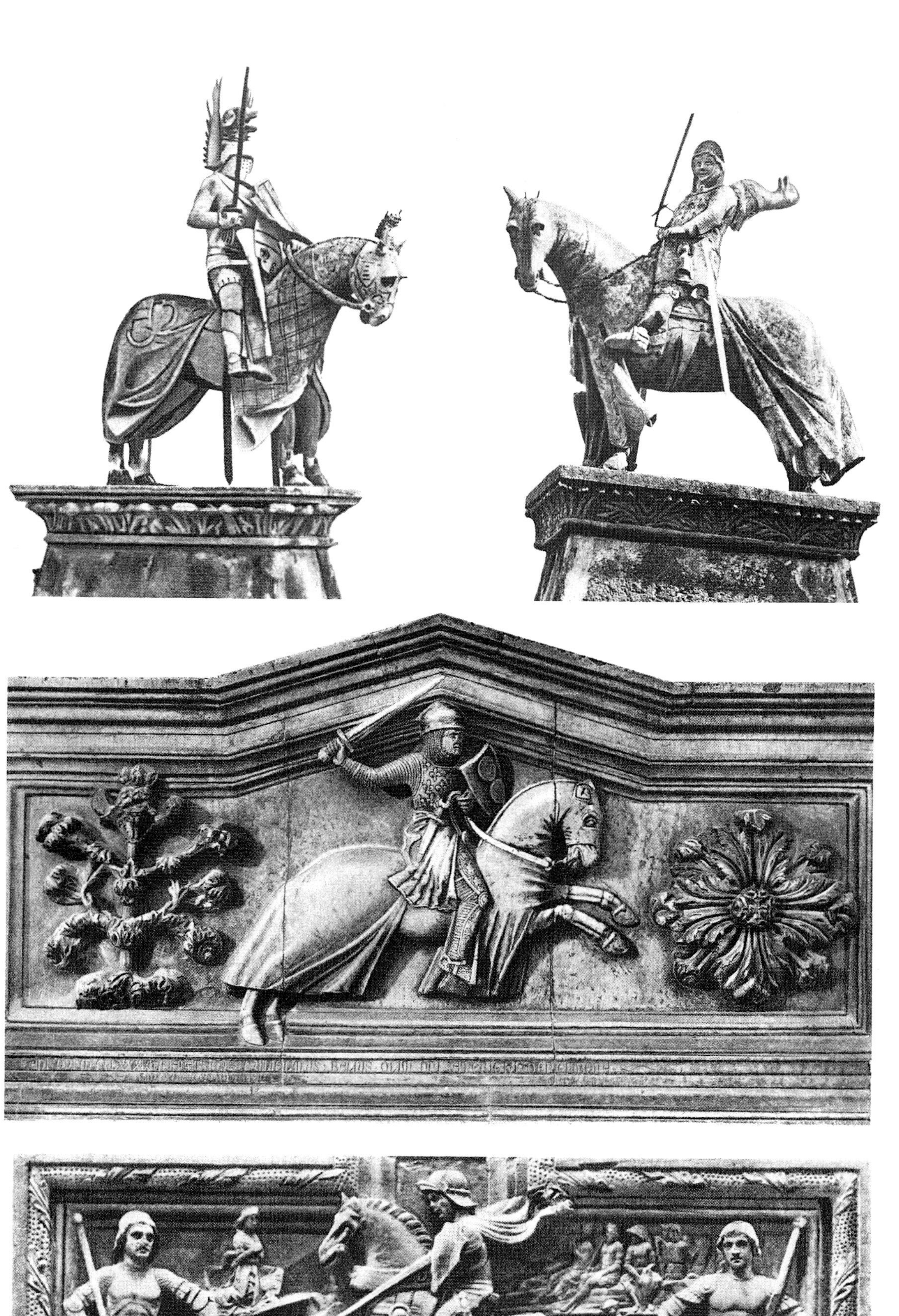

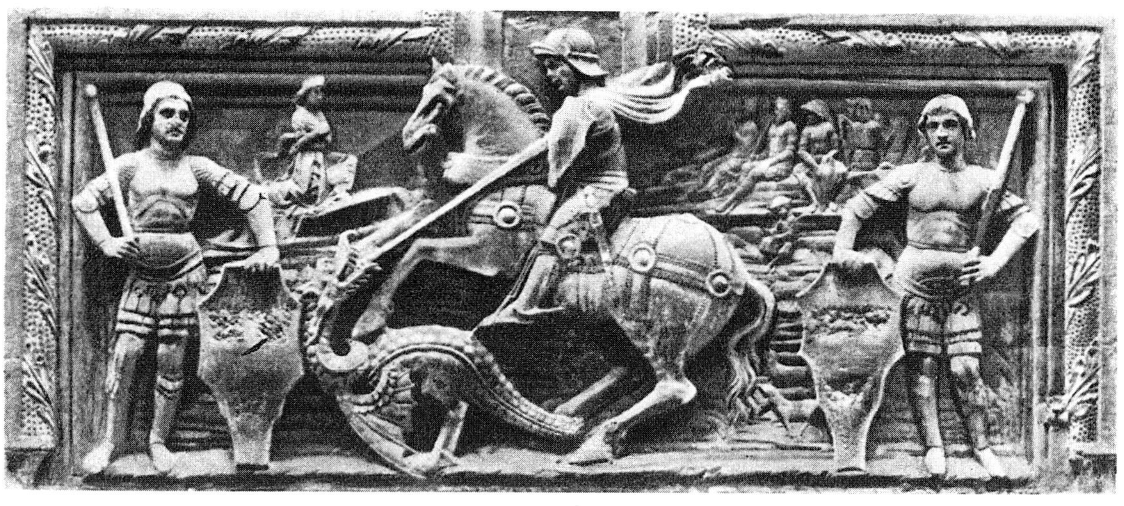

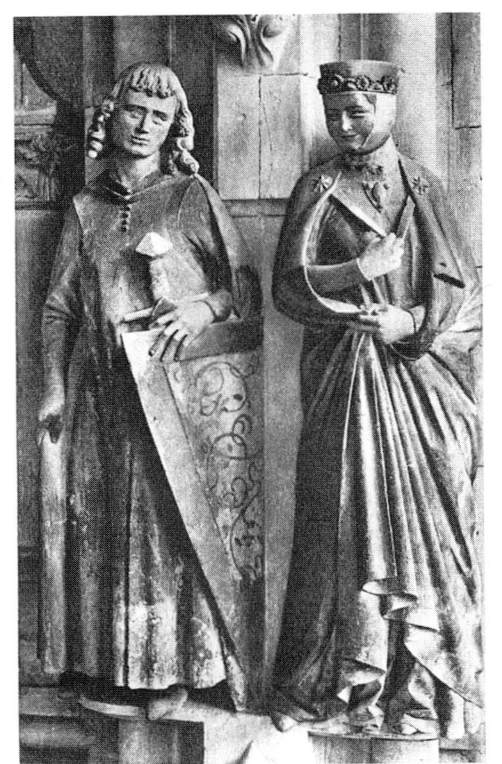

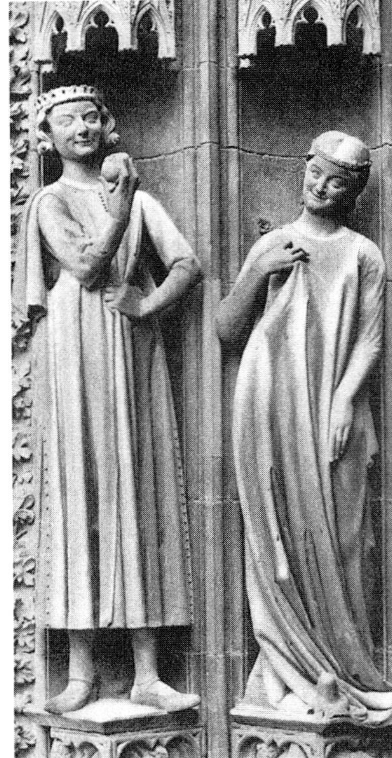

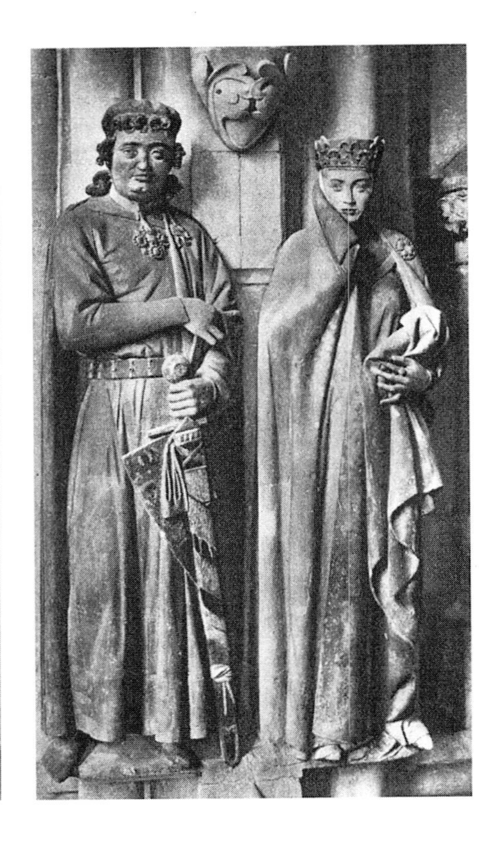

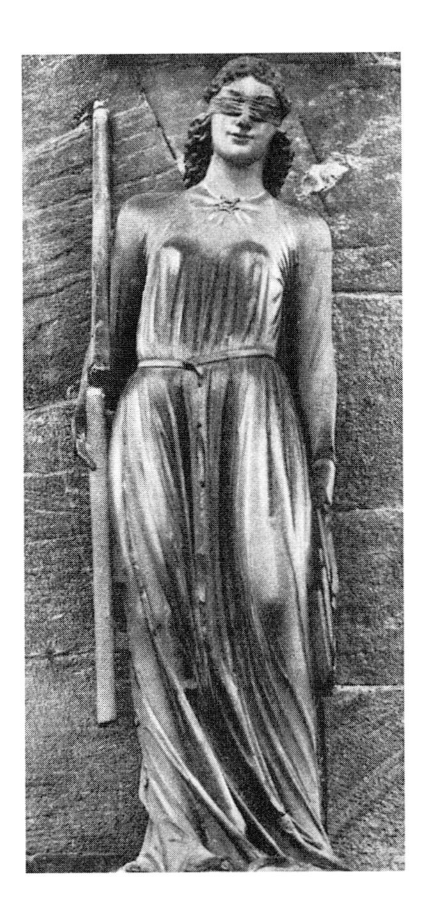

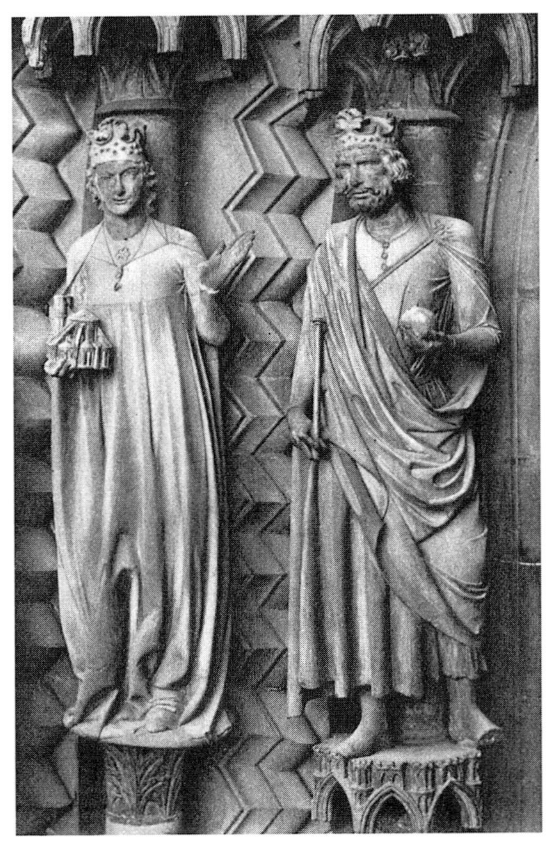

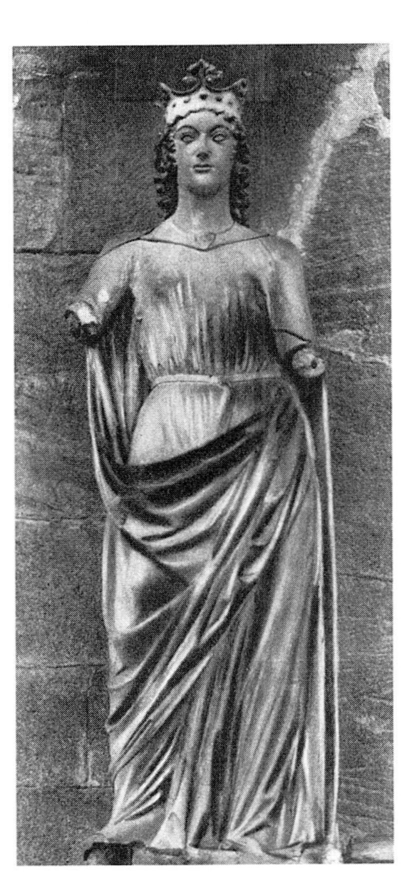

GERMANY
Naumburg, Strasburg, Bamberg

Costume of People of Rank
13th Century

ARMOURED KNIGHTS
Germany and Burgundy
14th Century

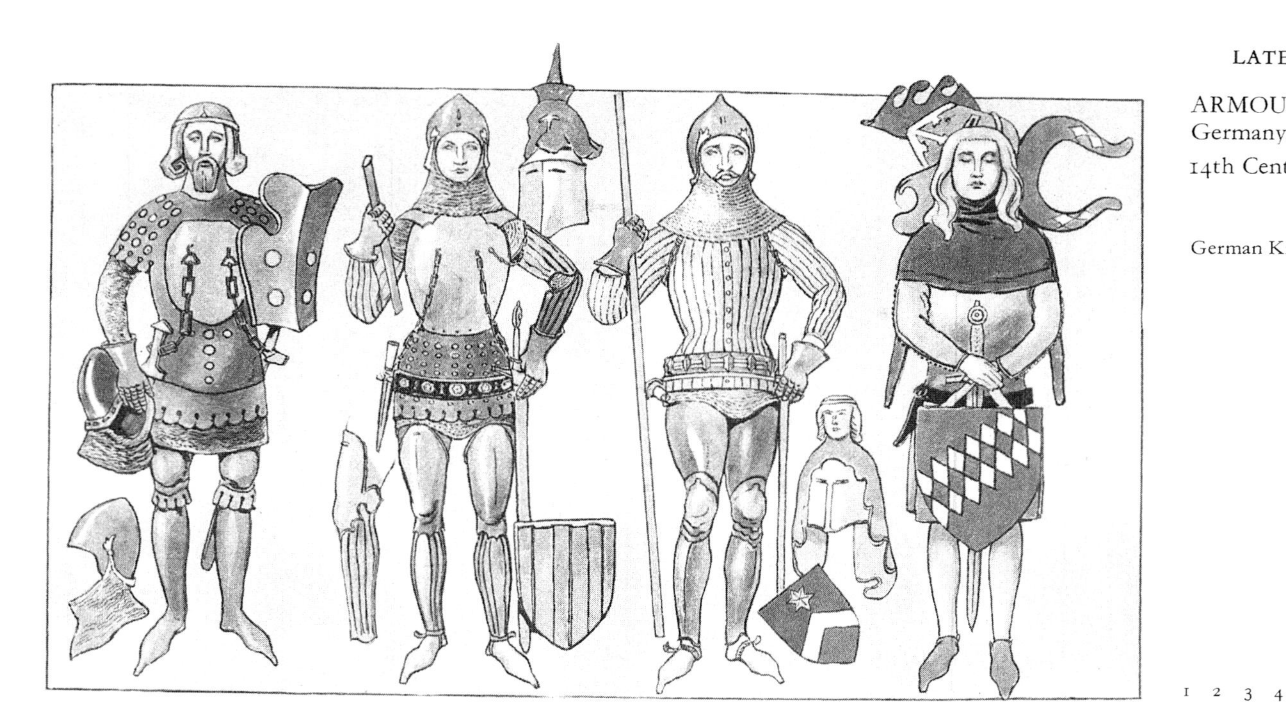

German Knights

1 2 3 4

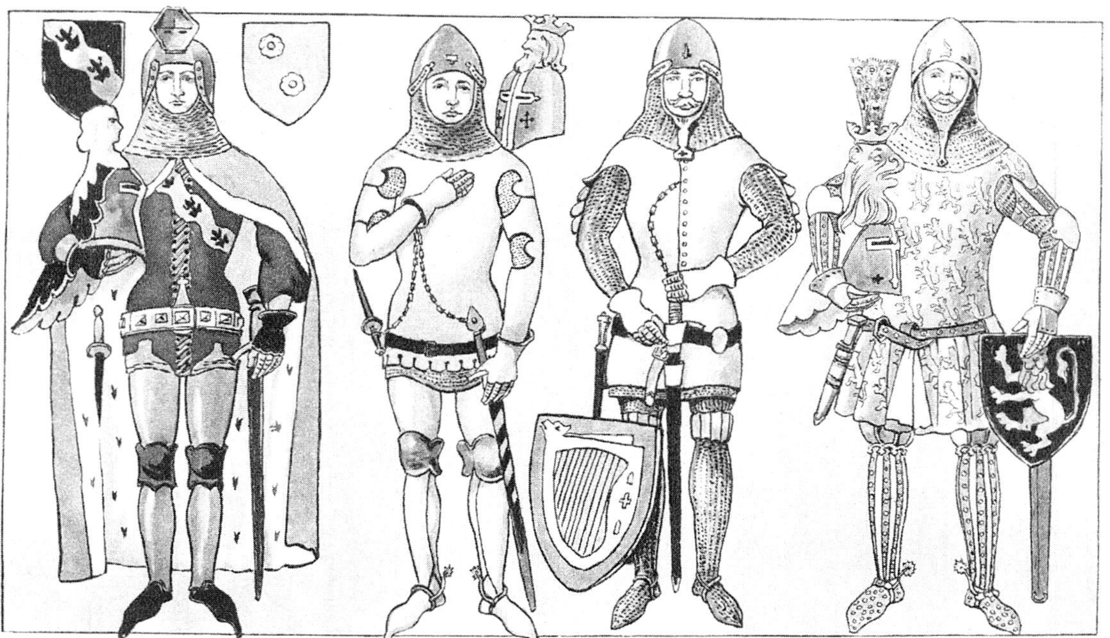

German Knights

5 6 7 8

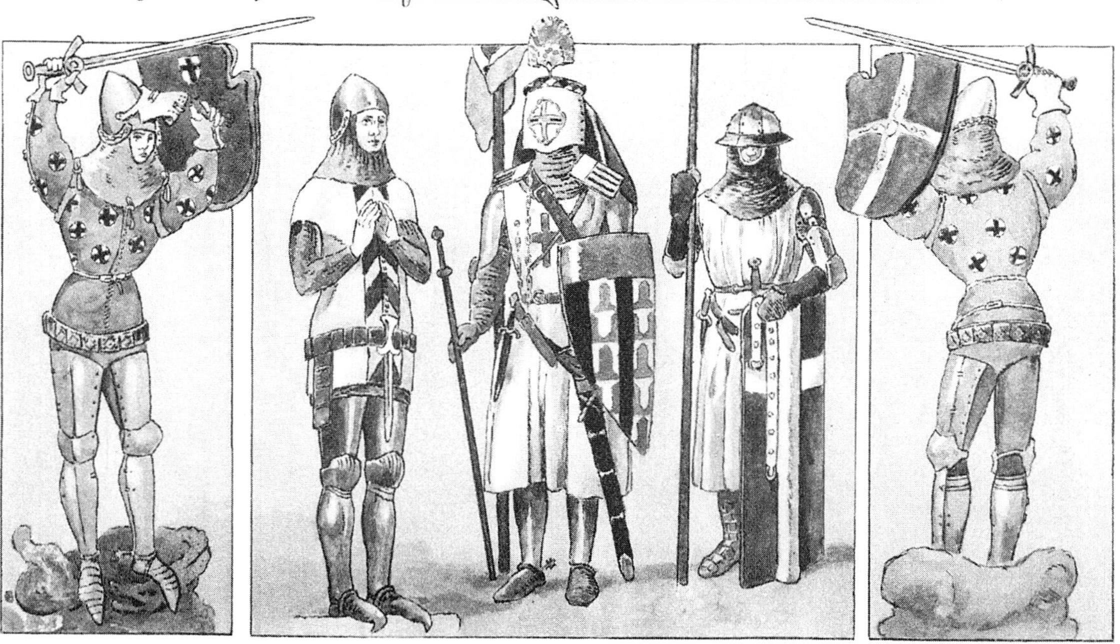

Burgundian Knights

9 10 11 12

KNIGHTS' ARMOUR

Armour, Helmets, Weapons

1–11

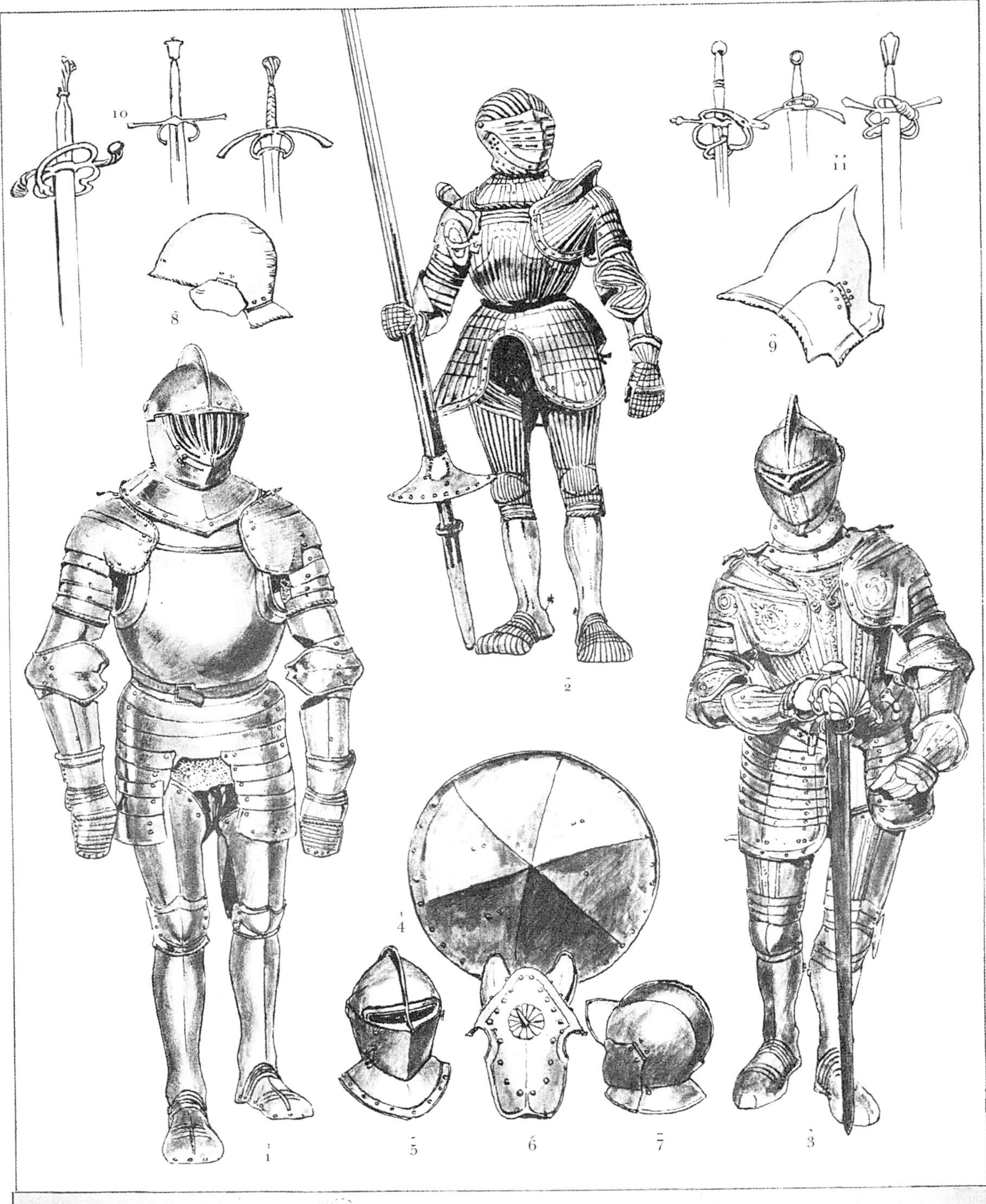

Tournament

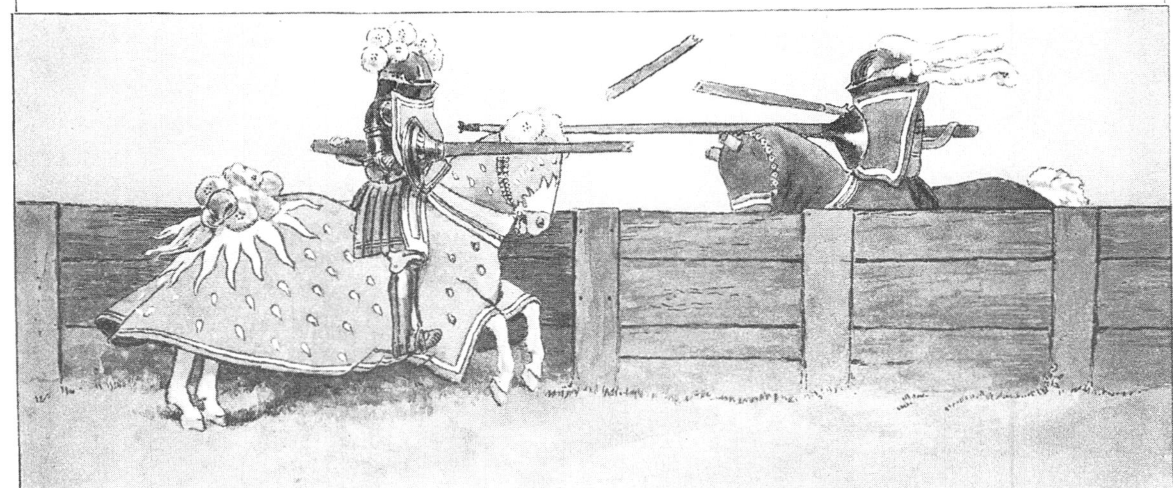

12 13

HELMETS AND WEAPONS
1000–1500

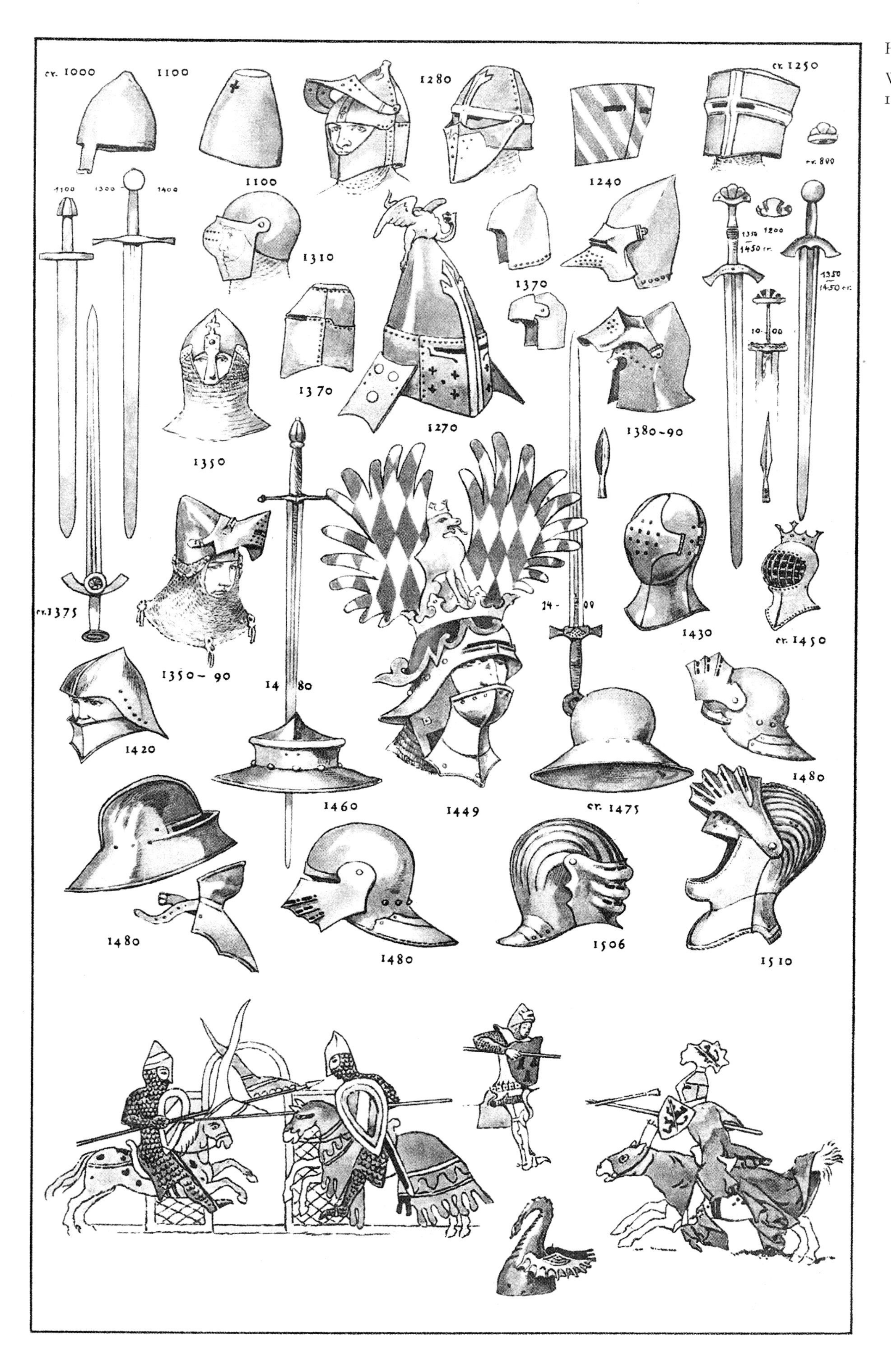

FRANCE
14th Century

Court dress

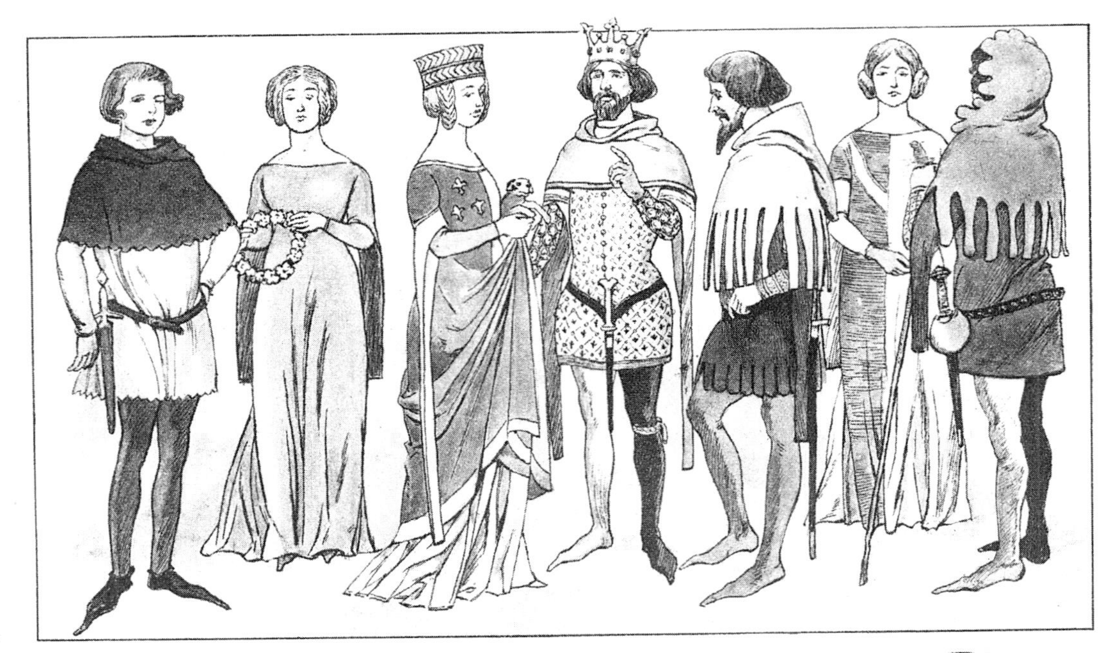

1 2 3 4 5 6 7

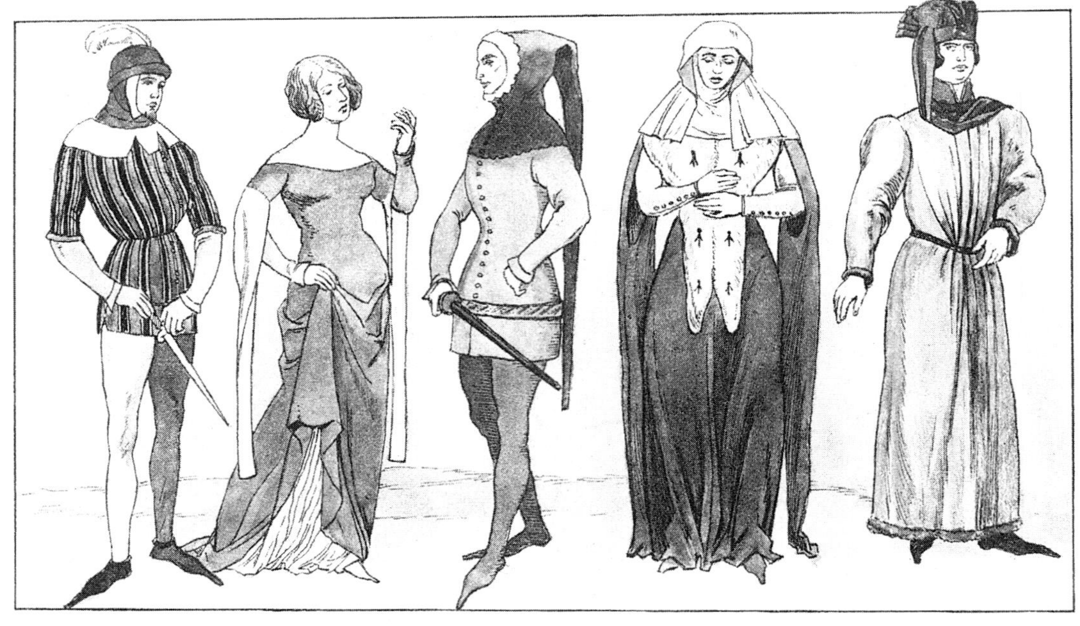

8 9 10 11 12

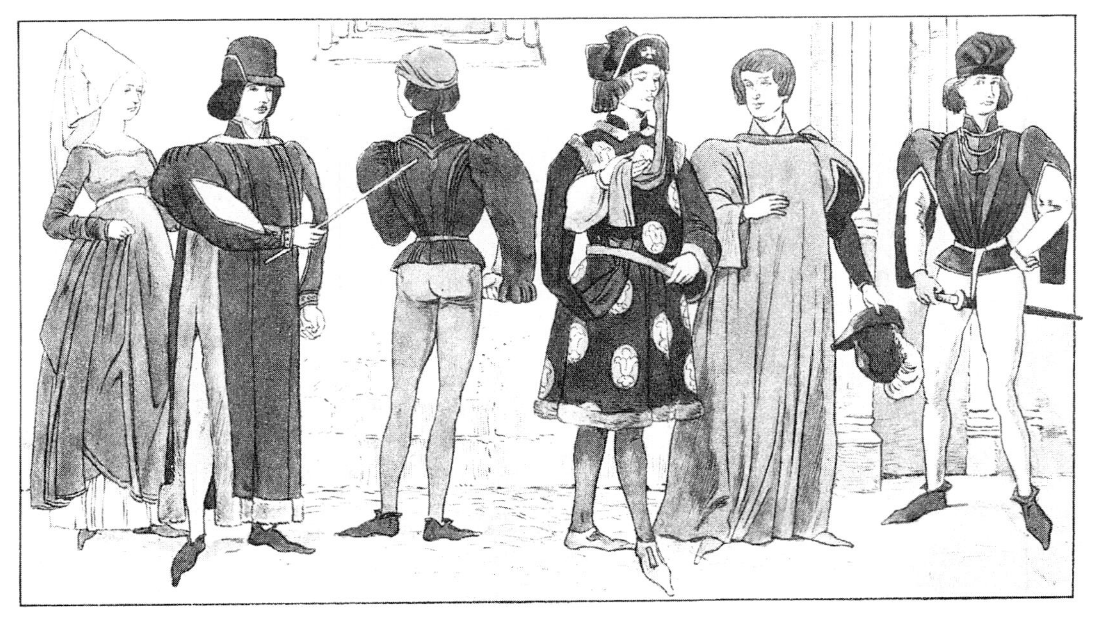

13 14 15 16 17 18

BURGUNDY
15th Century

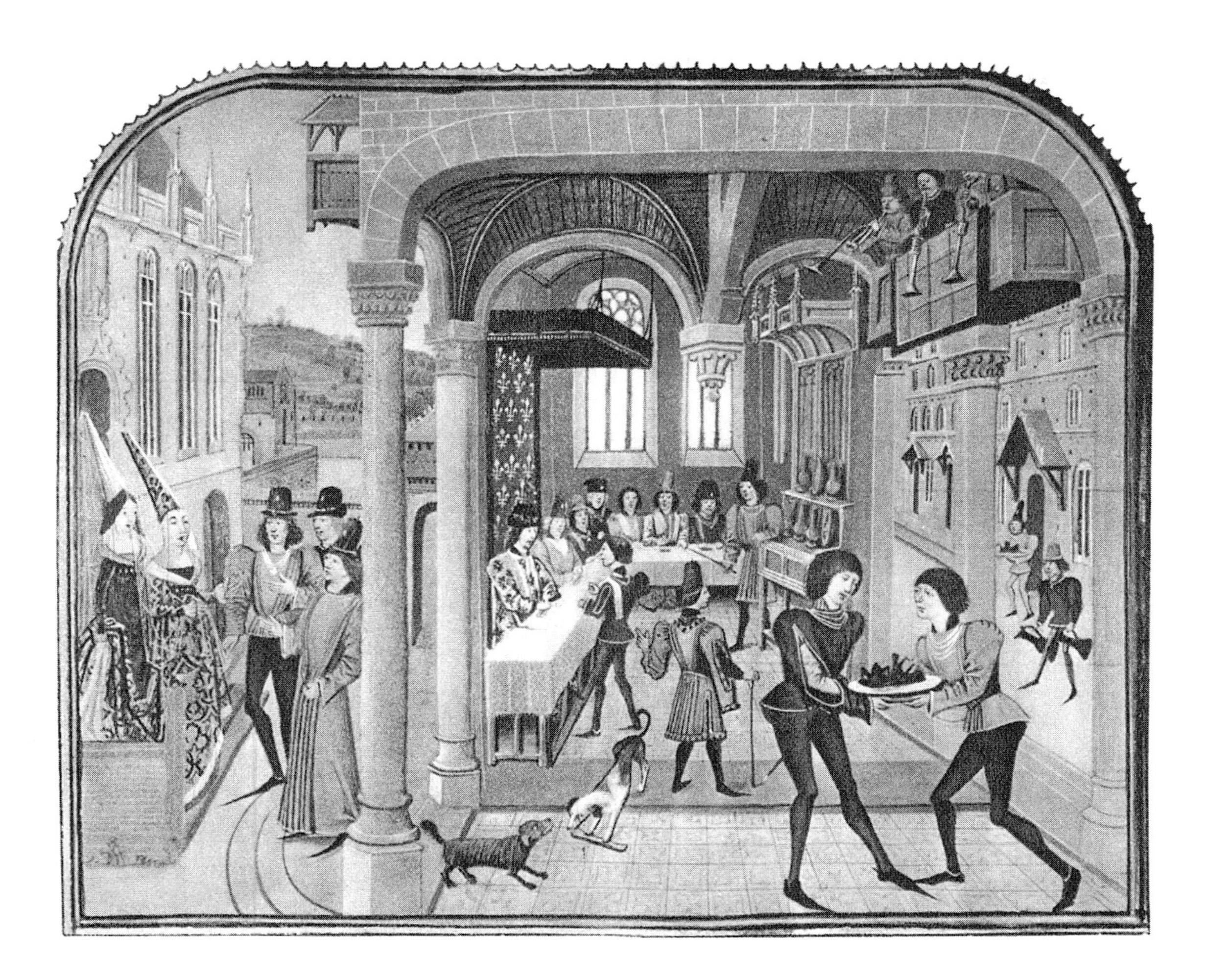

Banquet

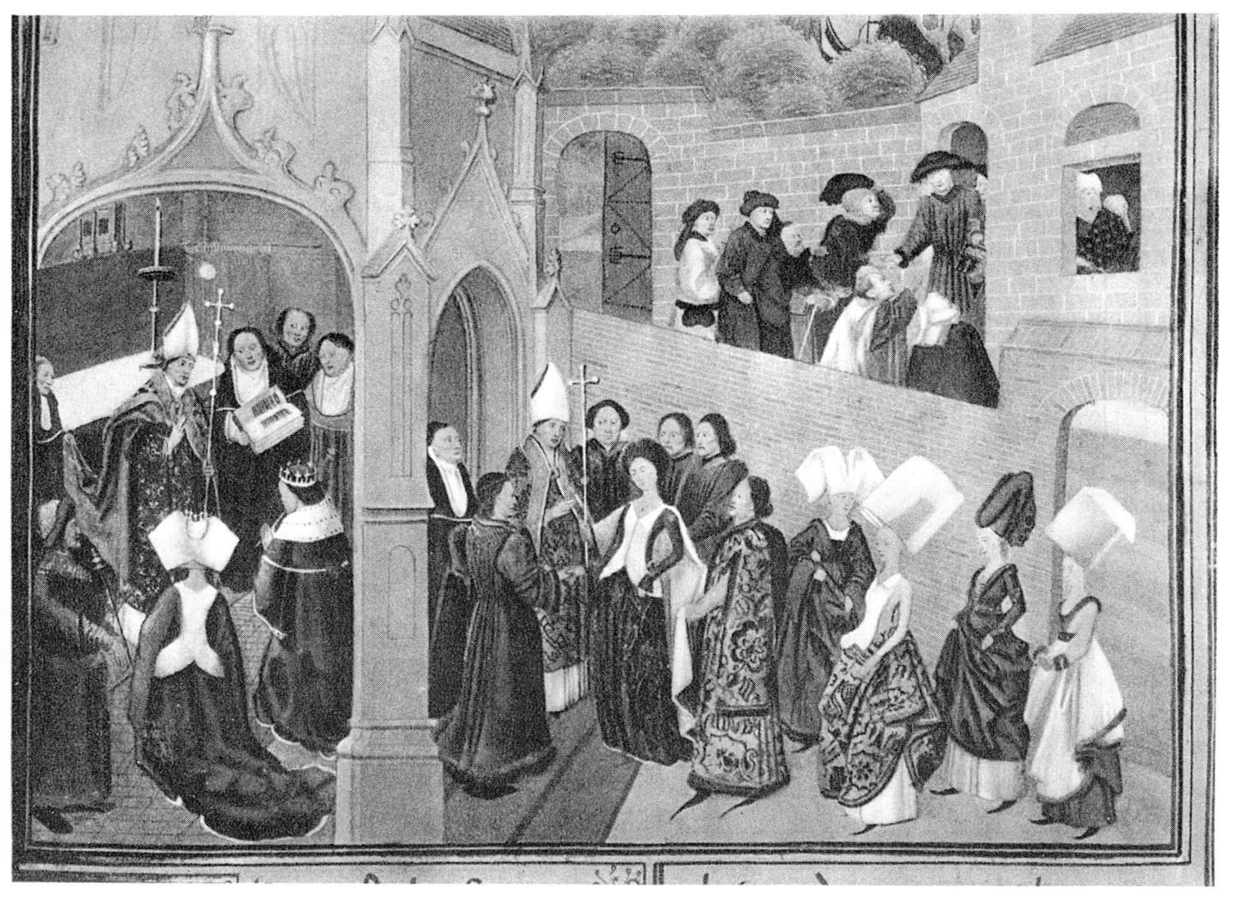

Coronation Ceremony

BURGUNDY
Head-dress and Hair Styles
15th Century

Women's Head-gear
Men's Hats
Men's Hair Styles

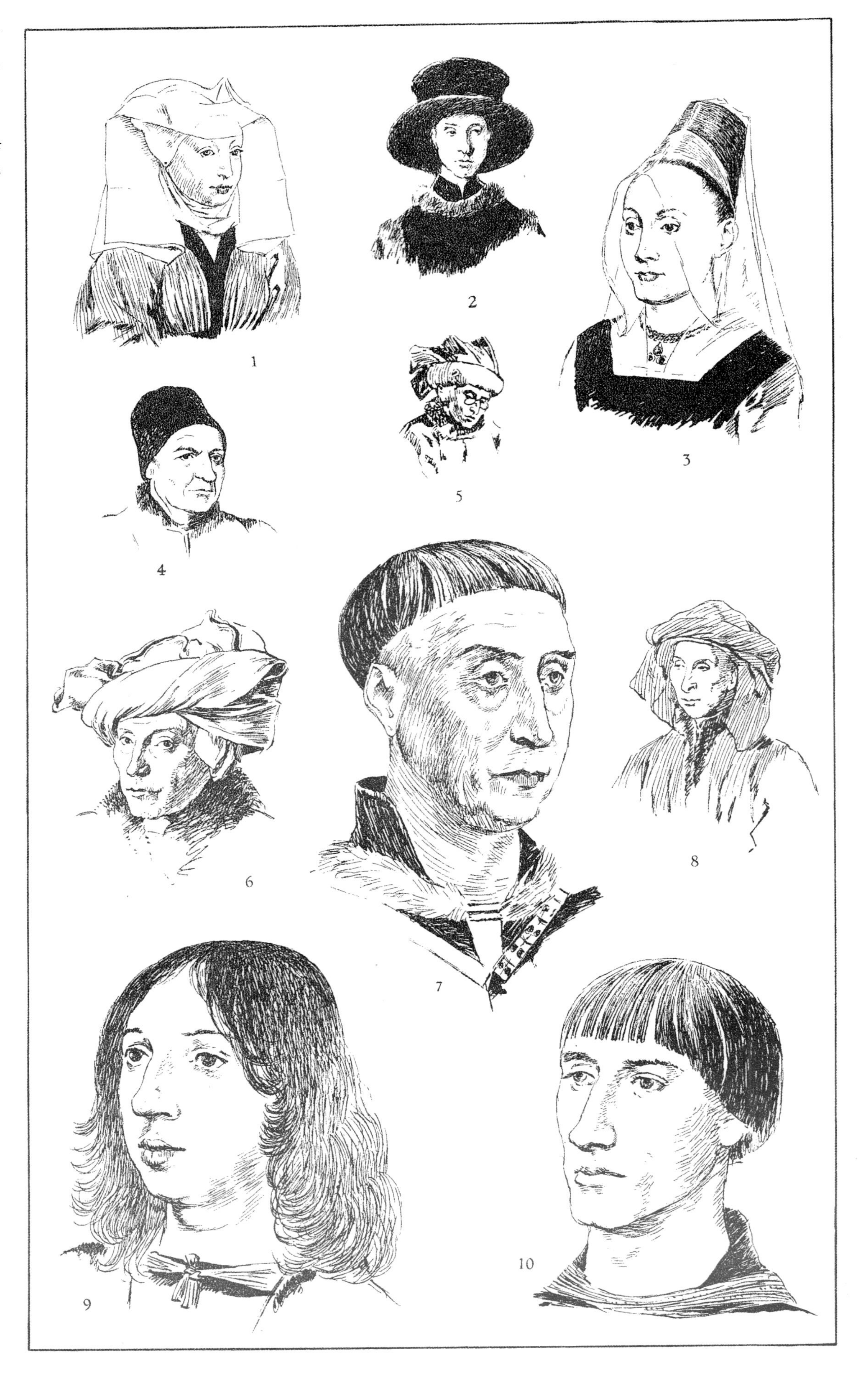

EUROPE
Footwear
14th and 15th Centuries

Pointed shoes and wooden

Sandals

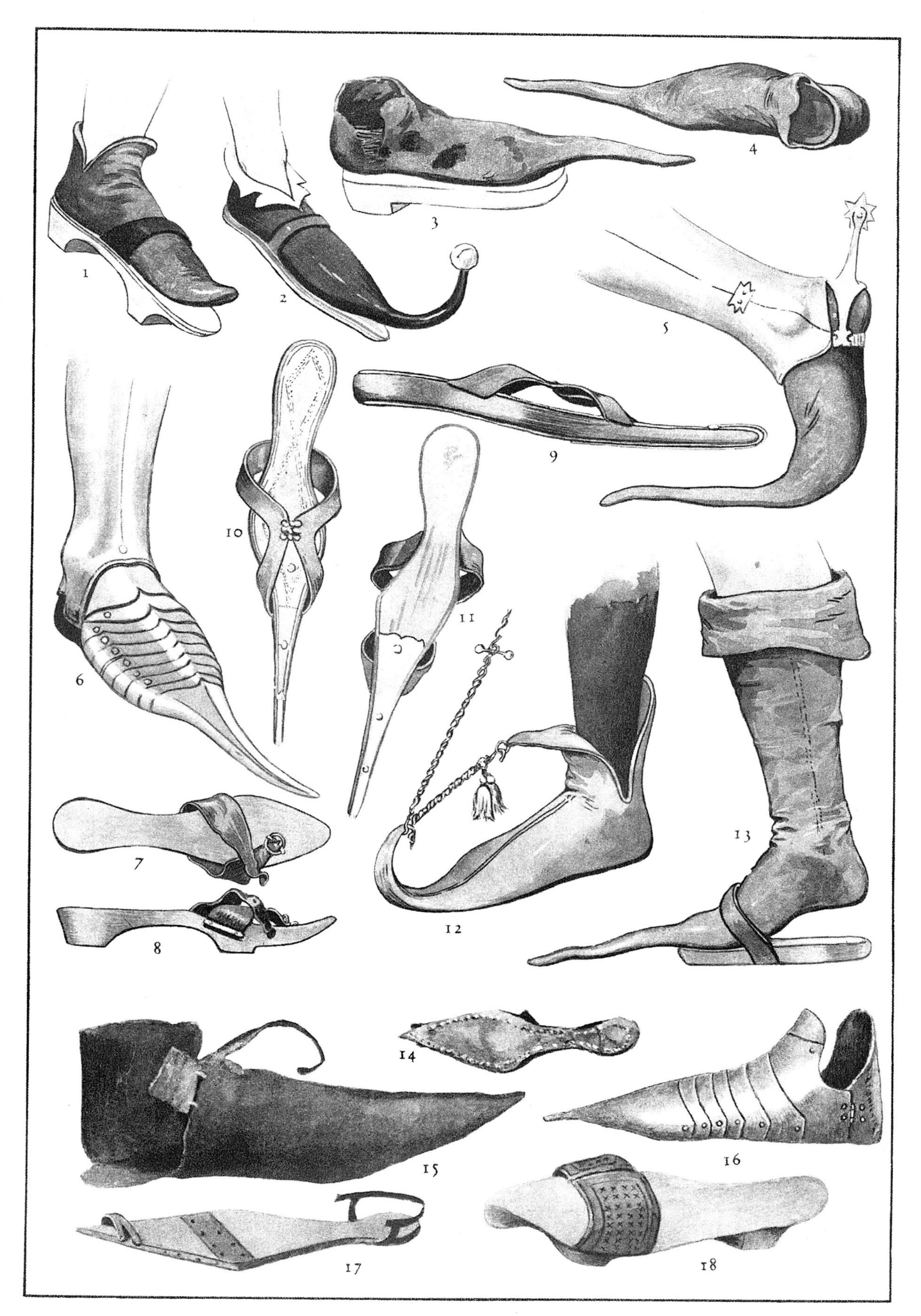

ITALY

1480–1490

Florentine Middle Class Life

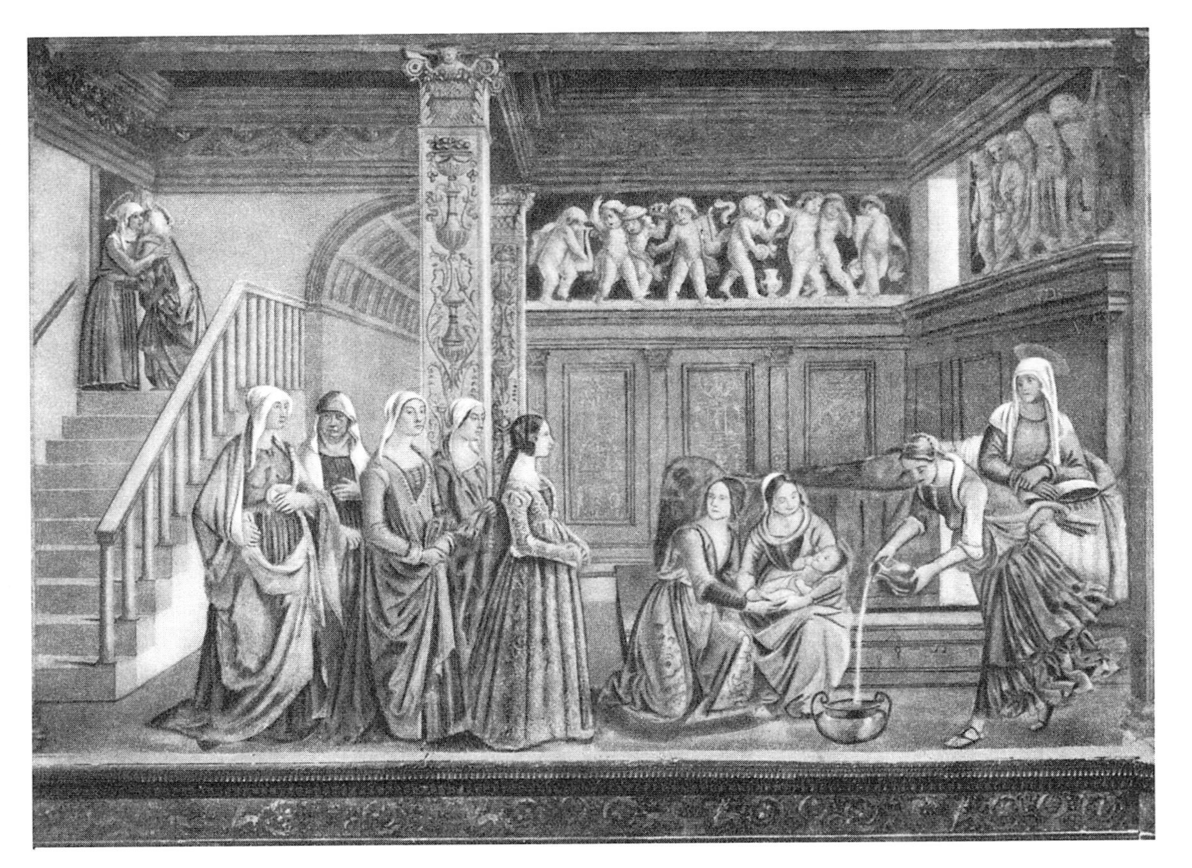

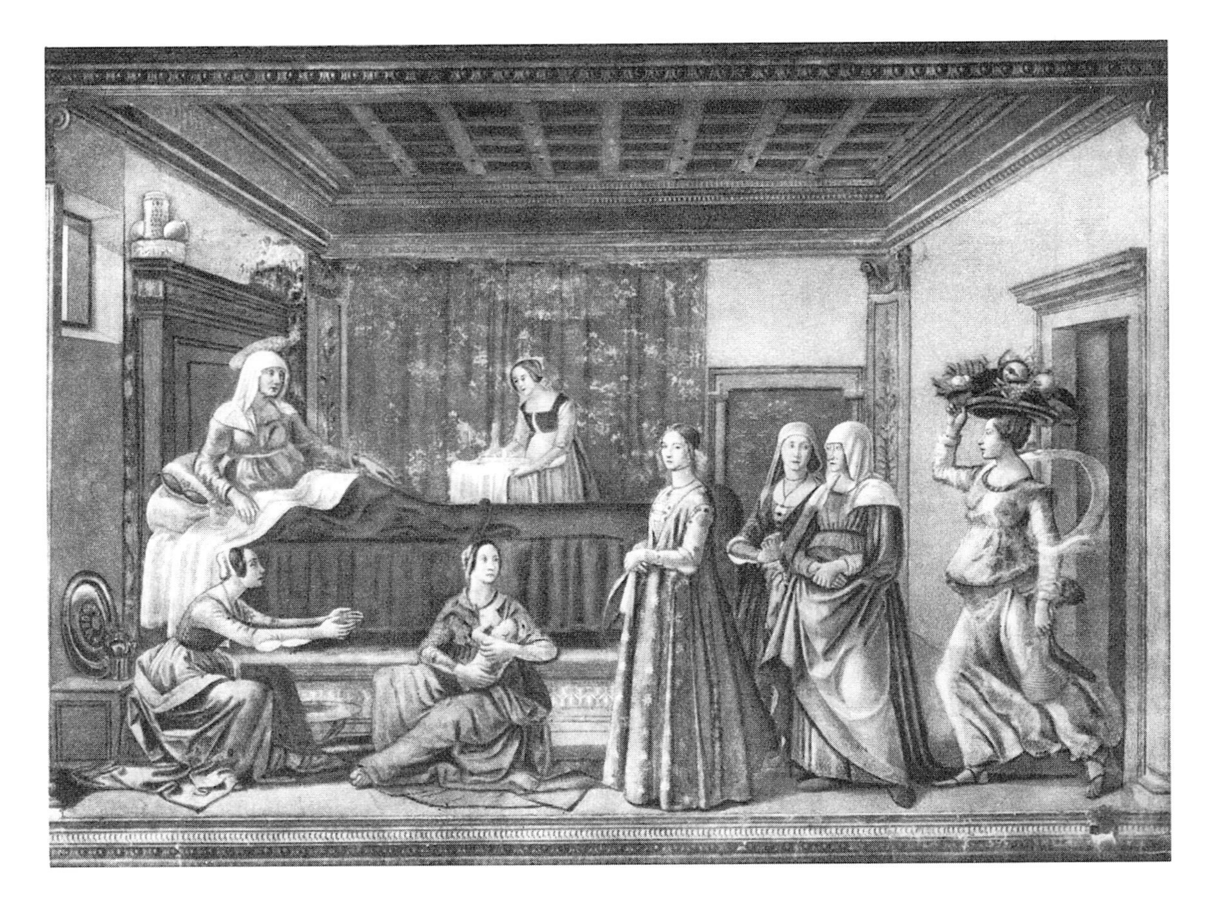

KNIGHTS' APPAREL
German

Tournament Apparel
1500–1515

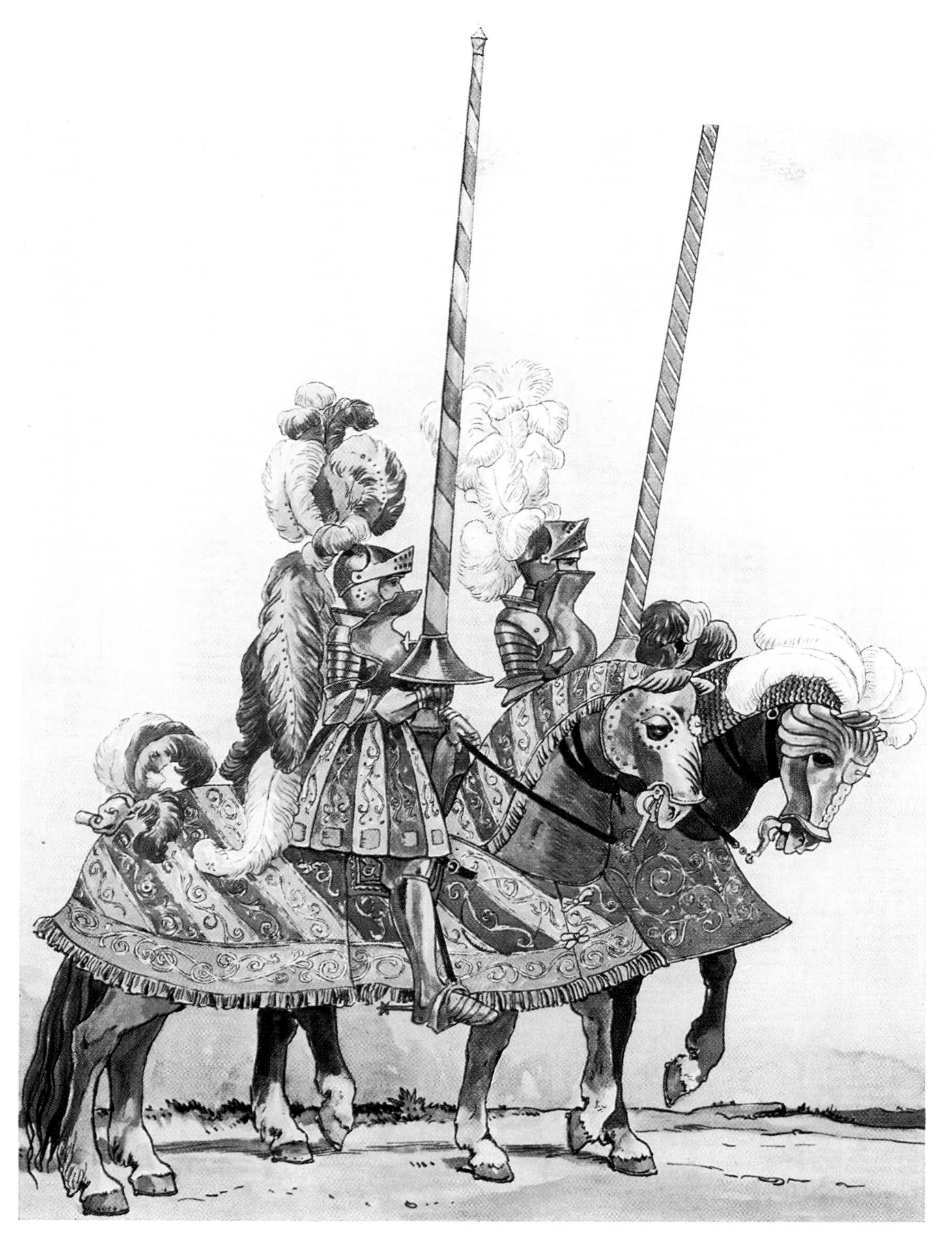

German Jousters about 1500

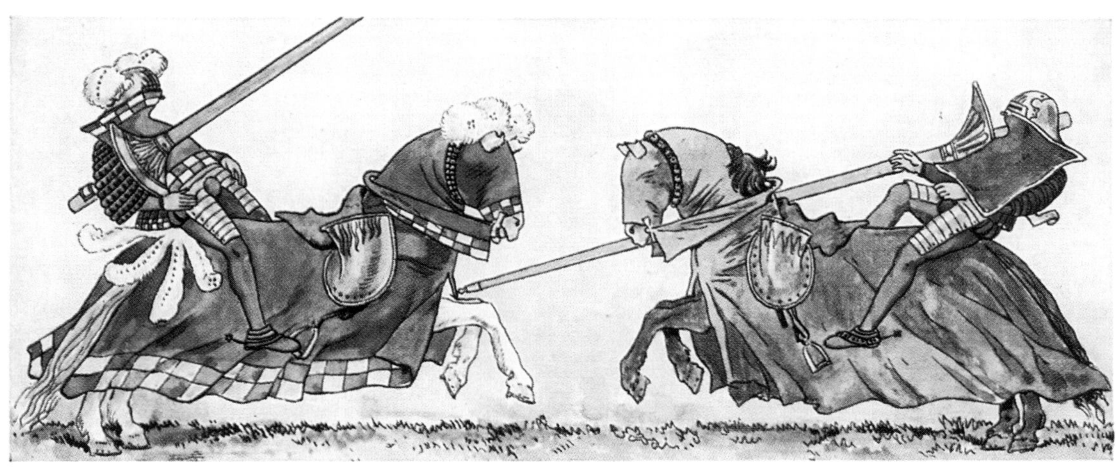

German Knights jousting about 1515

FRANCE
15th Century

Young Men of Rank

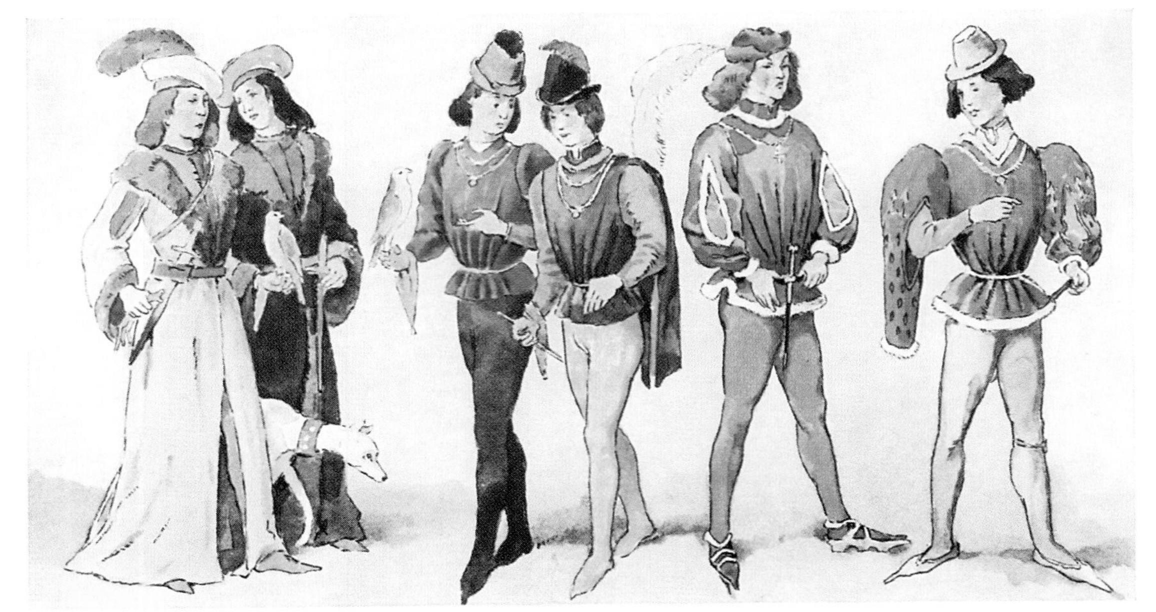

1 2 3 4 5 6

People of Rank

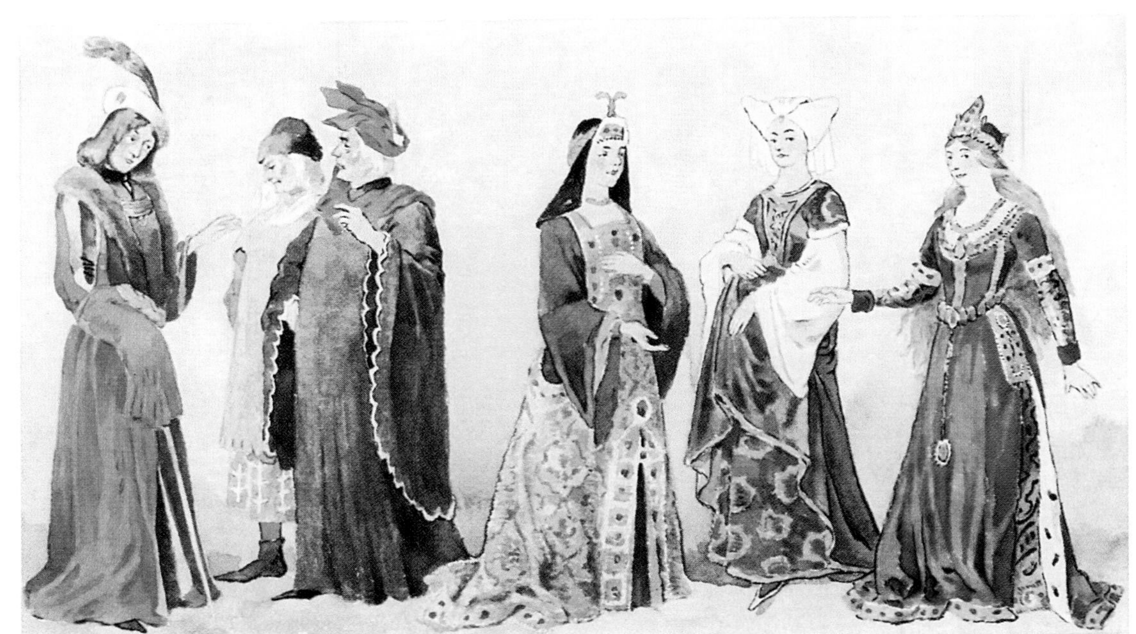

7 8 9 10 11 12

Ladies in Waiting

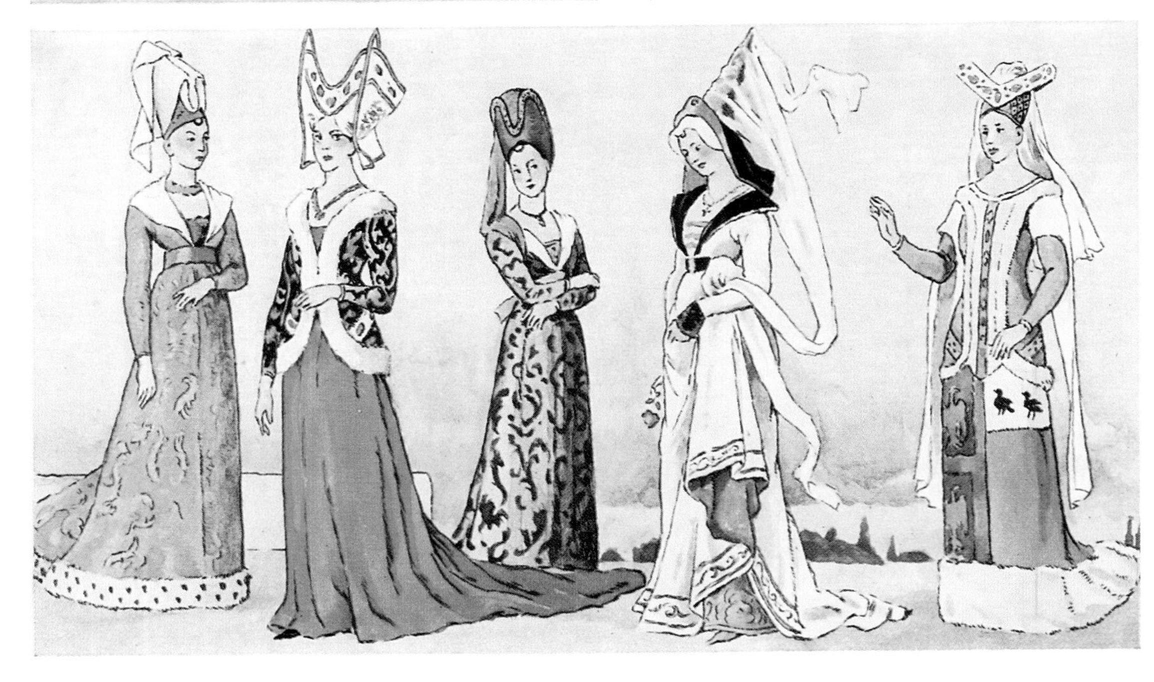

13 14 15 16 17

FRANCE
1485–1510

Court Dress

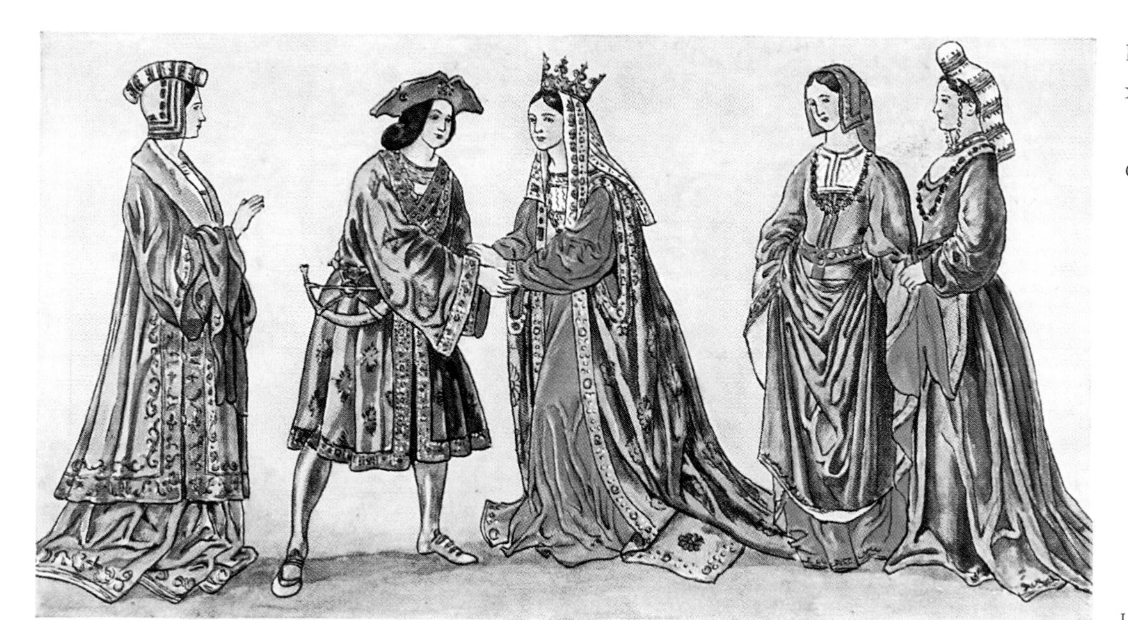

1 2 3 4 5

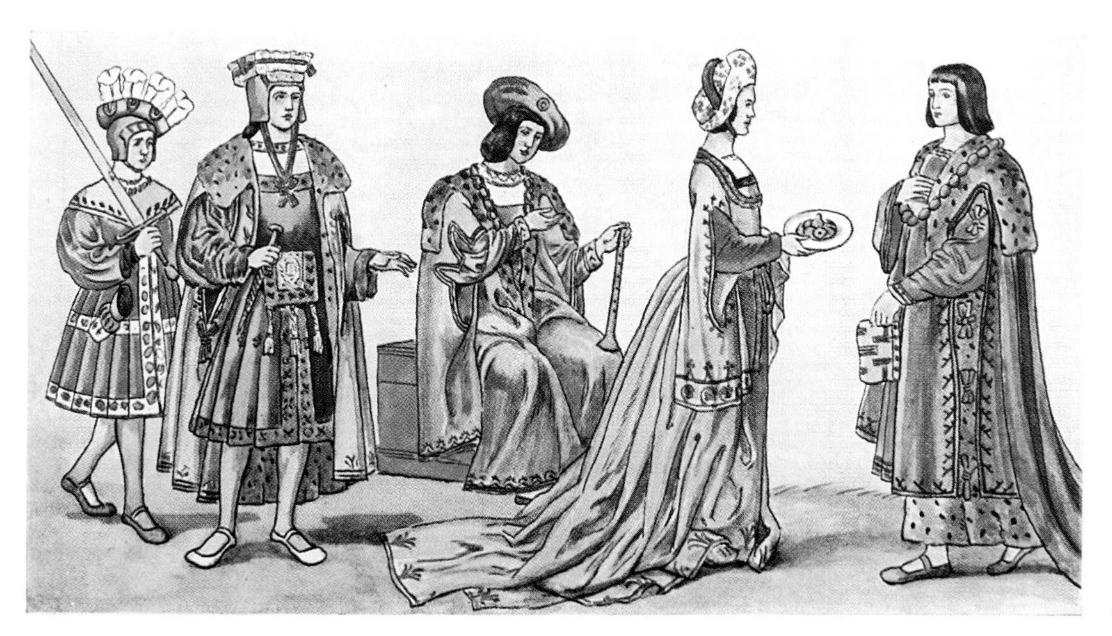

6 7 8 9 10

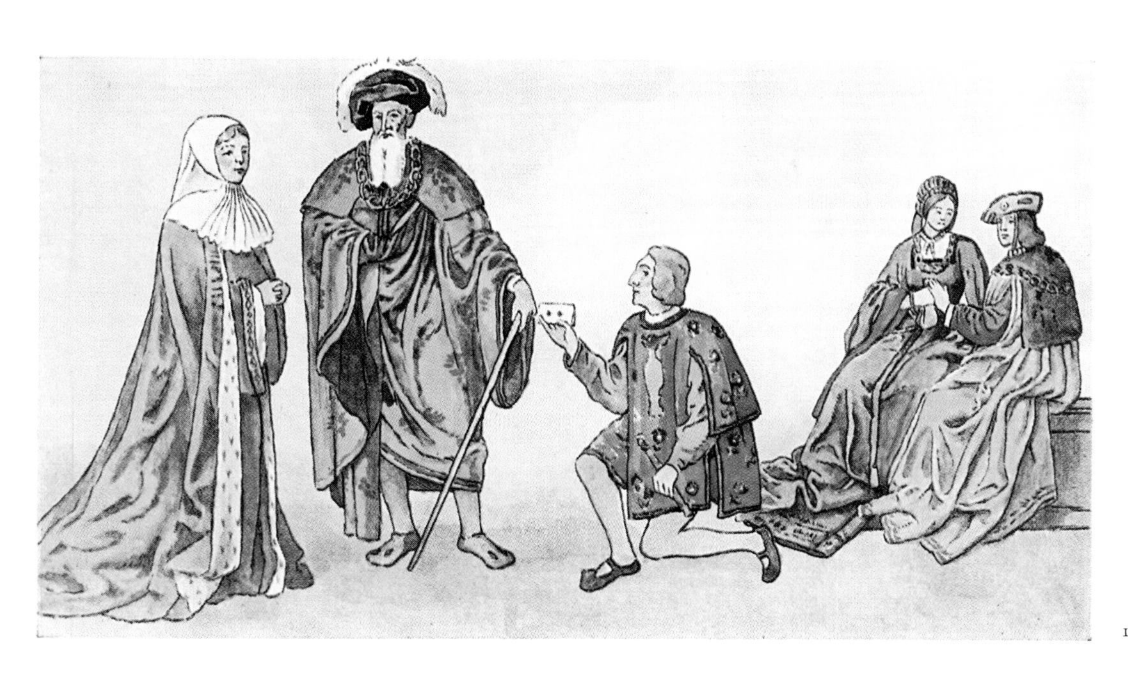

11 12 13 14 15

BURGUNDY
1425-1490

Court Dress

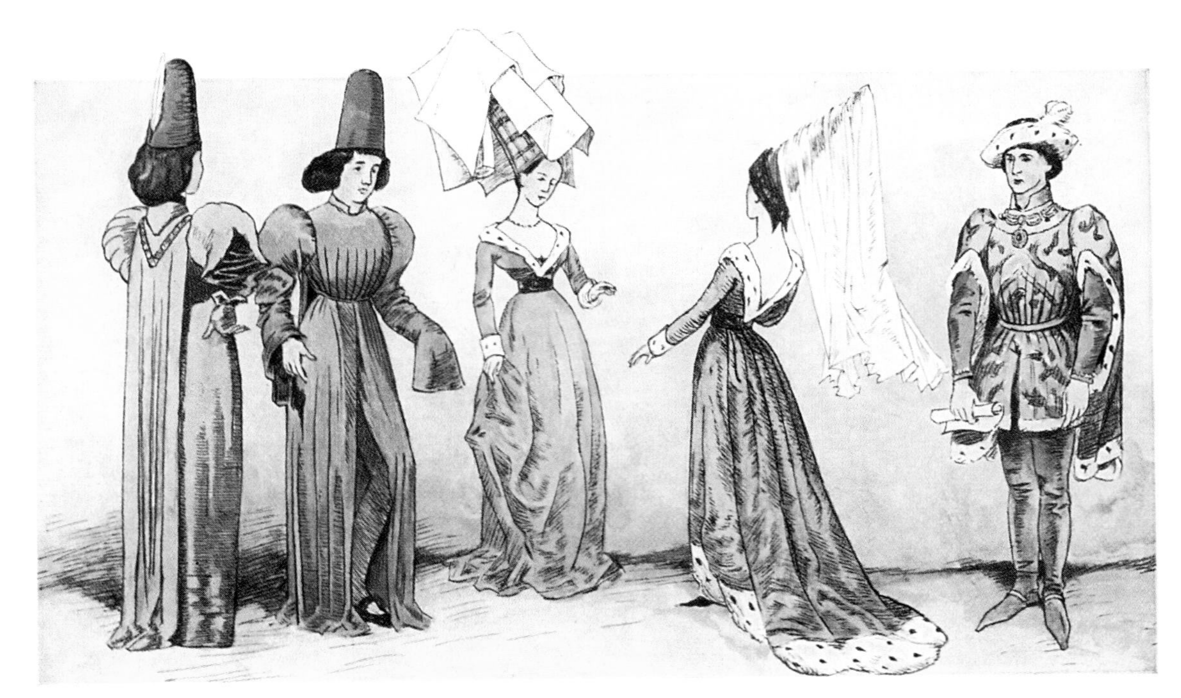

1 2 3 4 5

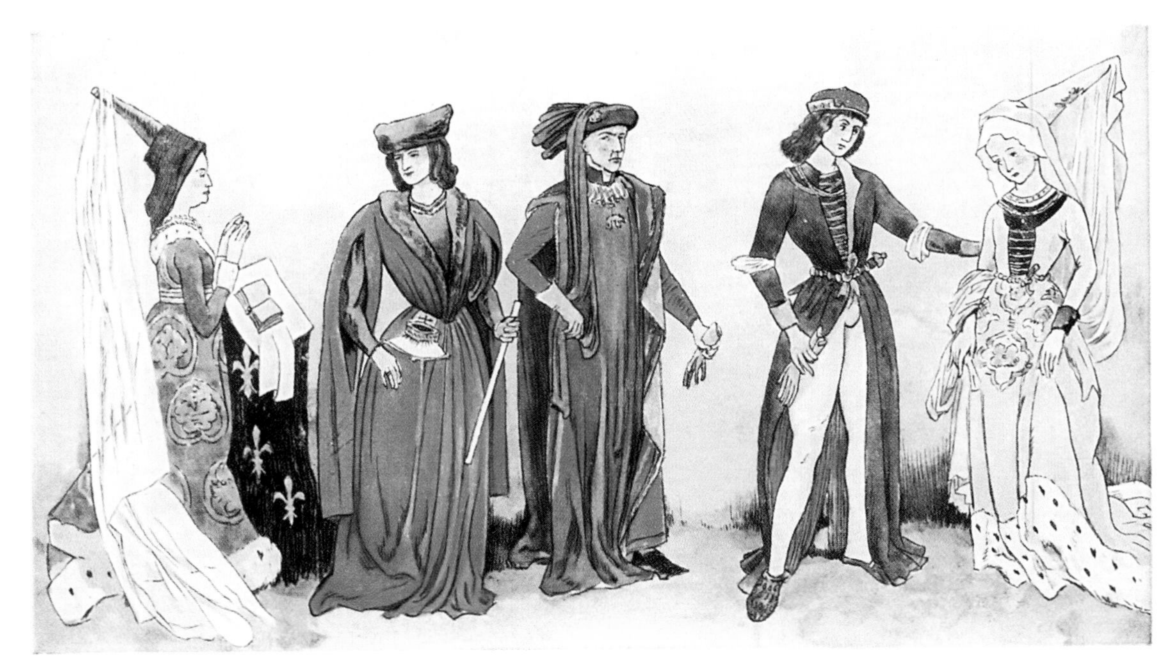

6 7 8 9 10

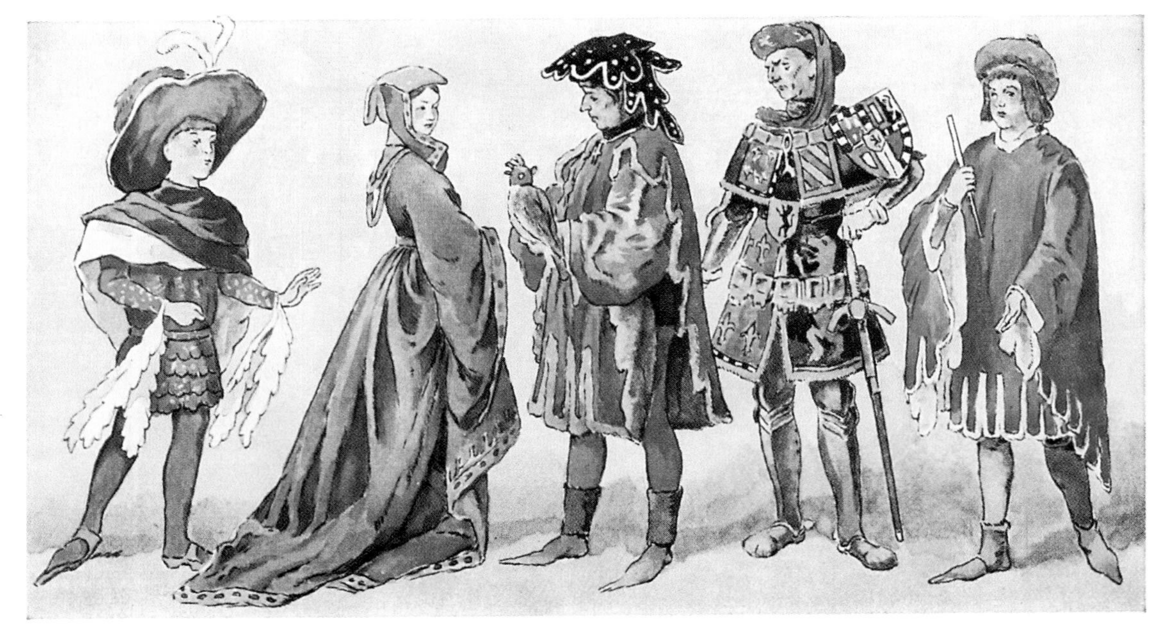

11 12 13 14 15

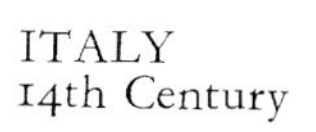

ITALY
14th Century

1310–1350

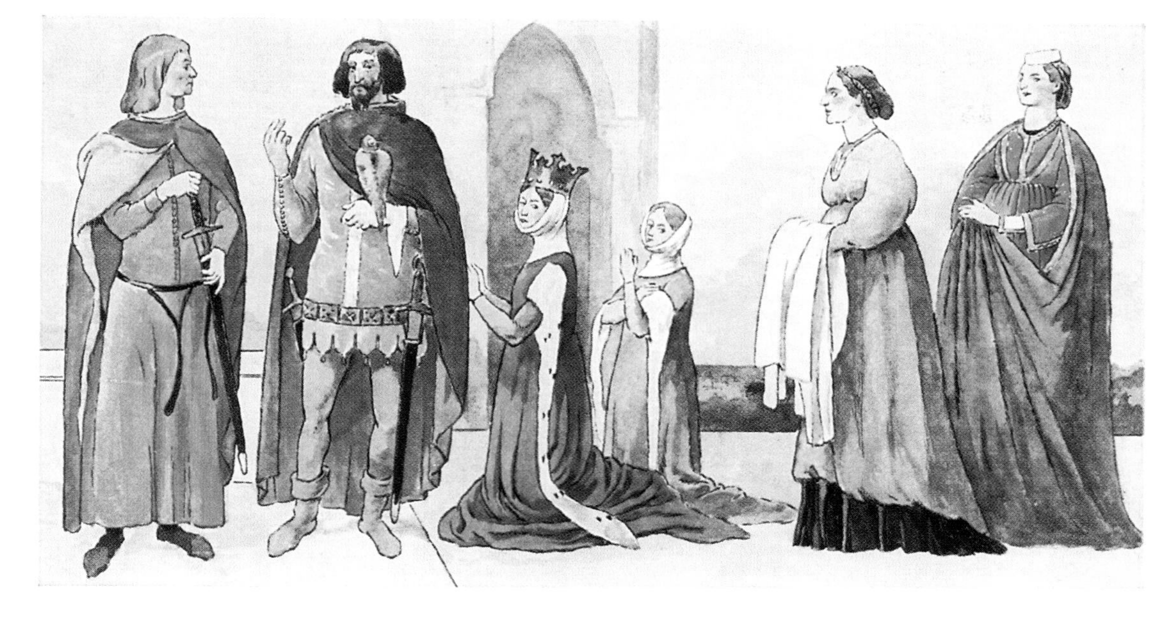

1 2 3 4 5 6

1325–1350

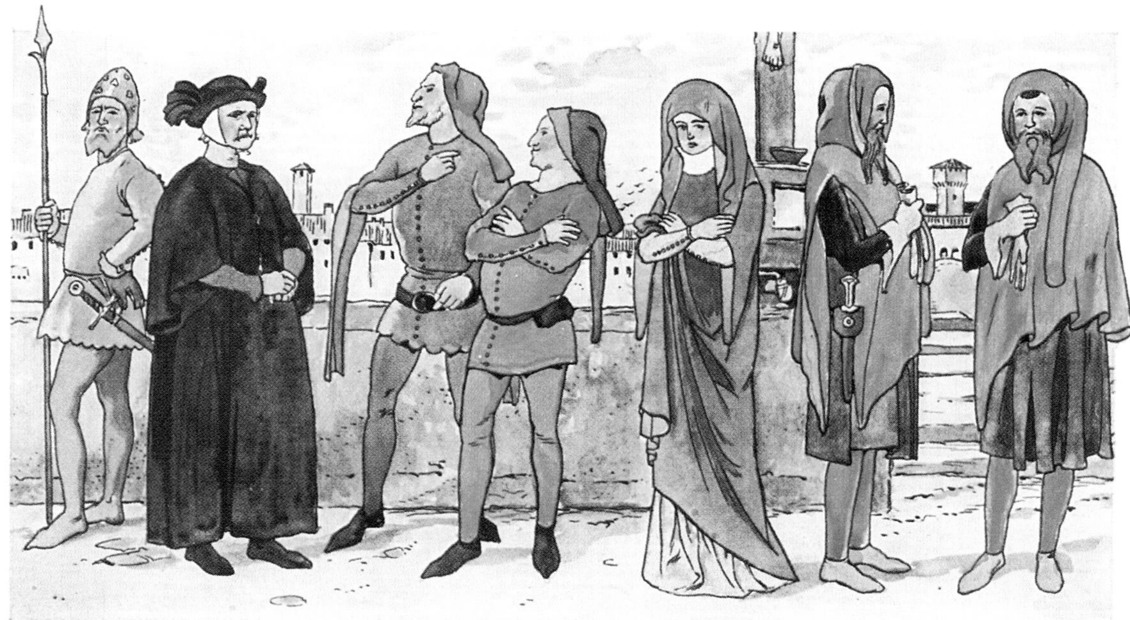

7 8 9 10 11 12 13

1340–1360

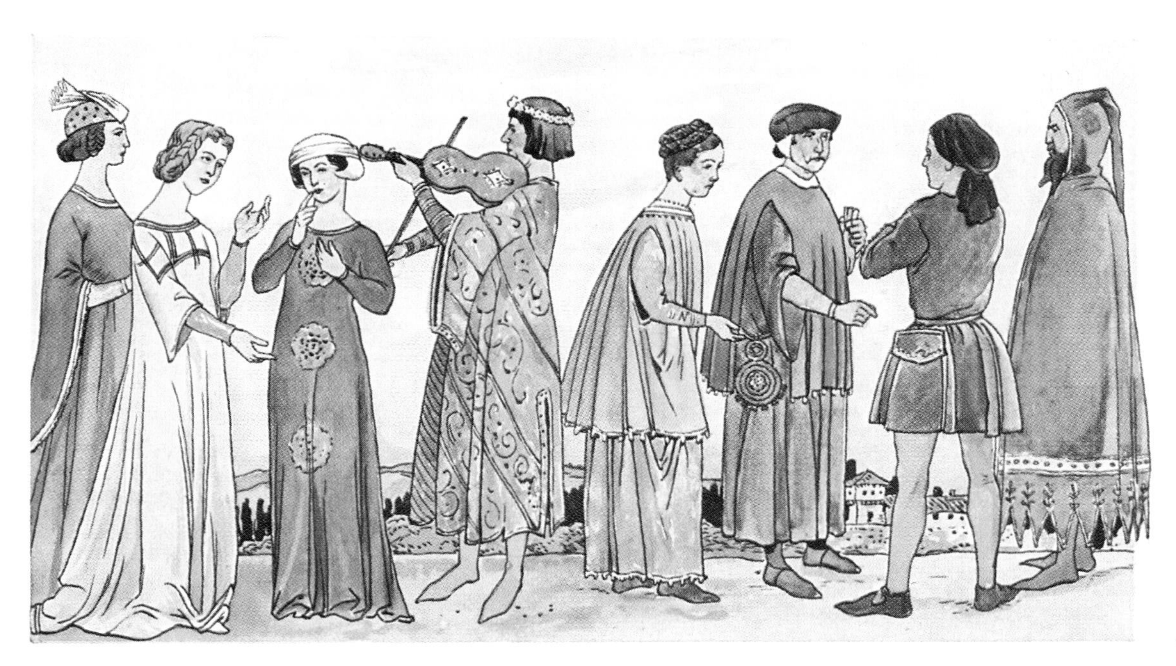

14 15 16 17 18 19 20 21

ITALY

1425–1480

Heralds, King

1 2 3 4 5 6 7 8

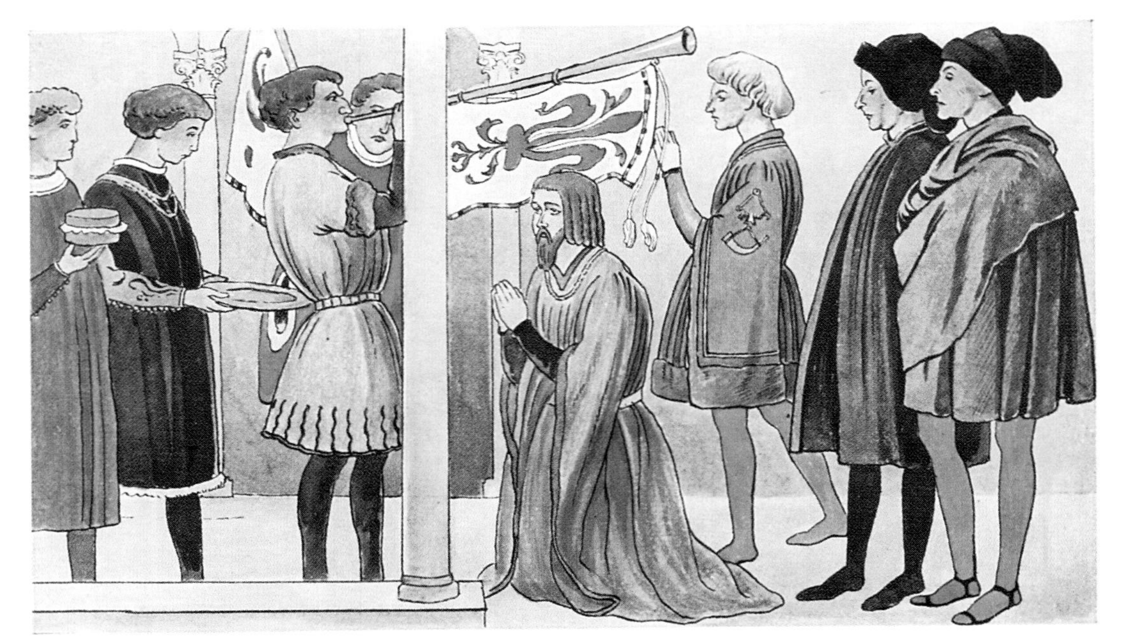

Man with a Falcon, Warriors

9 10 11 12 13 14 15

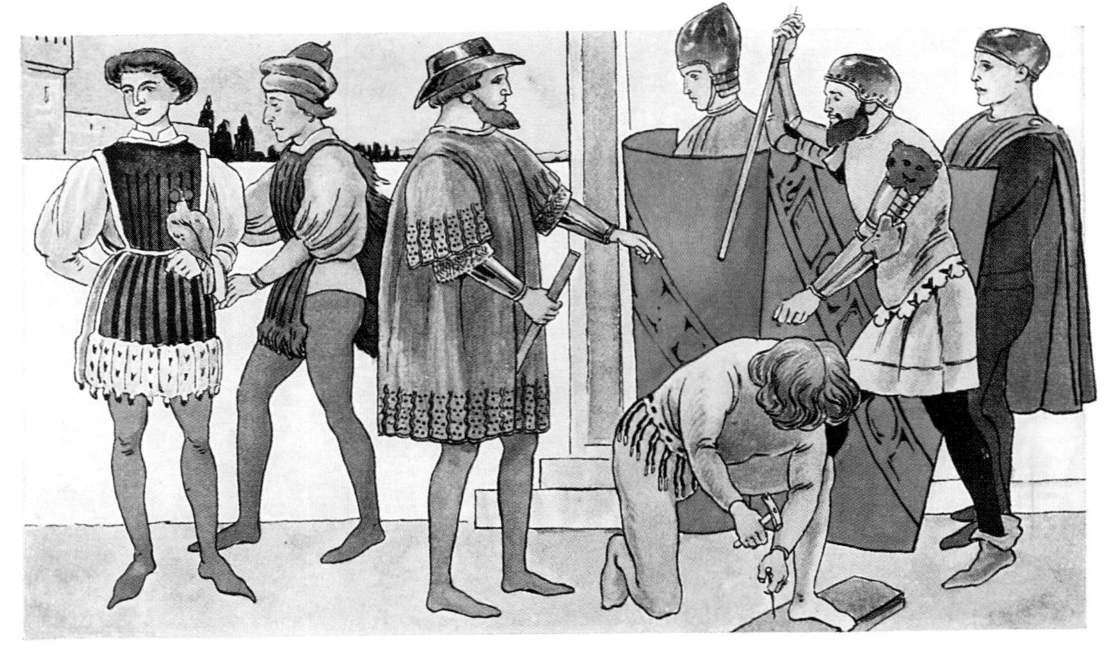

Costume of Men of Rank

16 17 18 19 20 21

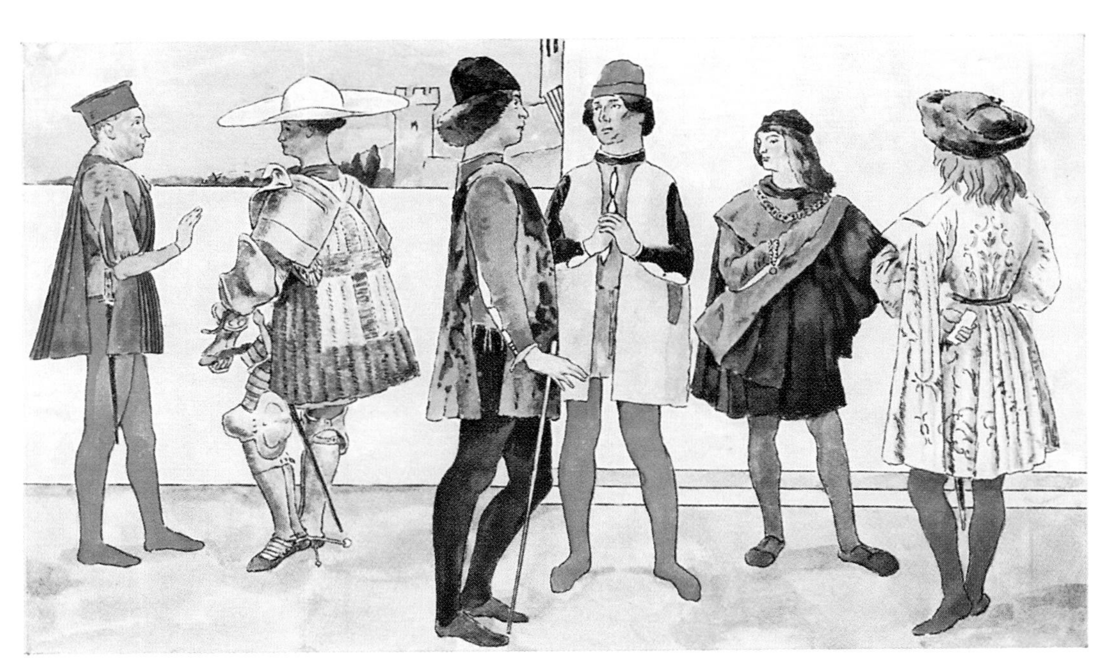

ITALY
15th Century

Northern Italy

1435–1440

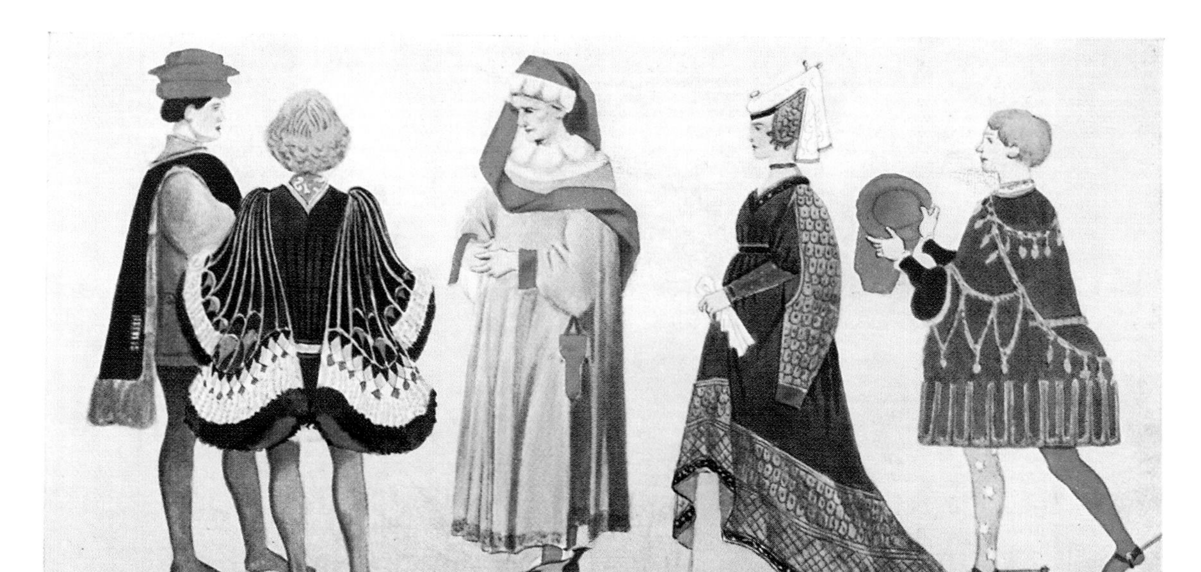

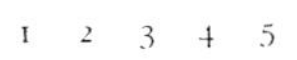

1 2 3 4 5

Northern Italy

1450

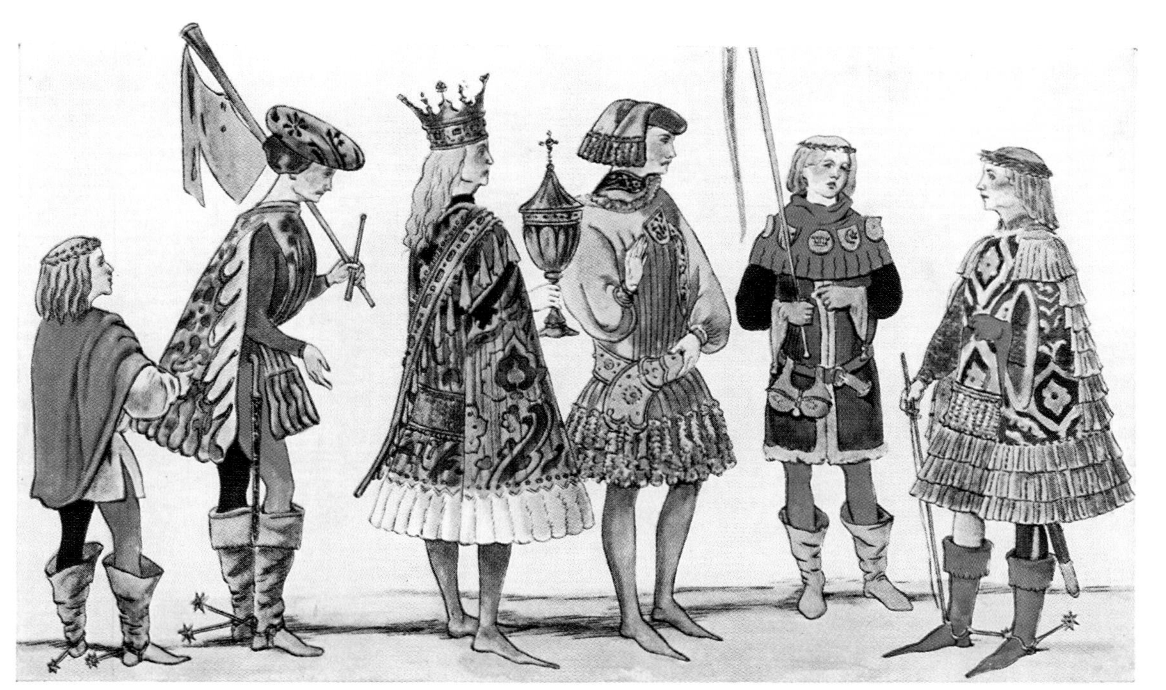

6 7 8 9 10 11

Venice about 1485

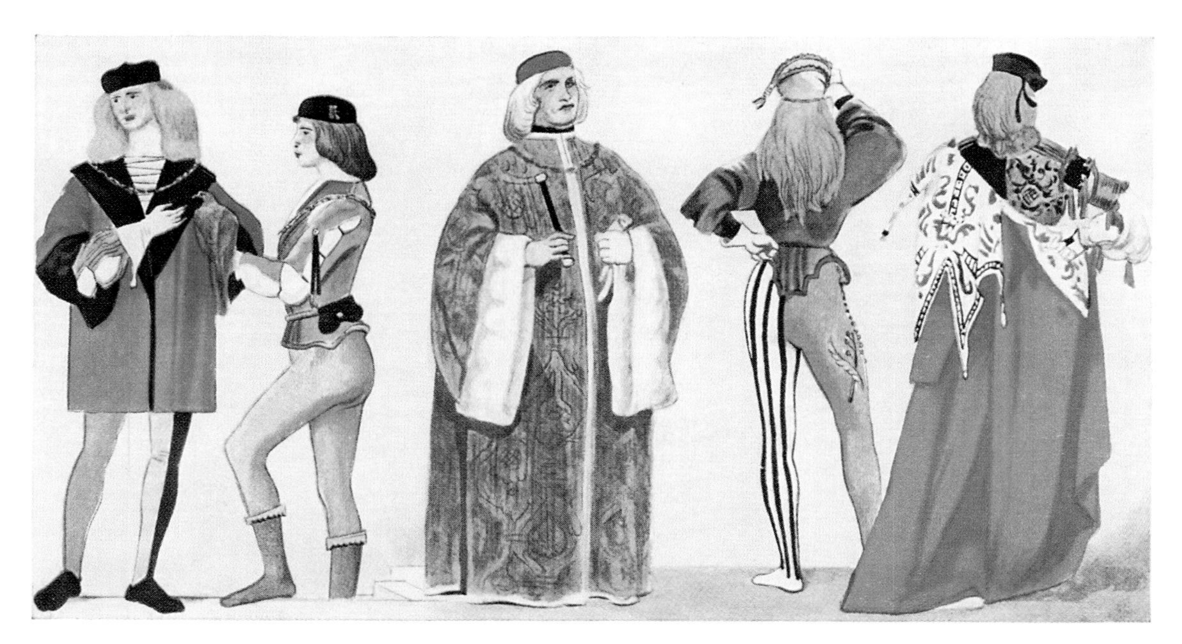

12 13 14 15 16

ITALY
1350–1500

14th Century

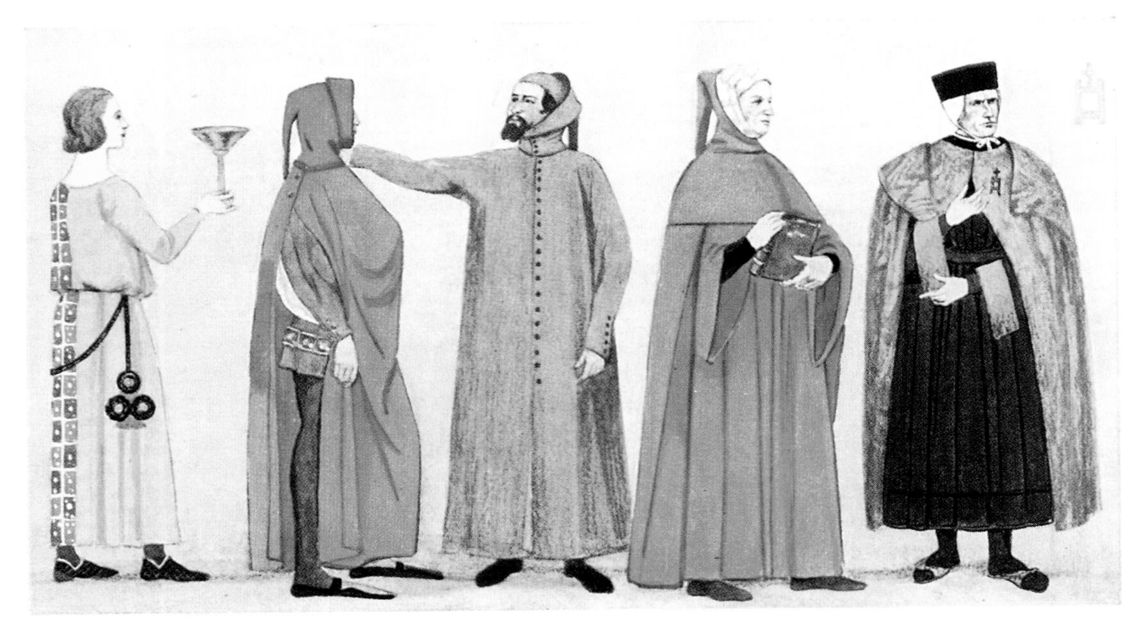

1 2 3 4 5

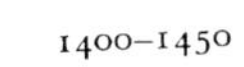

1400–1450

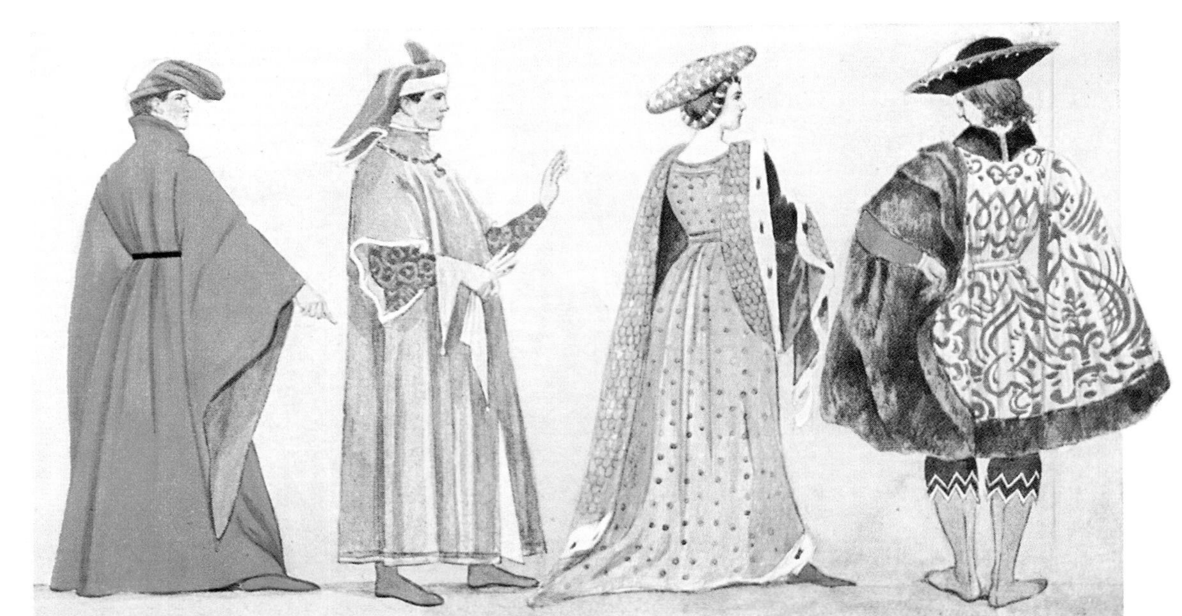

6 7 8 9

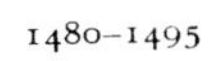

1480–1495

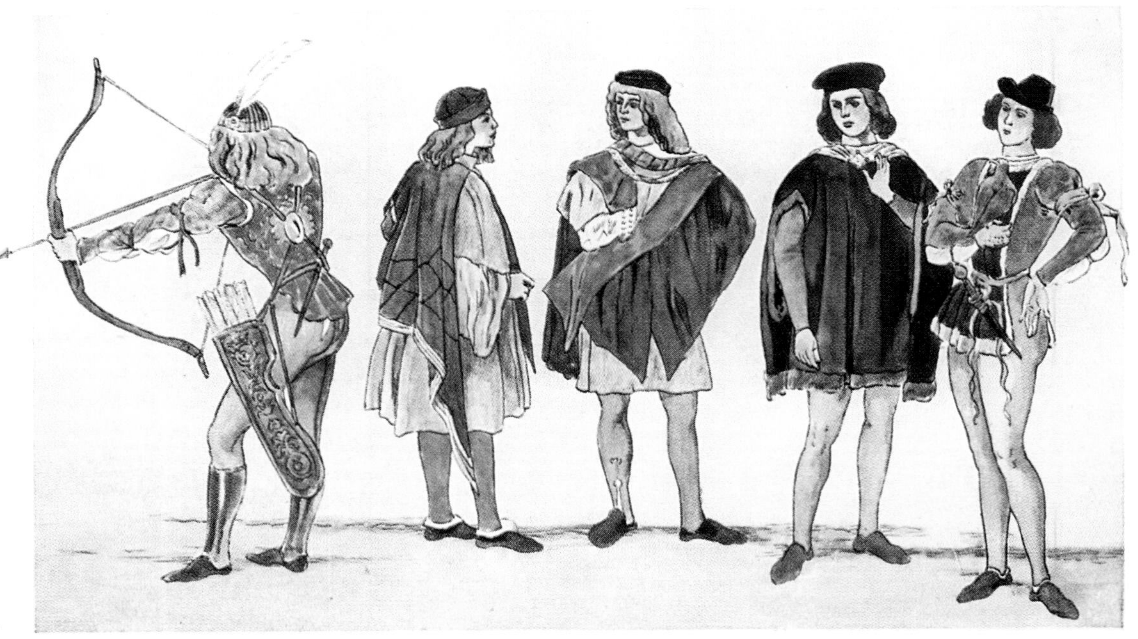

10 11 12 13 14

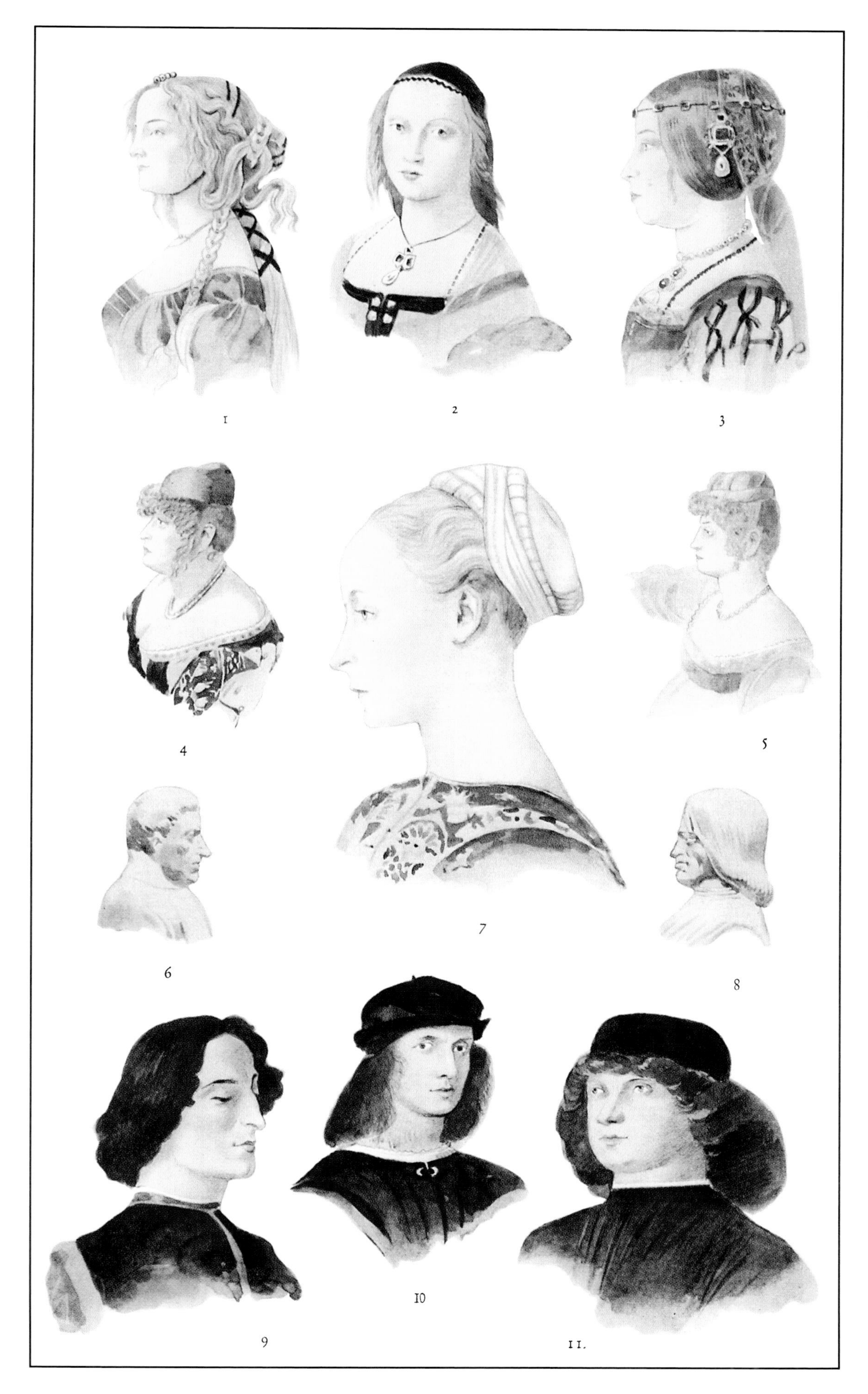

ITALY

Head-dresses

and Hair Styles 1470–1500

GERMANY
End of 15th Century

Craftsmen and Burghers

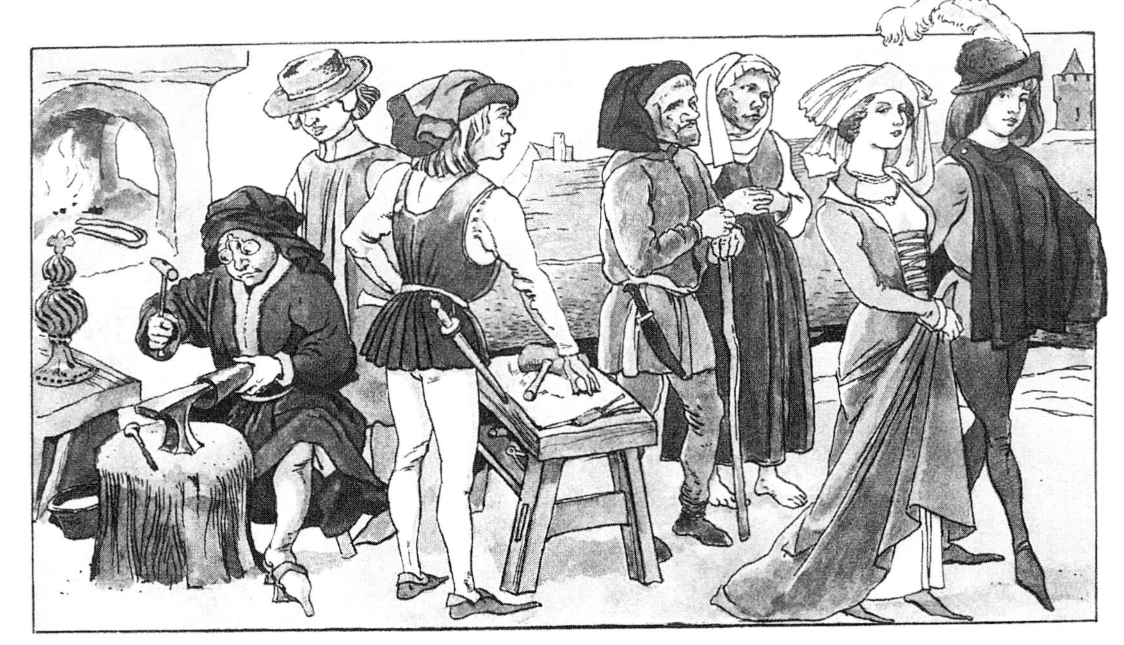

1 2 3 4 5 6 7

Dancing Costume, etc.

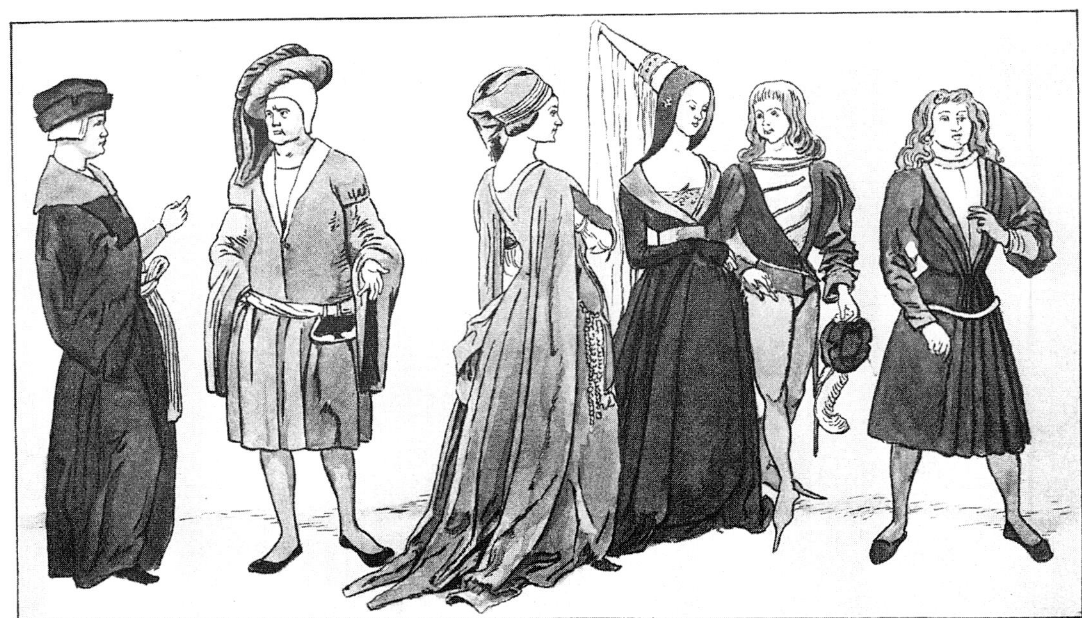

8 9 10 11 12 13

Peasants, Mercenaries, Jew

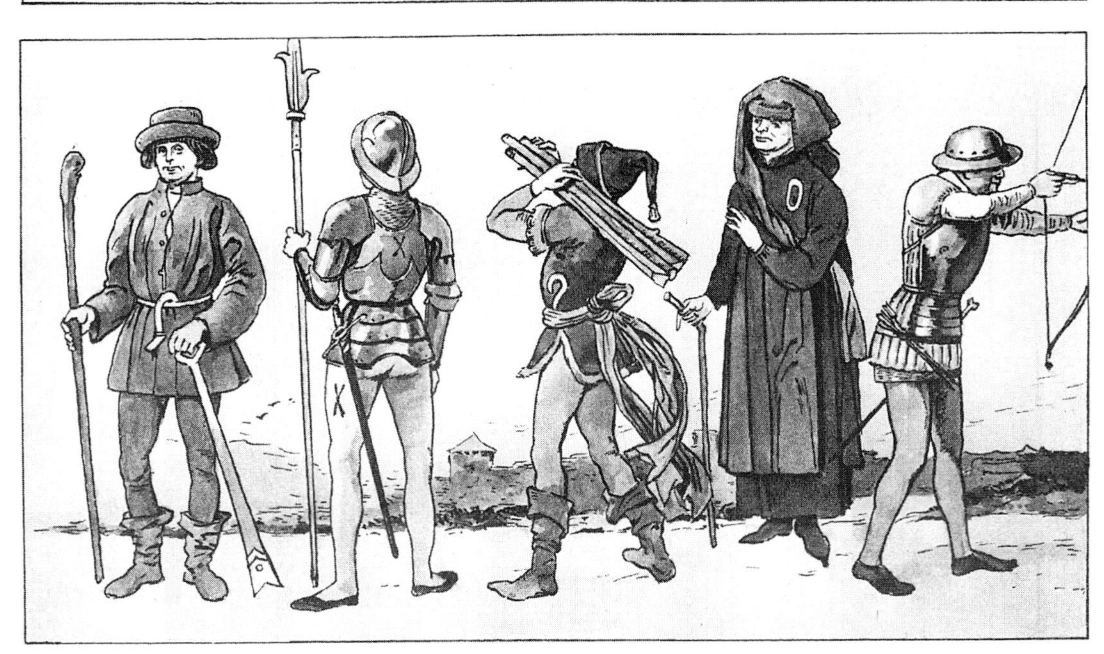

14 15 16 17 18

SPAIN
13th–15th Century

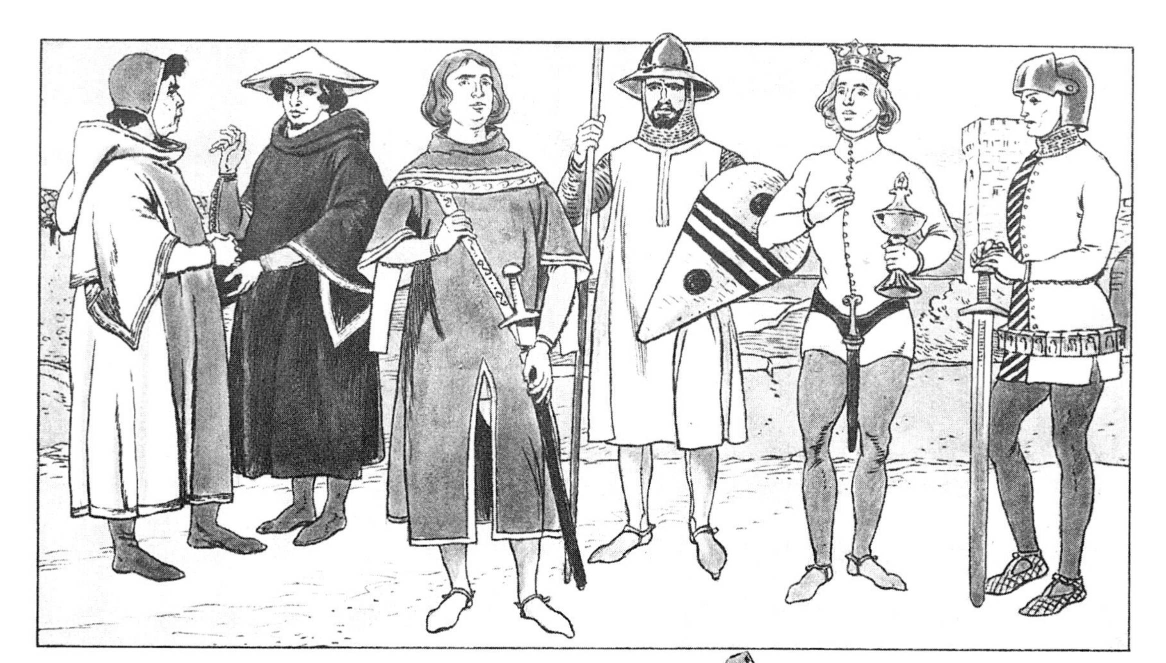

Burghers and Knights

1 2 3 4 5 6

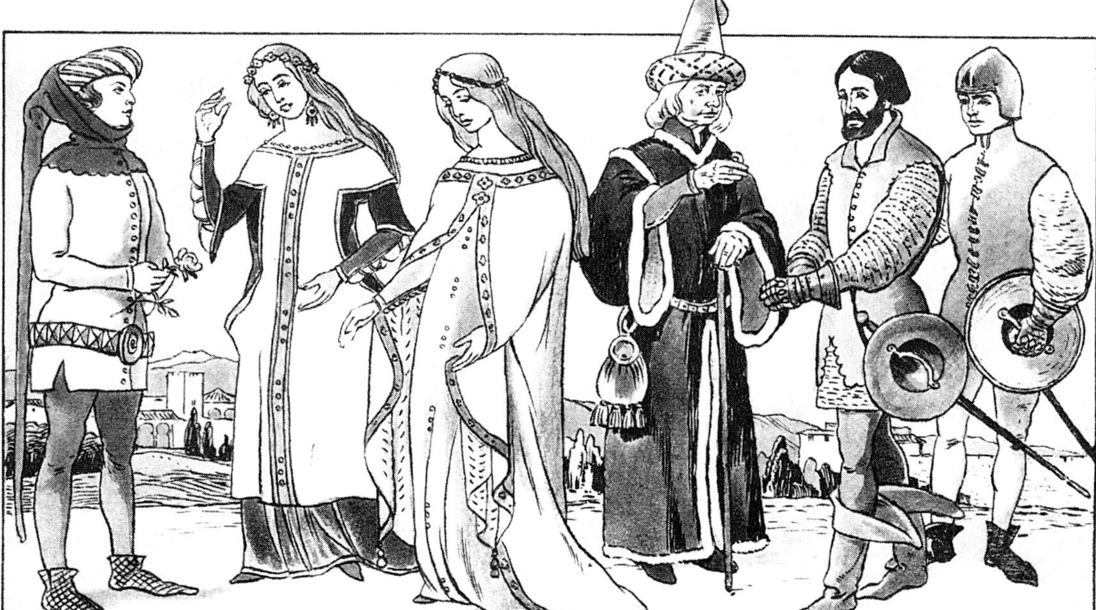

Court Dress

7 8 9 10 11 12

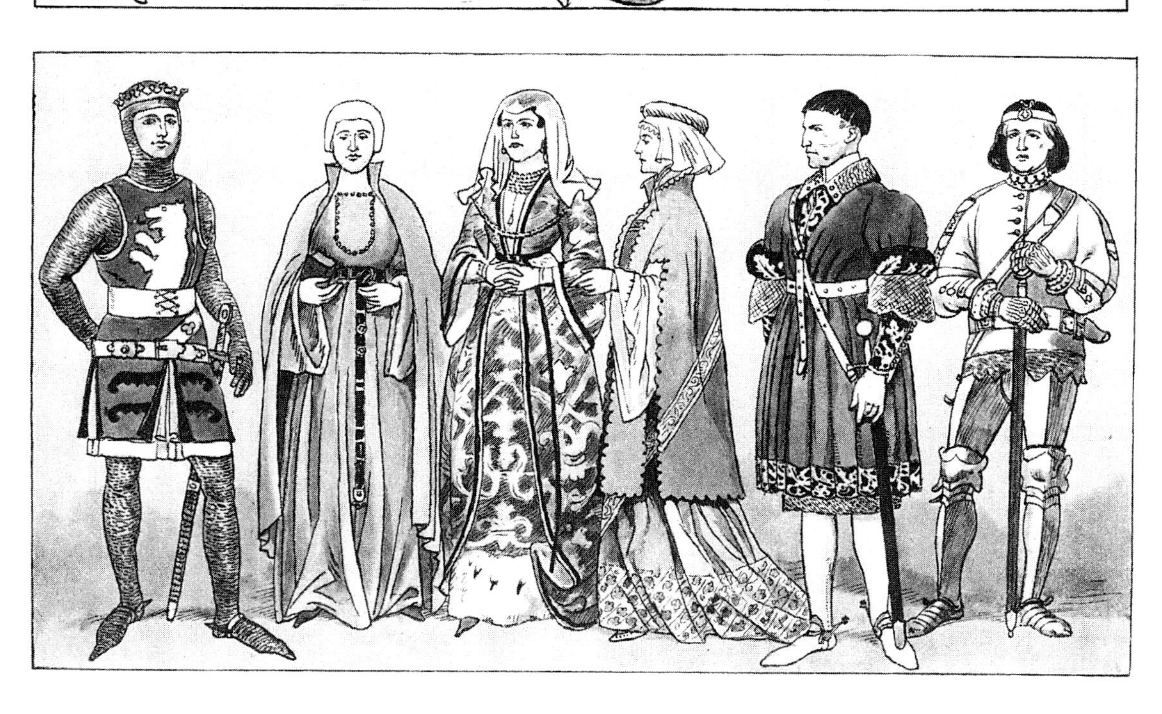

Famous People

13 14 15 16 17 18

GERMANY
1500–1525

Citizens and Peasants

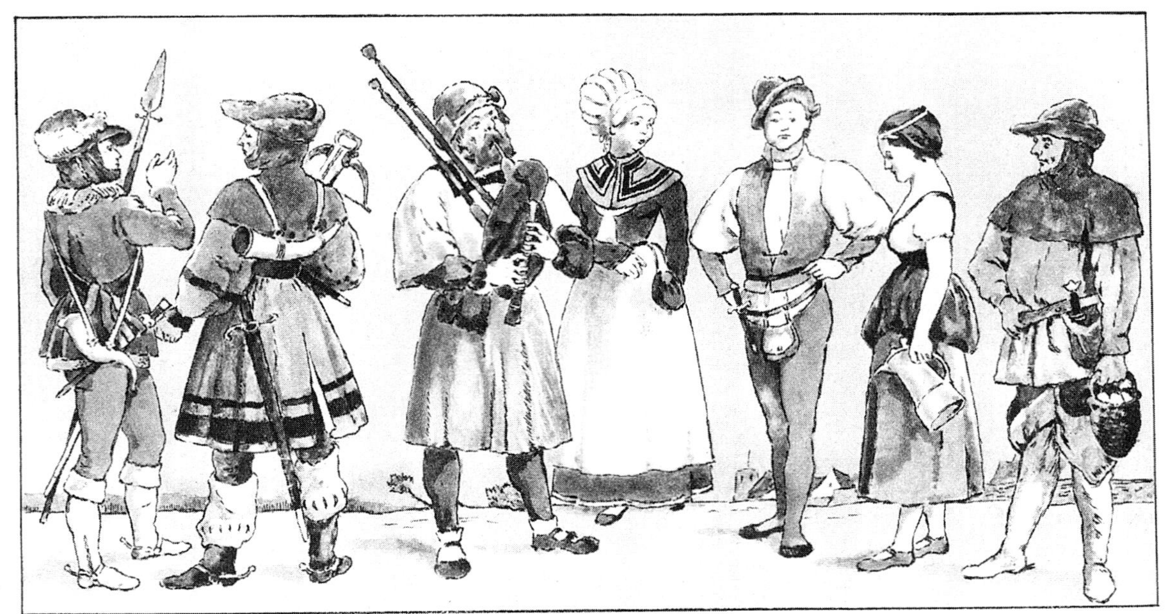

1 2 3 4 5 6 7

Peasants

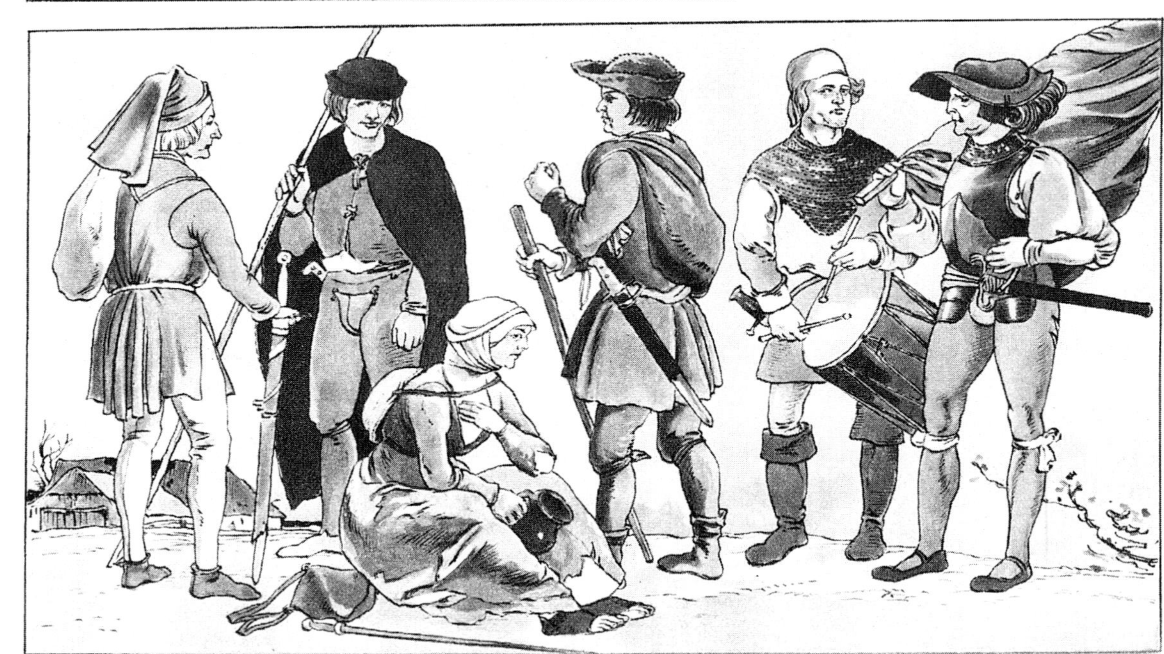

8 9 10 11 12 13

Vagrants

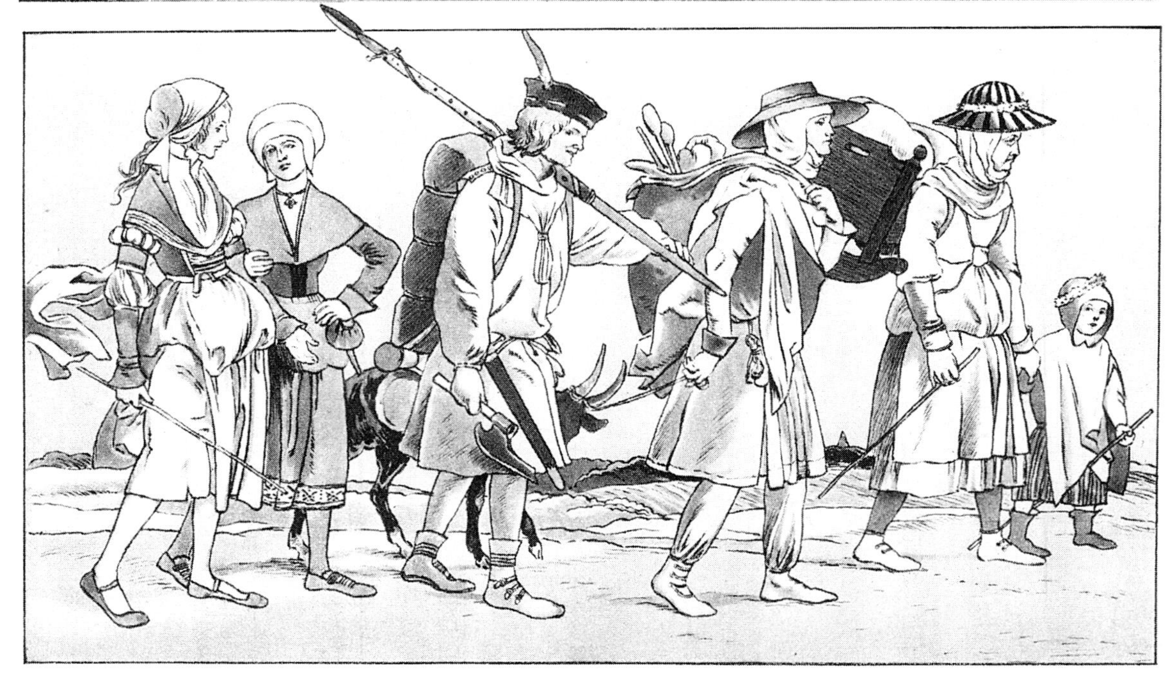

14 15 16 17 18 19

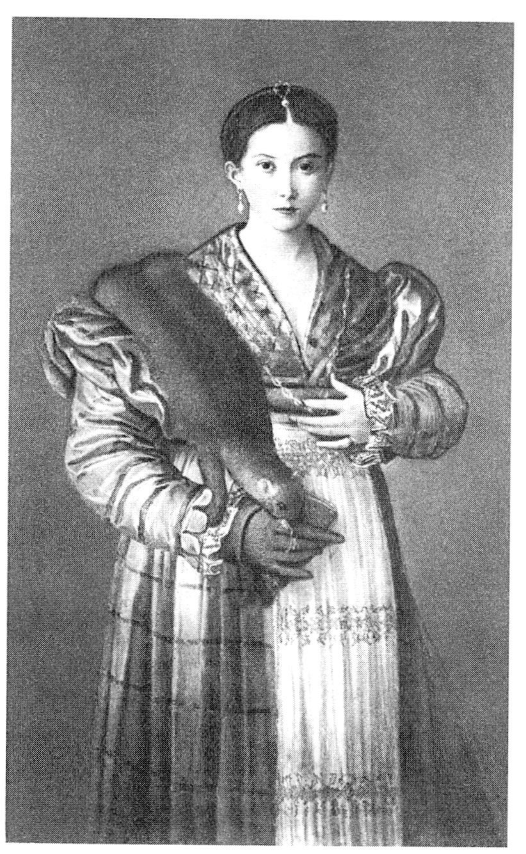

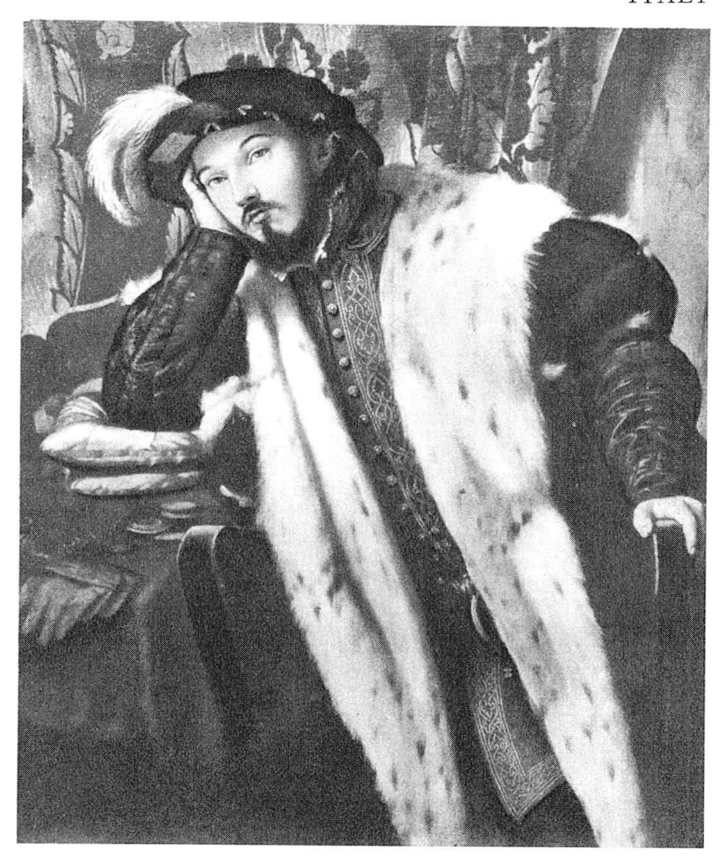

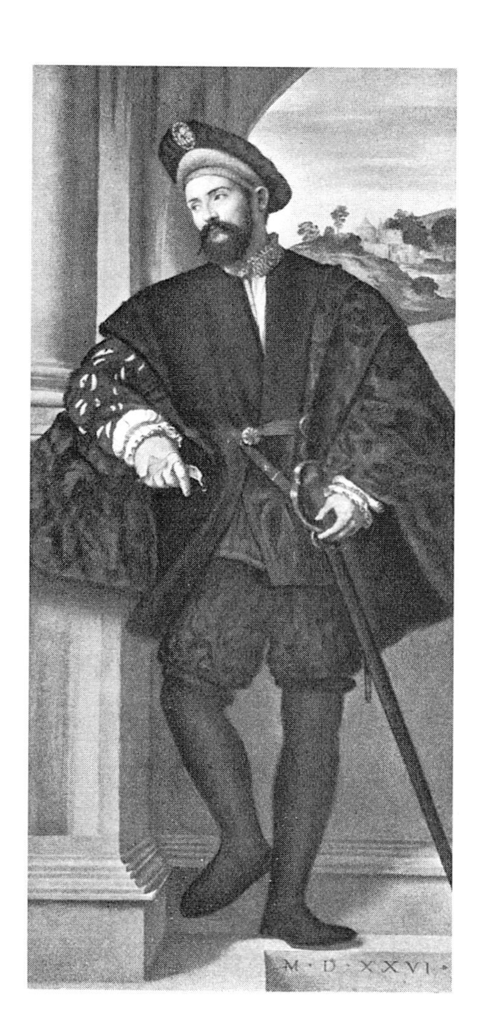

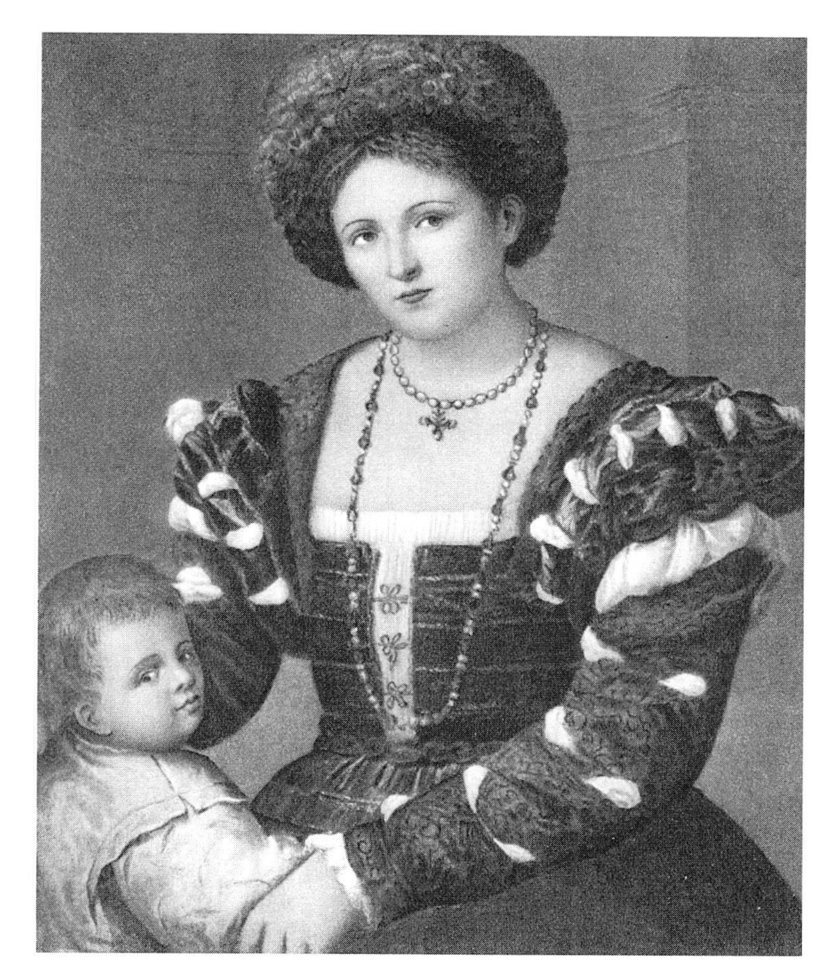

Patricians 1520–1530

GERMANY
Head-dress
1500–1550

Flat Bonnet and Long Hair

Flat Bonnet
and Scholer's Cap

Women's Bonnets
and Net-hood

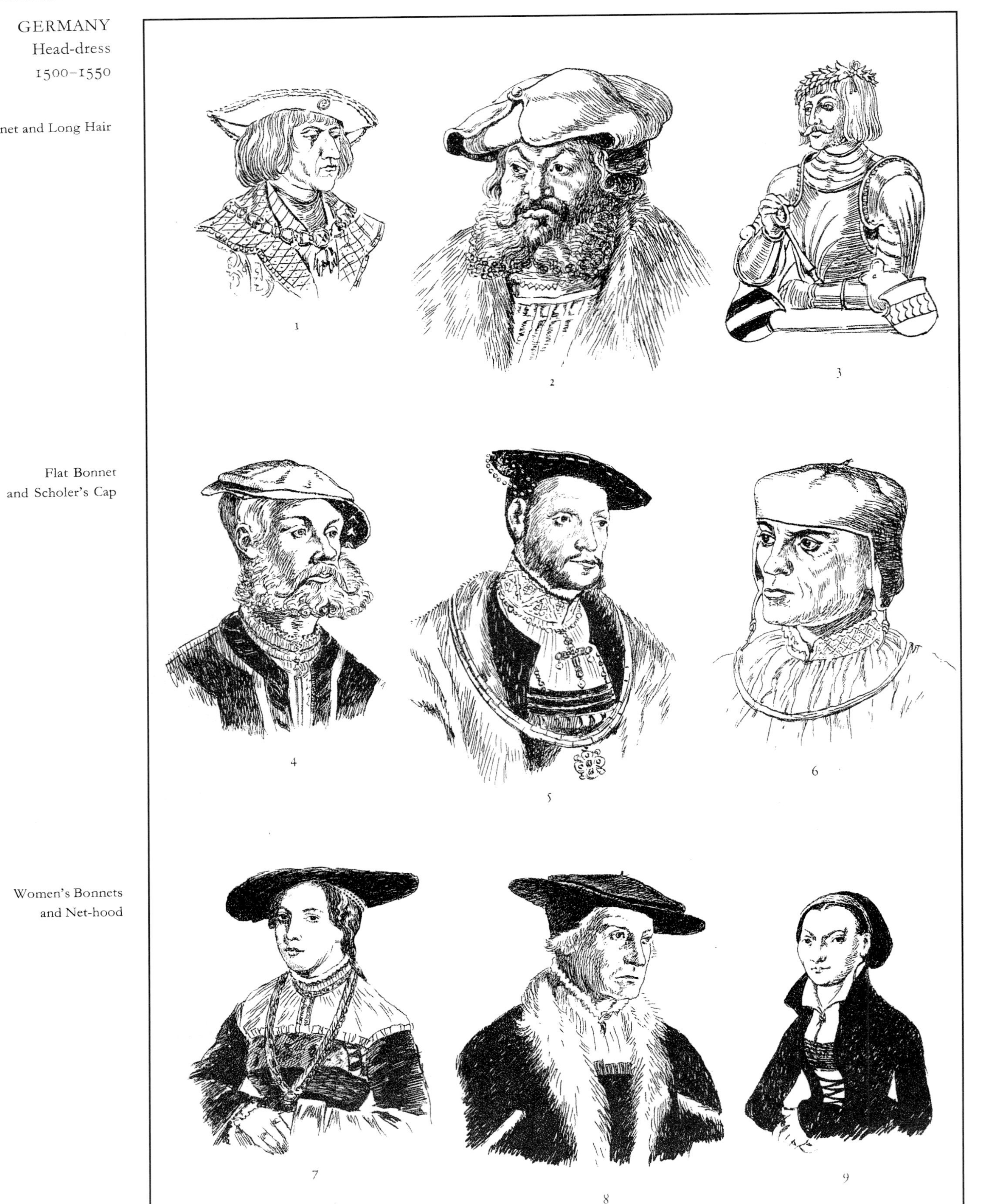

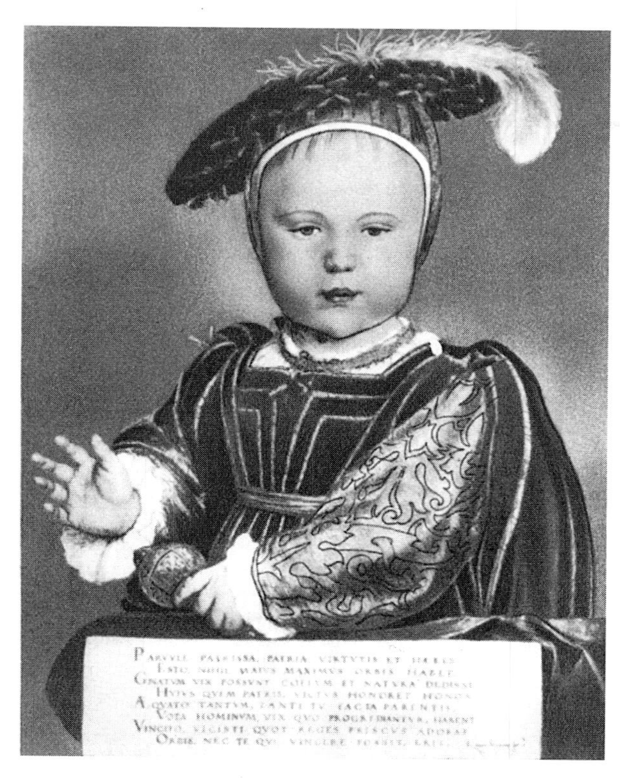

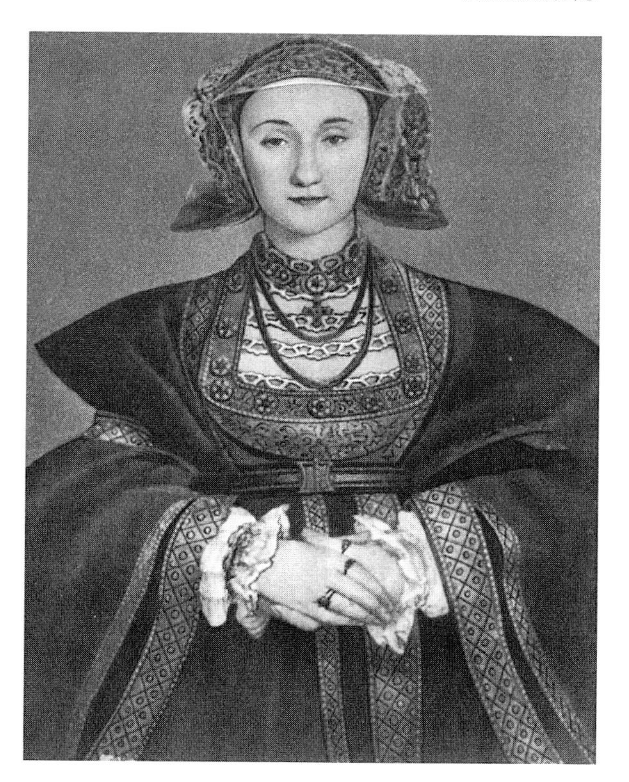

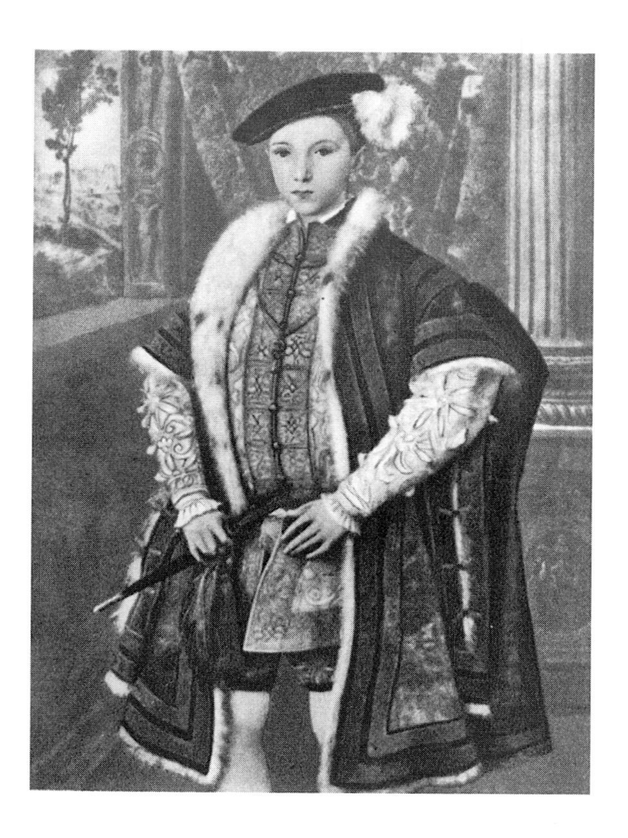

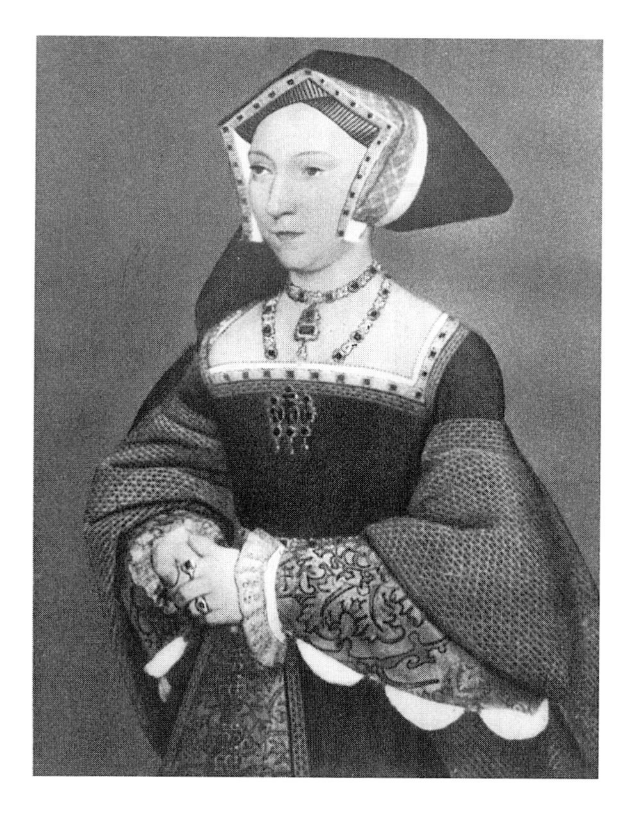

Time of Henry VIII.

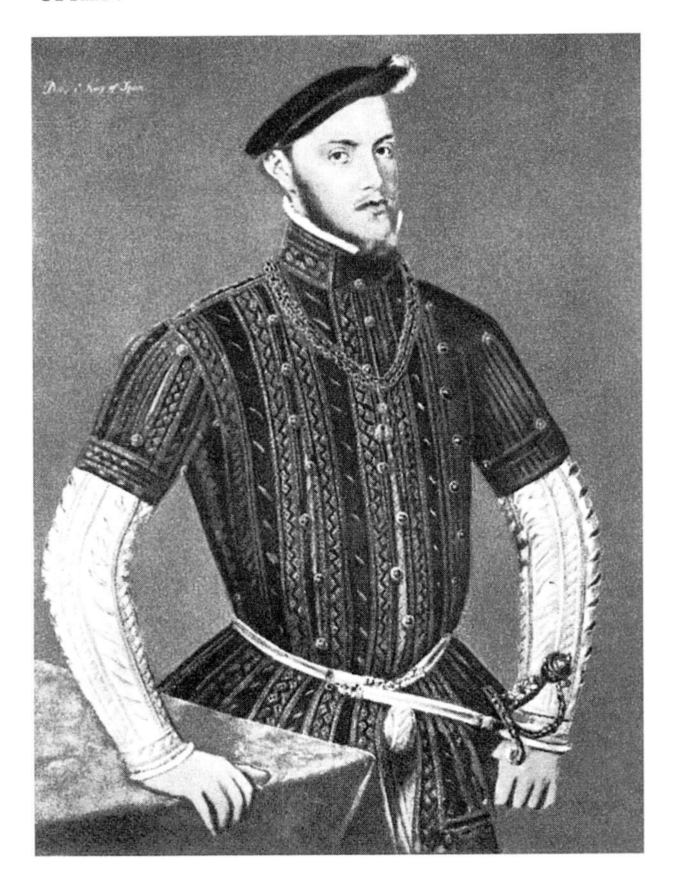

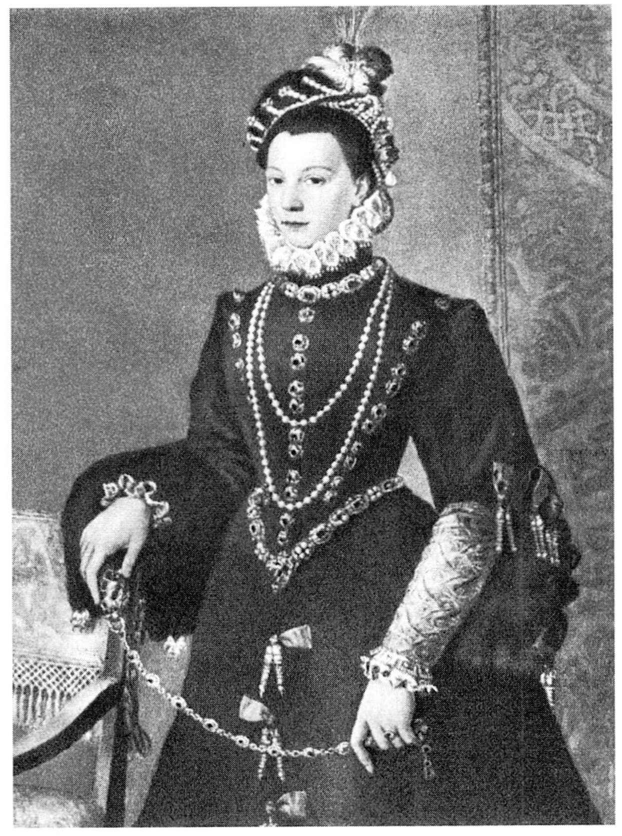

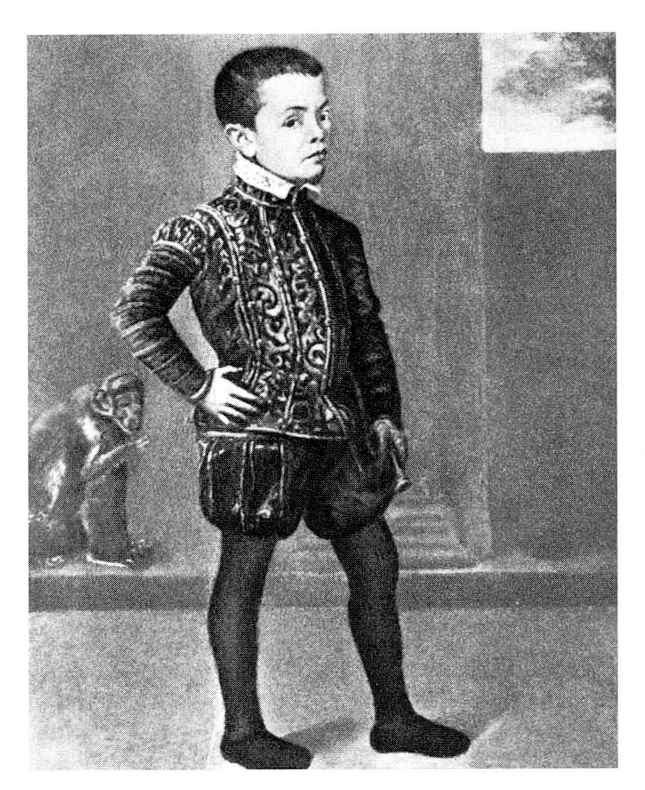

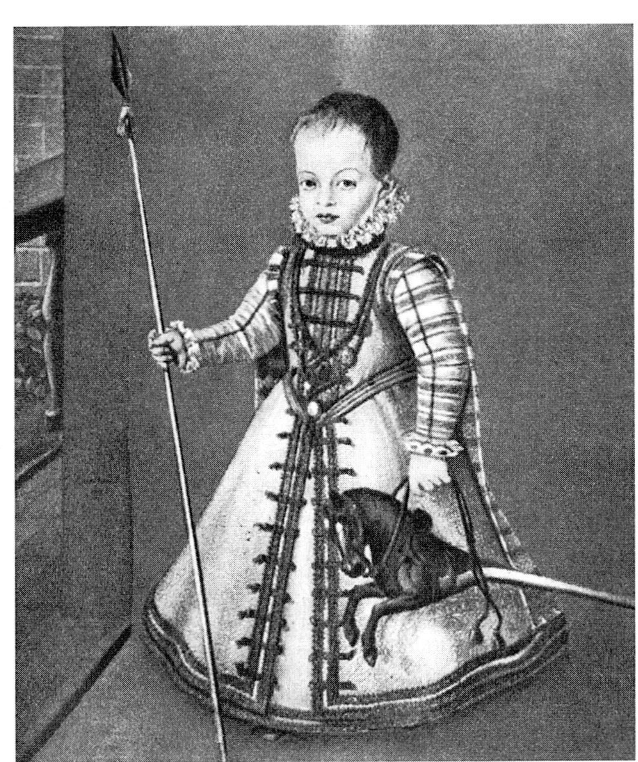

Time of Philip II. 1556–1598

GERMANY
1510–1550

German Citizens of all Ranks

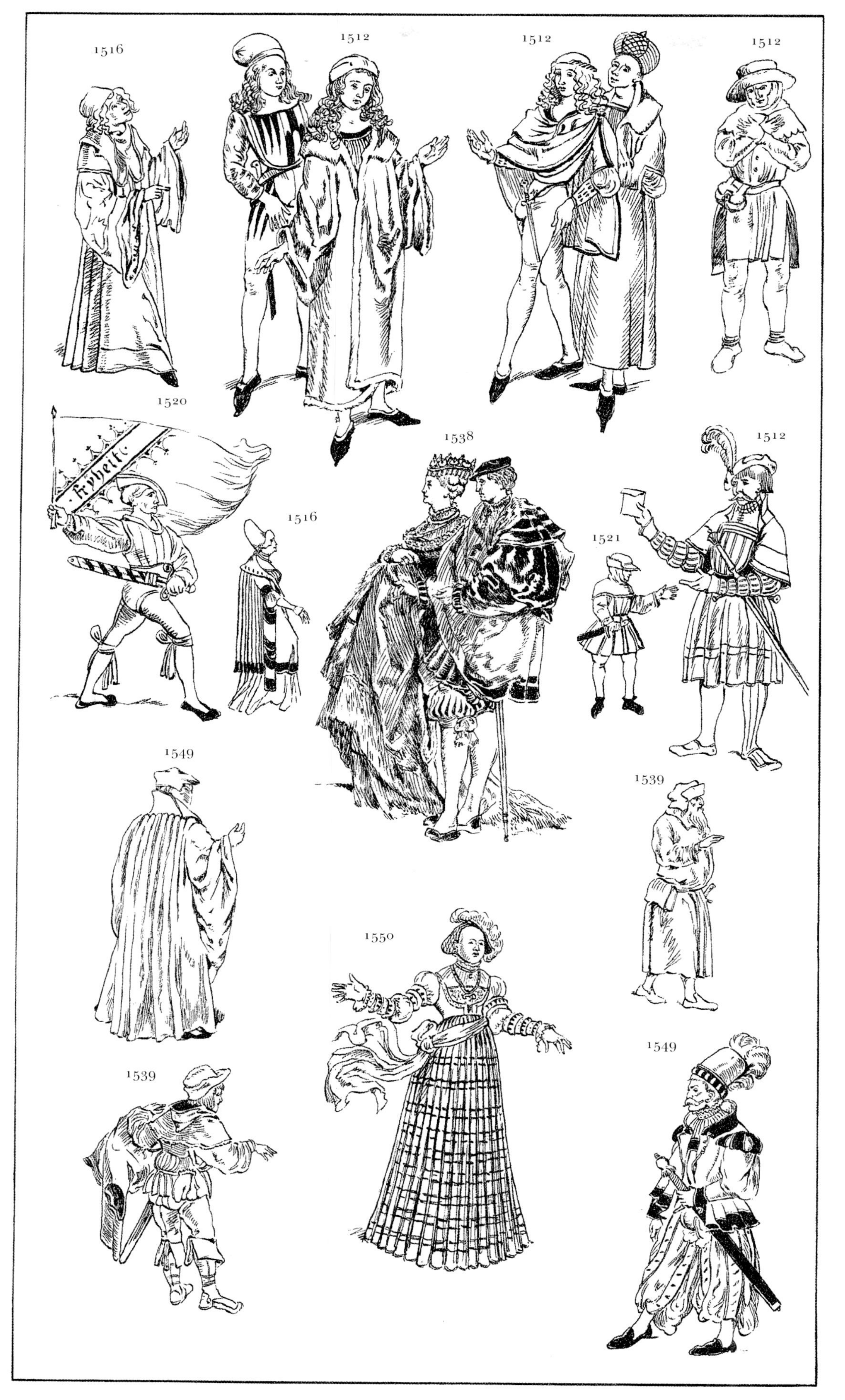

ITALY
Head-dress
and Hair Styles
1500–1550

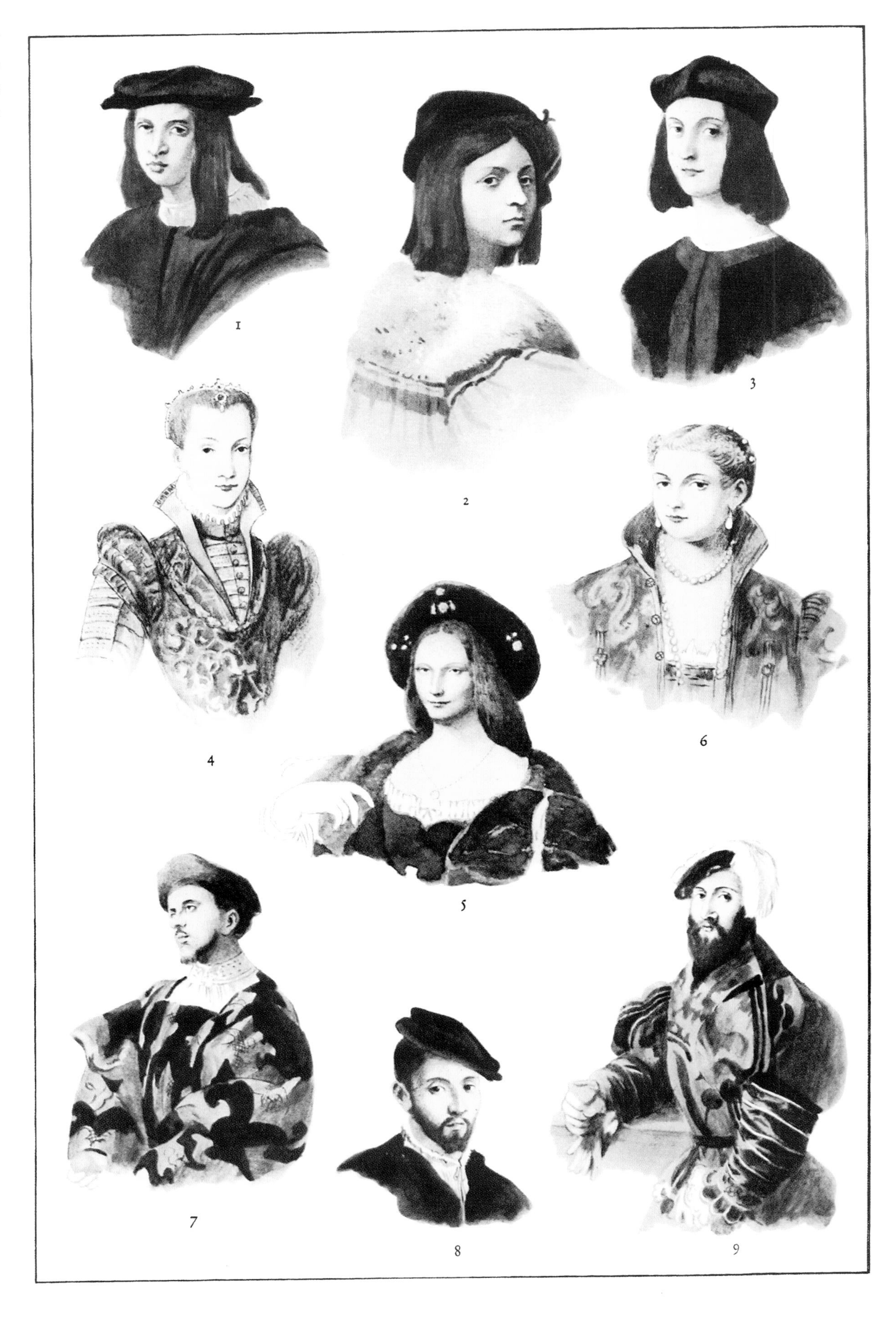

ITALY

Early Renaissance
1460–1500

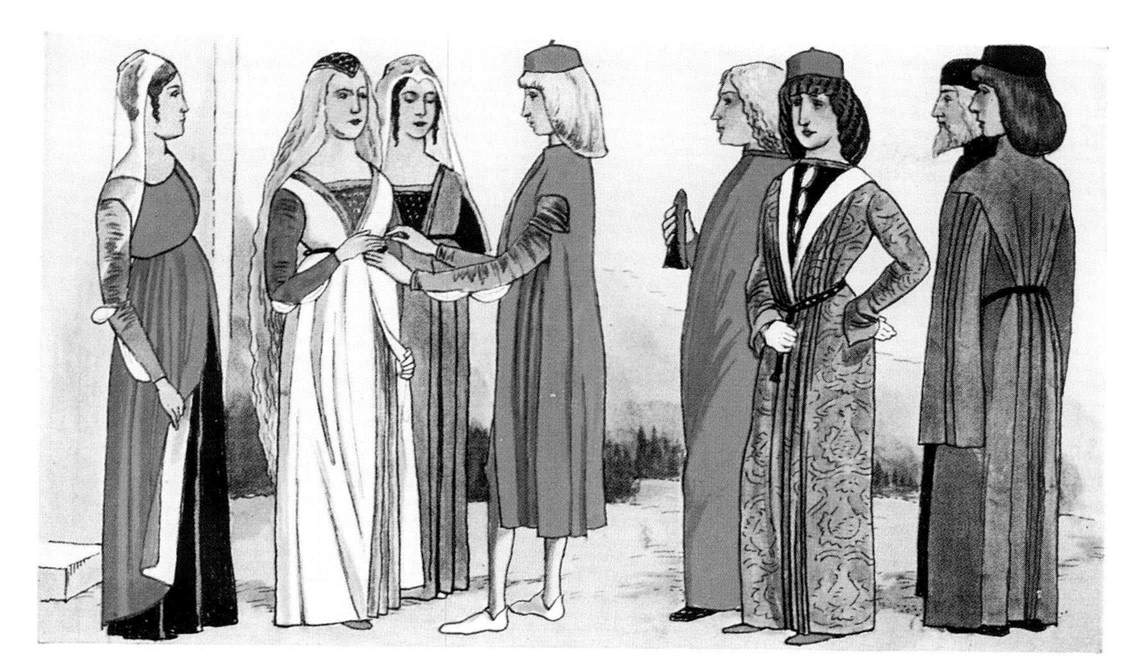

Ferrarra 1460–1470

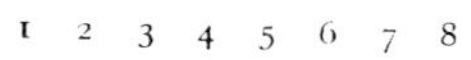

1 2 3 4 5 6 7 8

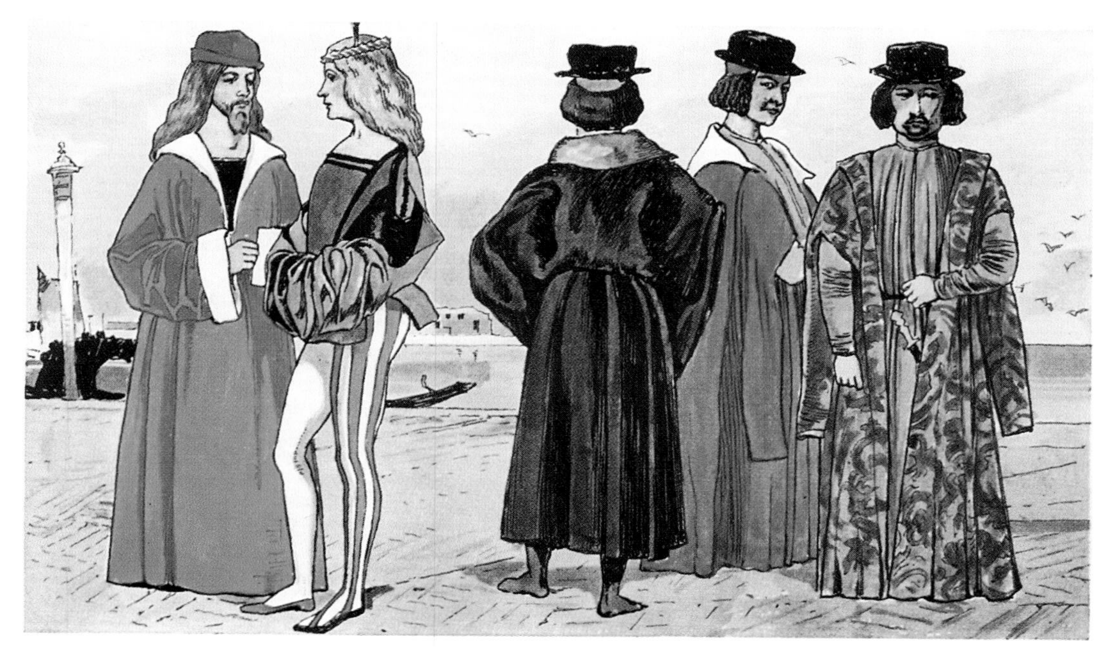

Venice 1495

9 10 11 12 13

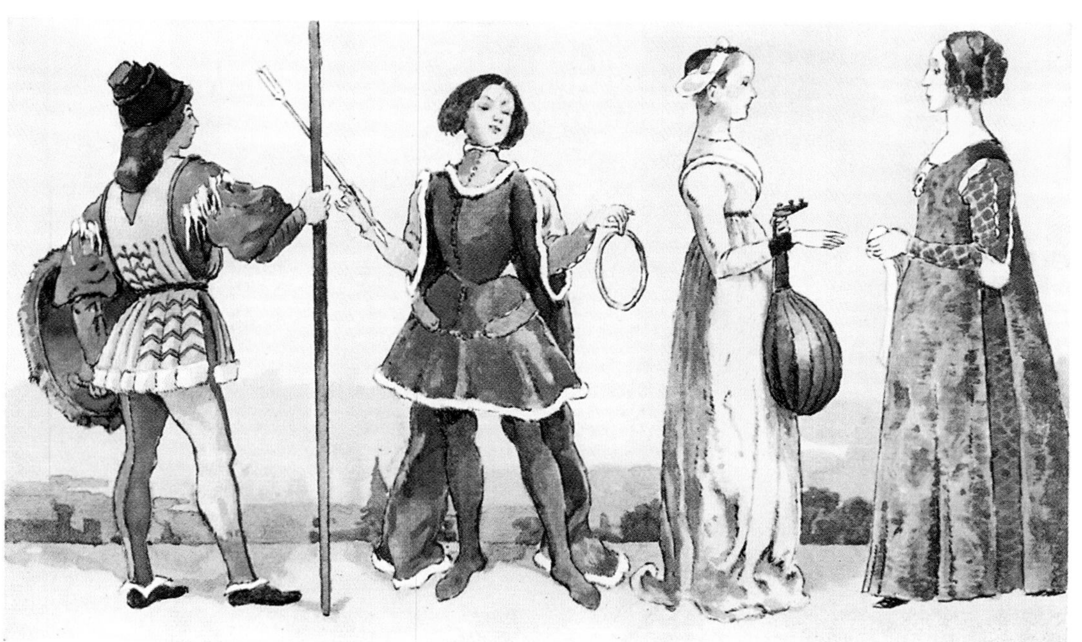

Ferrarra 1470
Florence 1490

14 15 16 17

ITALY
about 1500

Venice
Doge and his Retinue

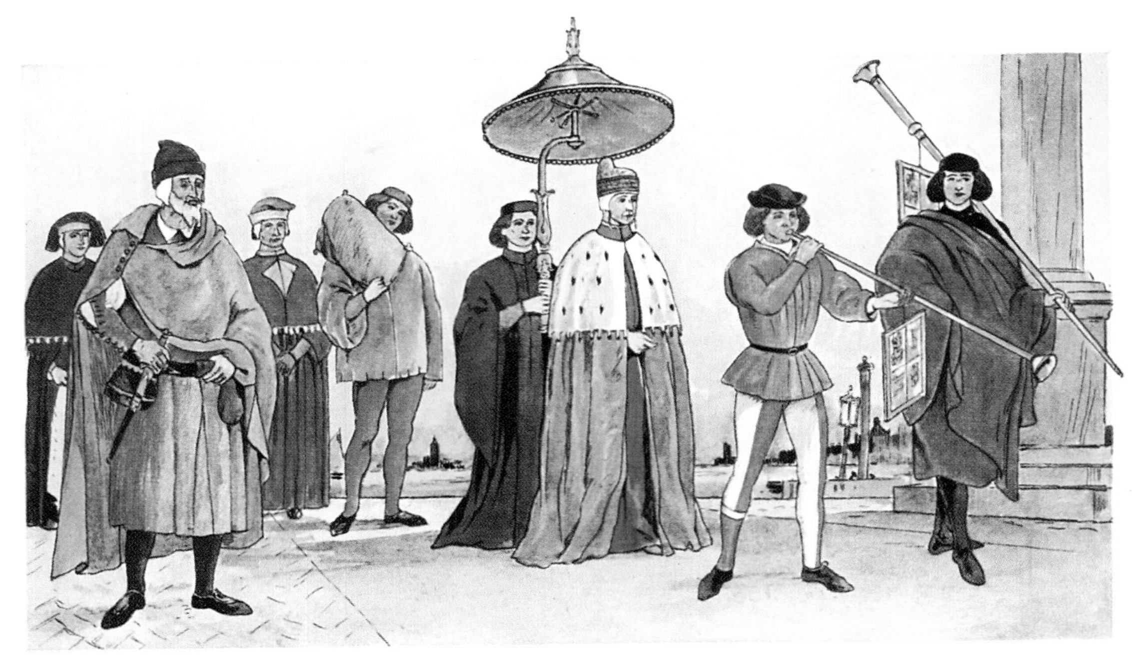

1 2 3 4 5 6 7 8

Northern Italy
1505–1508

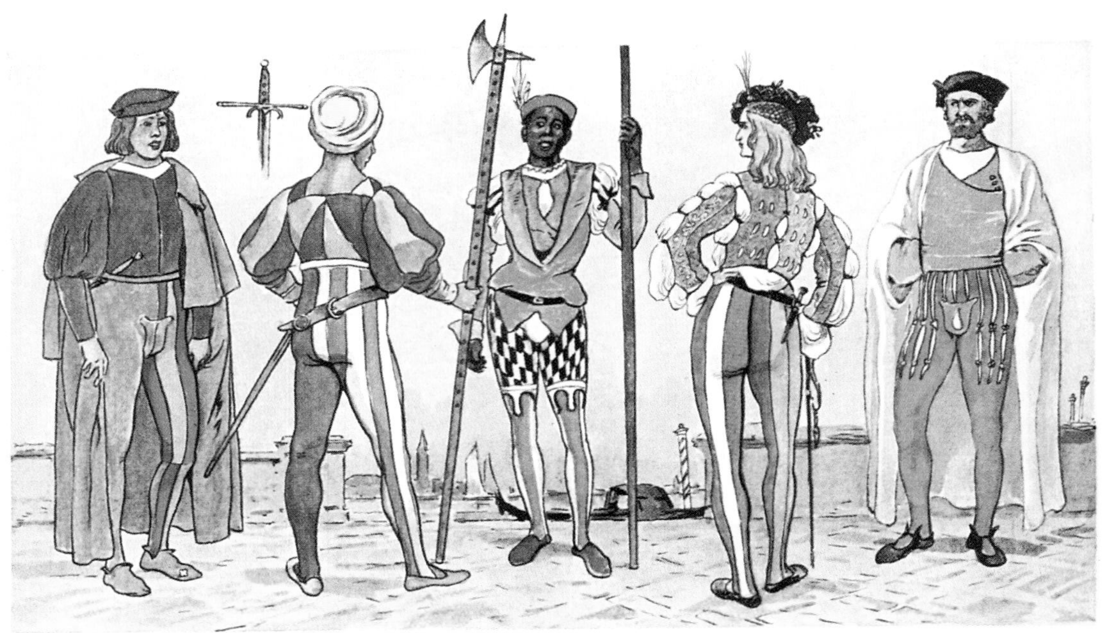

9 10 11 12 13

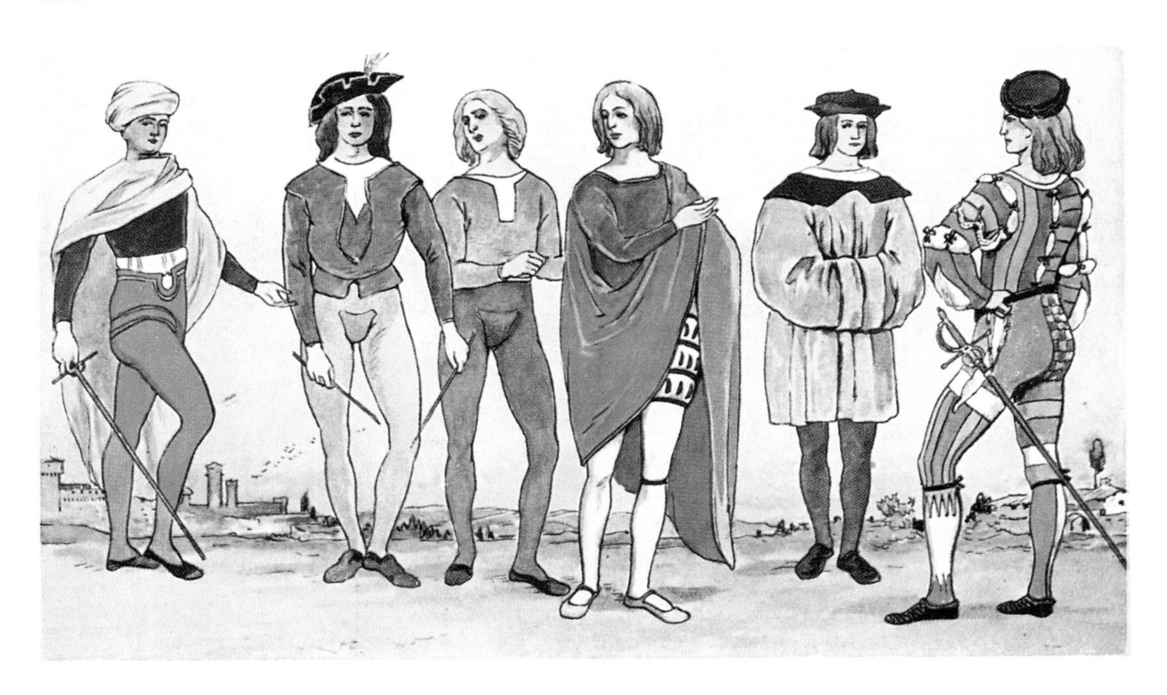

14 15 16 17 18 19

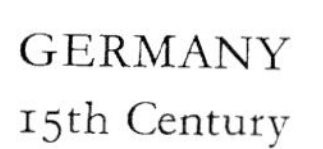

GERMANY
15th Century

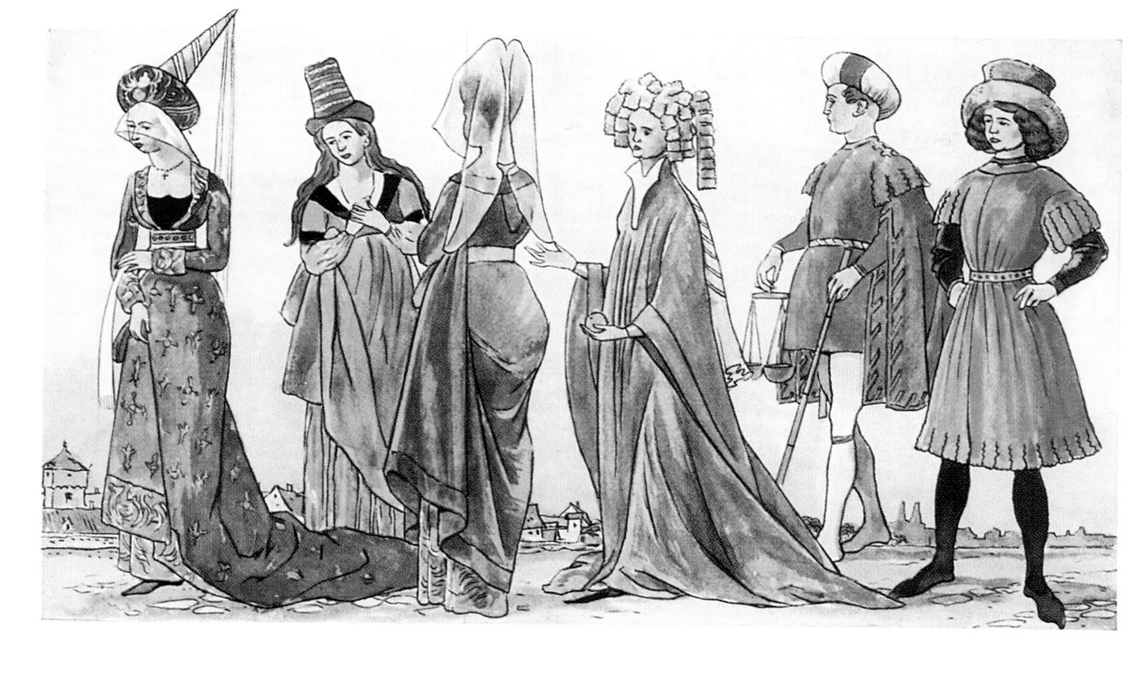

1410–1460

1 2 3 4 5 6

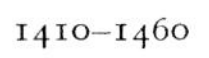

1410–1460

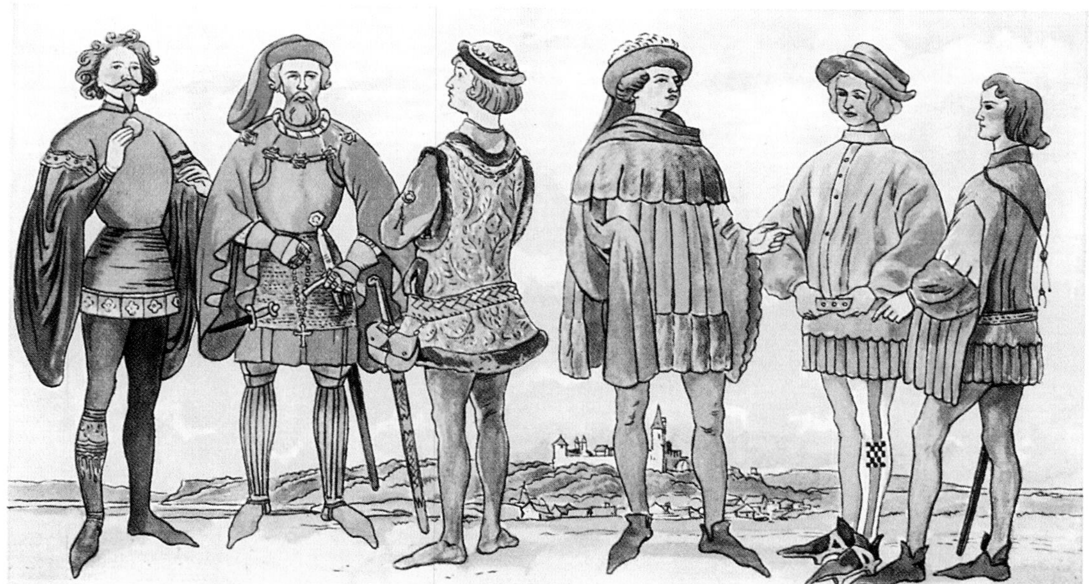

7 8 9 10 11 12

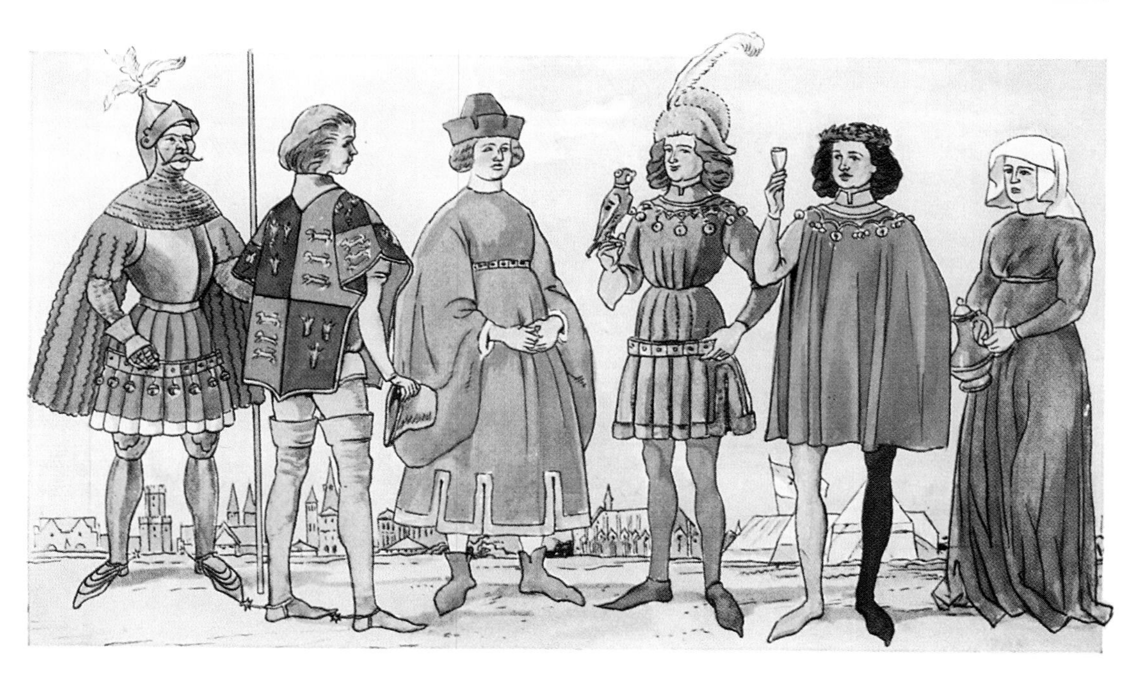

1450-1470

13 14 15 16 17 18

GERMANY
16th Century
Mercenaries

1500–1520

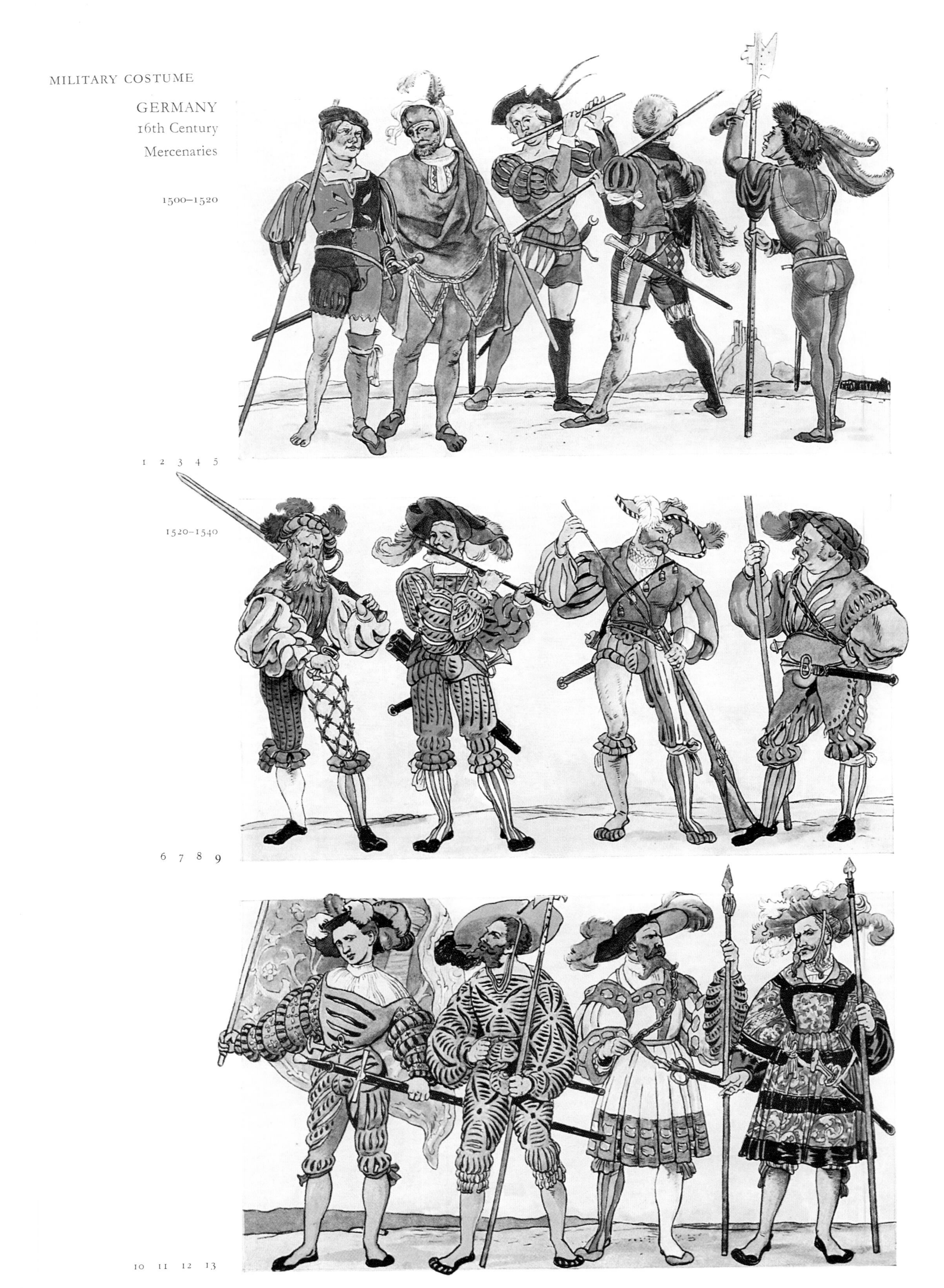

1 2 3 4 5

1520–1540

6 7 8 9

10 11 12 13

GERMANY
16th Century
Mercenaries

1540–1550

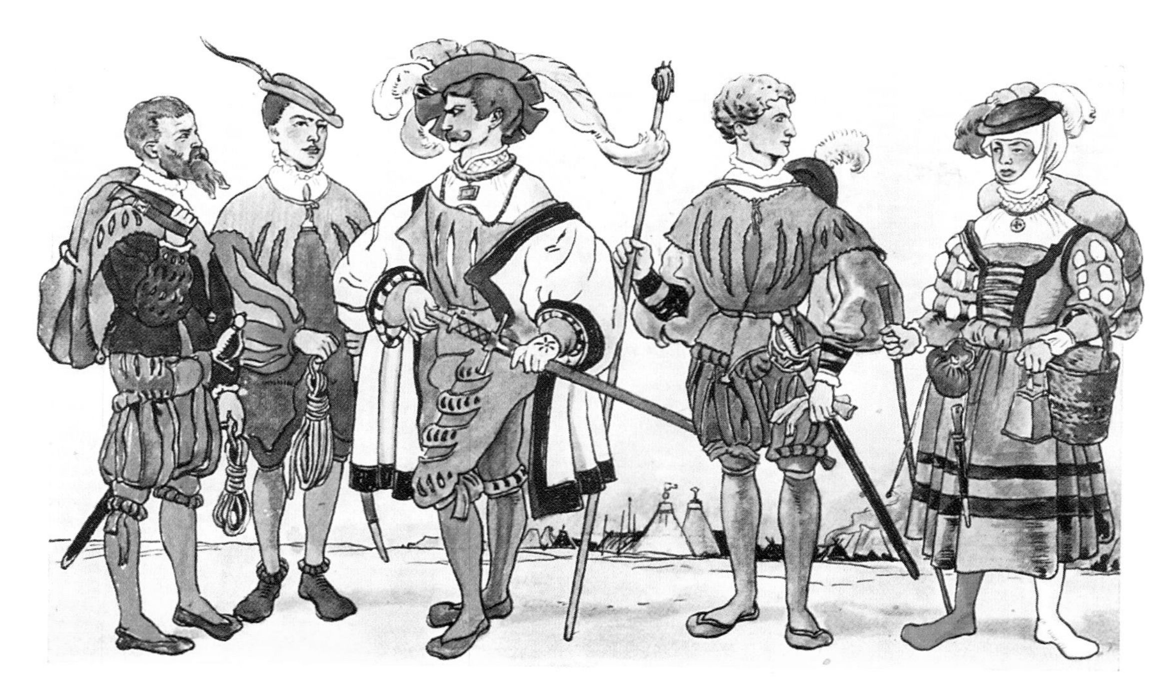

1 2 3 4 5

1550

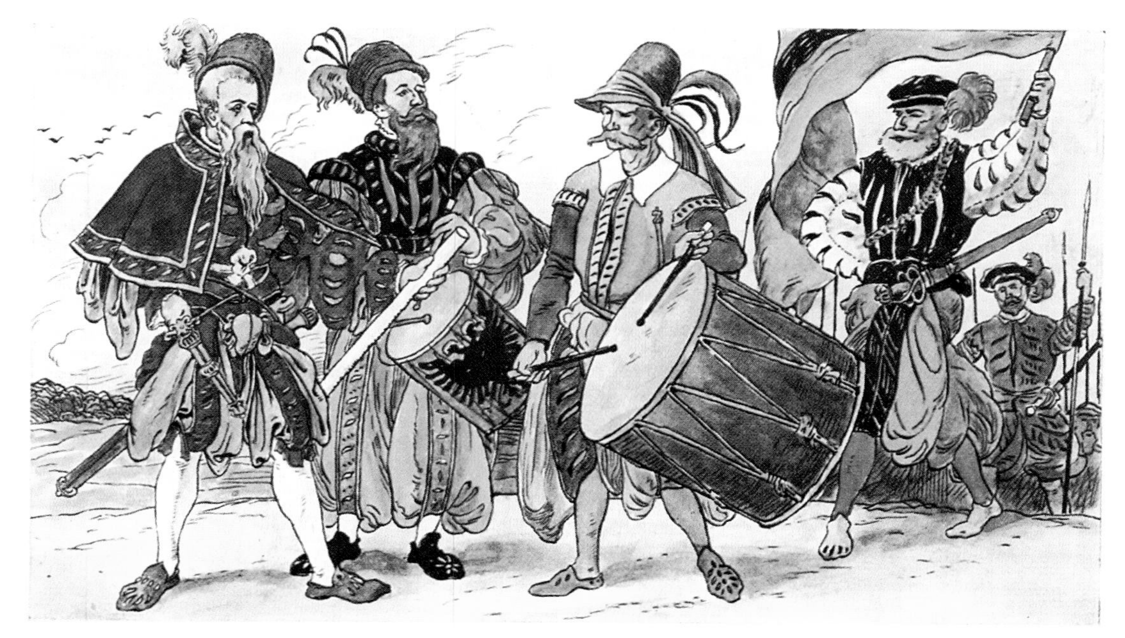

6 7 8 9 10

1560

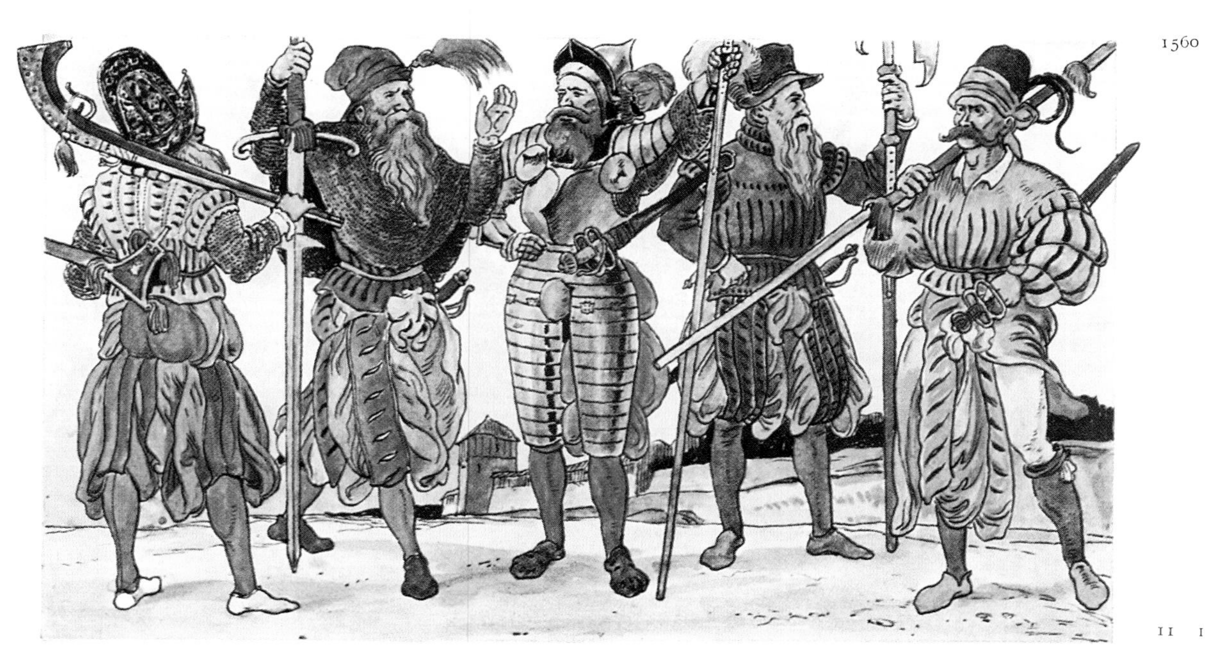

11 12 13 14 15

GERMANY
1500–1530

Nuremberg Middle Class Women

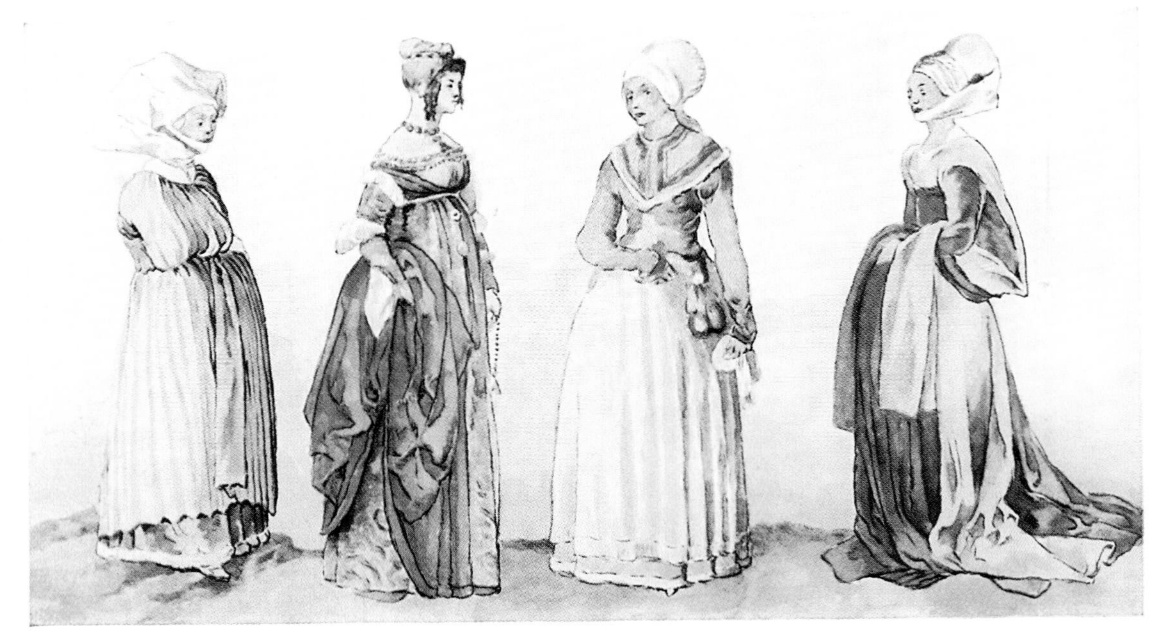

1 2 3 4

Basle Middle Class Women

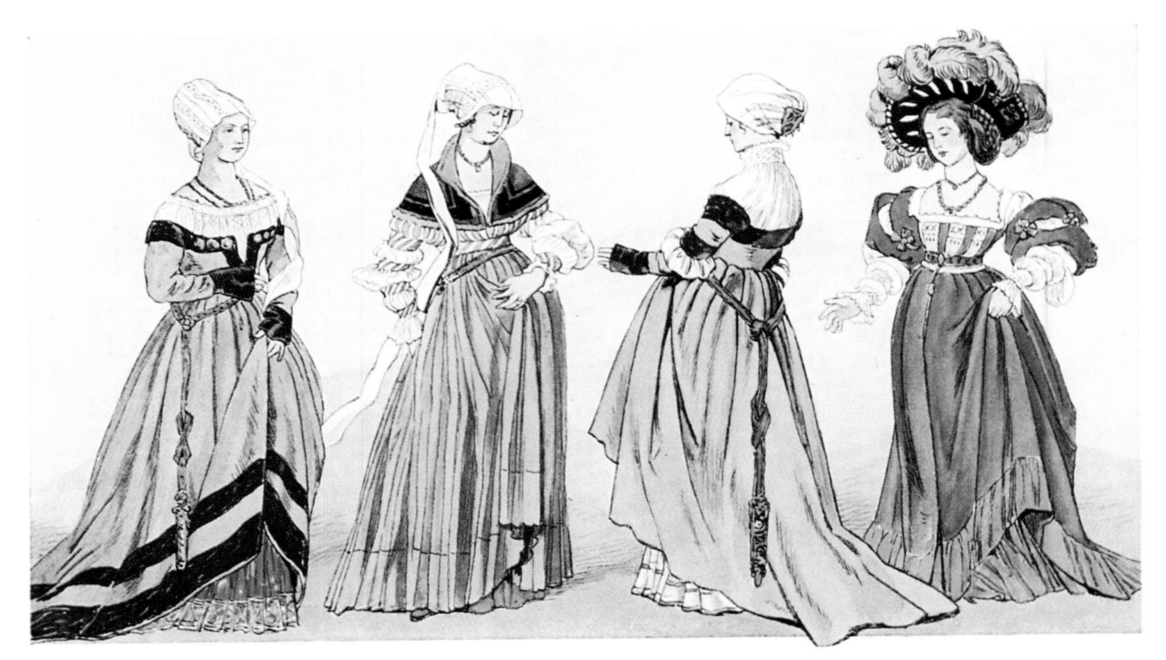

5 6 7 8

Men's Furlined Mantle,
Pleated Coat

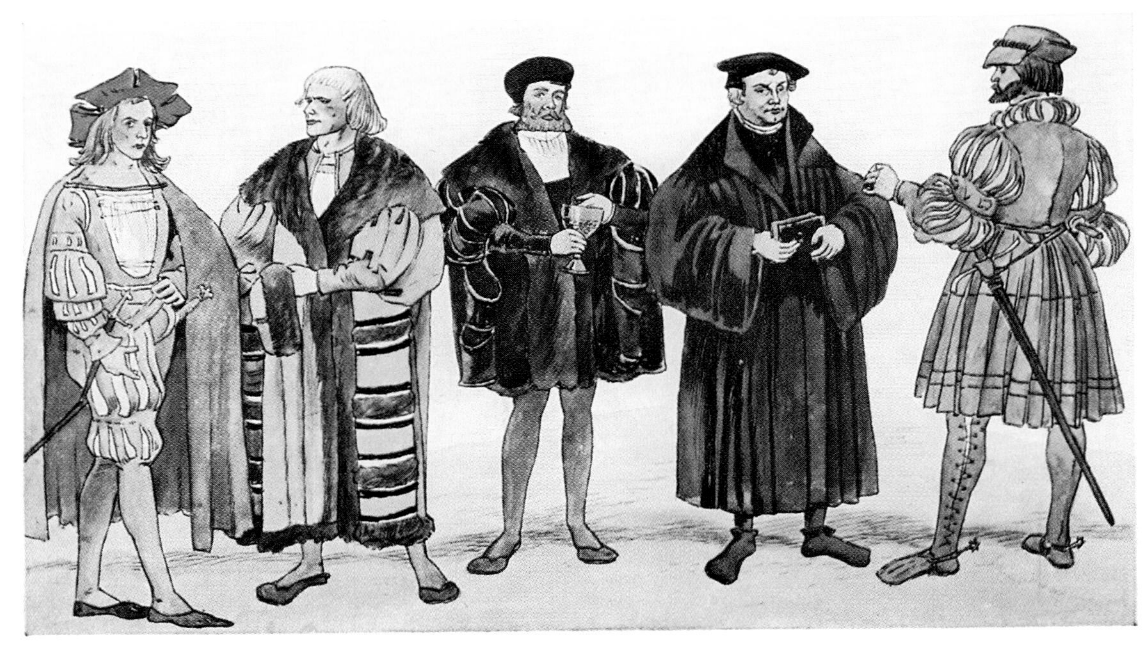

9 10 11 12 13

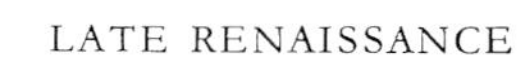

GERMANY
1550–1600

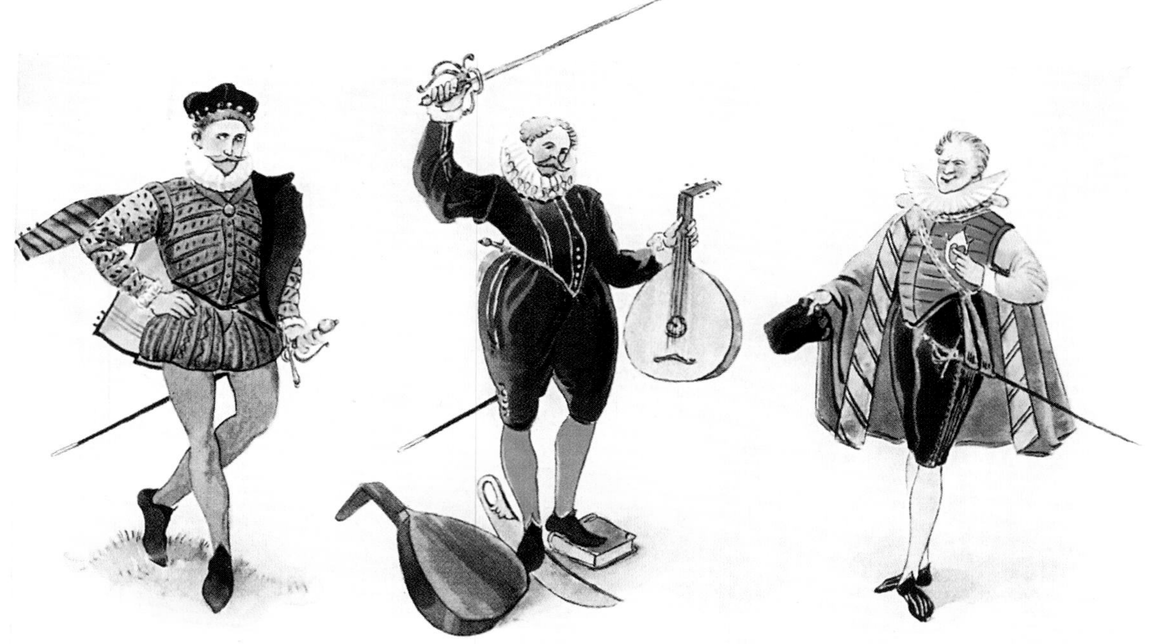

Spanish Fashion in Germany
1590–1595

1 2 3

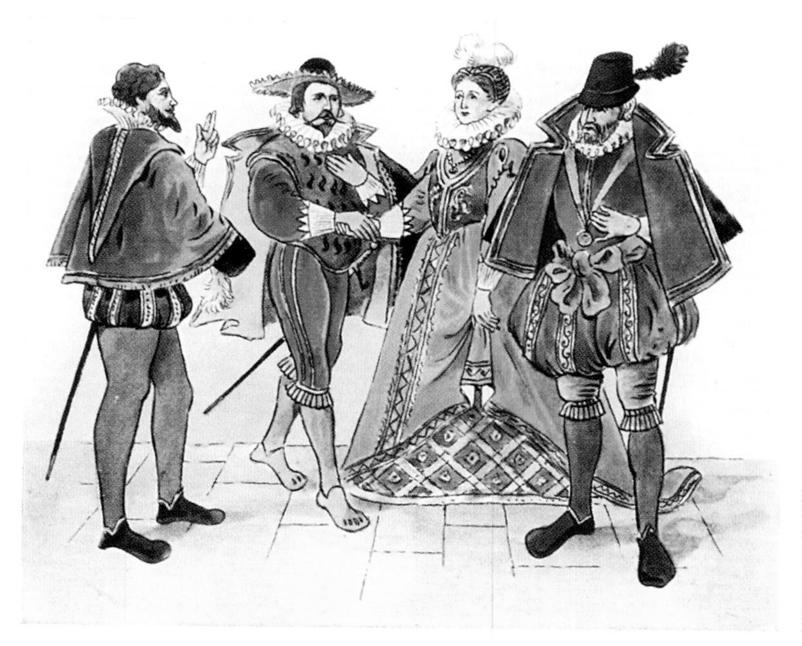

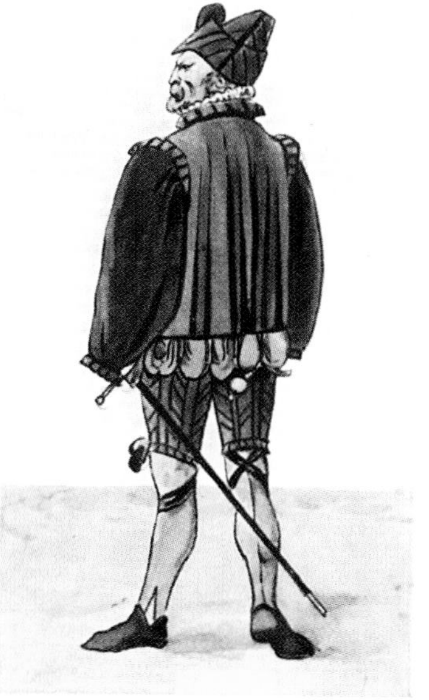

Betrothal Ceremony 1585

4 5 6 7 8

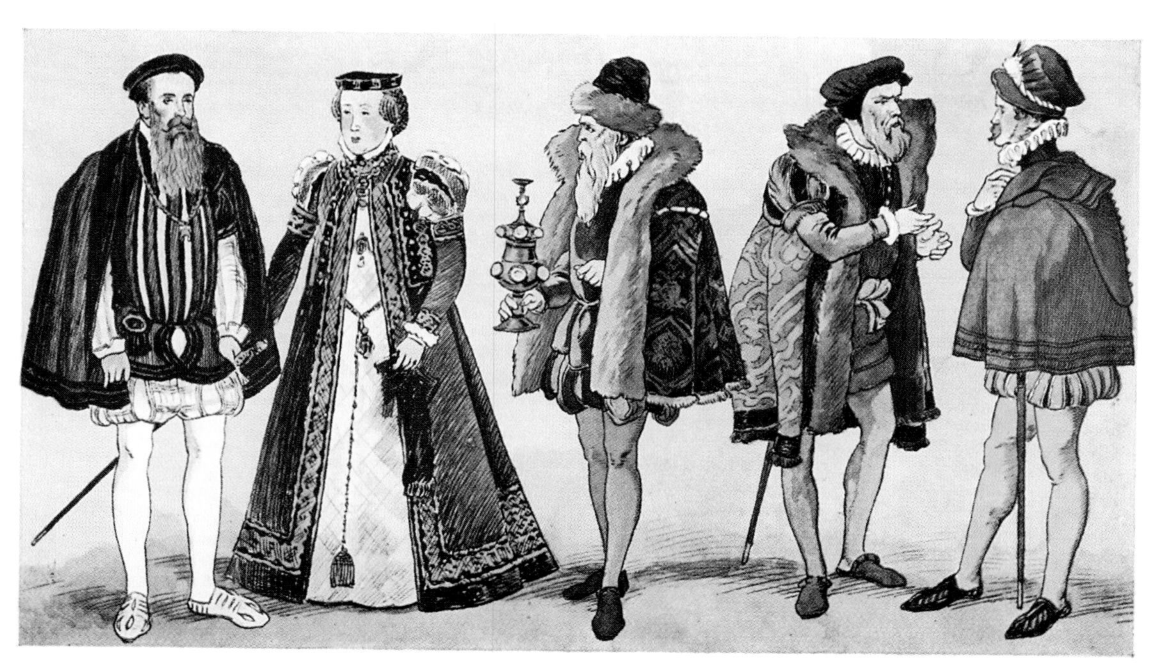

Duke Albrecht V. of Bavaria
and People of Rank

9 10 11 12 13

SPAIN AND PORTUGAL 1500–1540

Spanish Princes and Discoverers

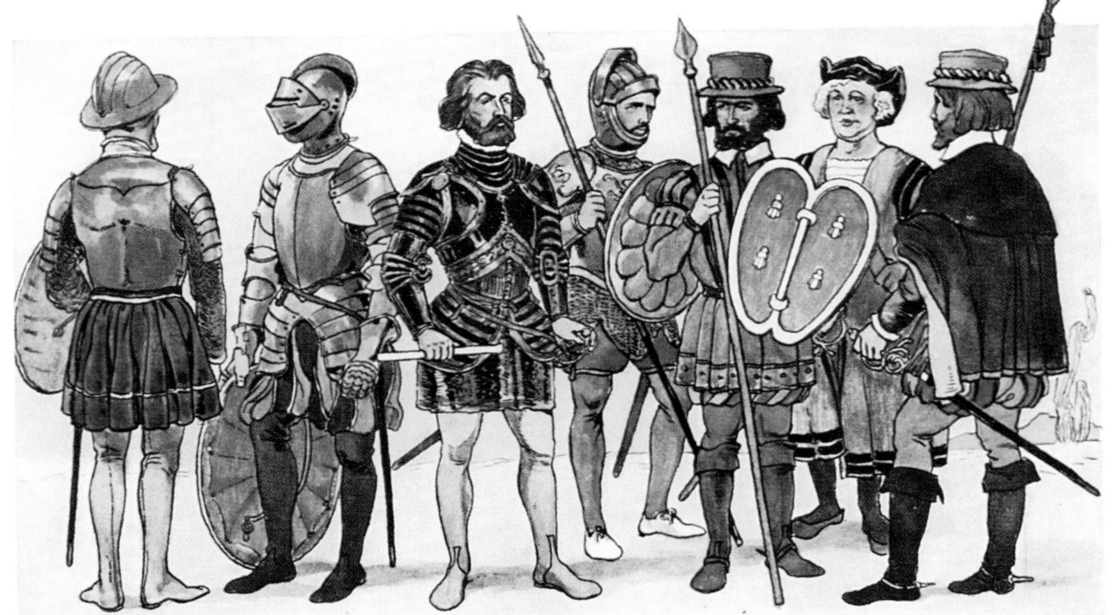

1 2 3 4 5 6 7

Portuguese Discoverers

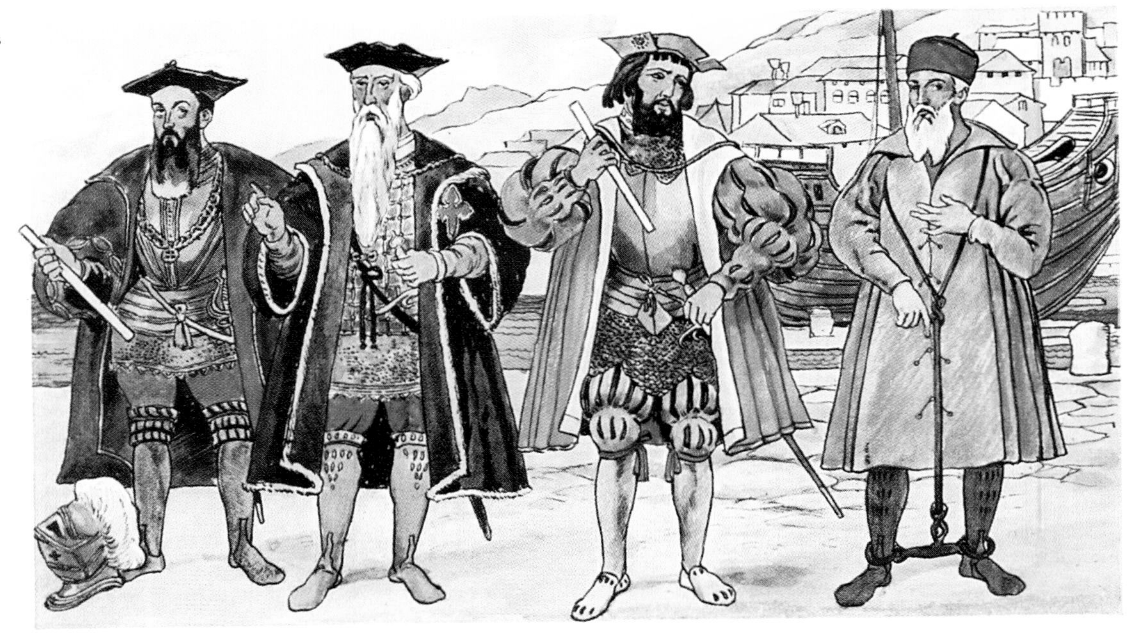

8 9 10 11

Spanish Moors, 15th Century

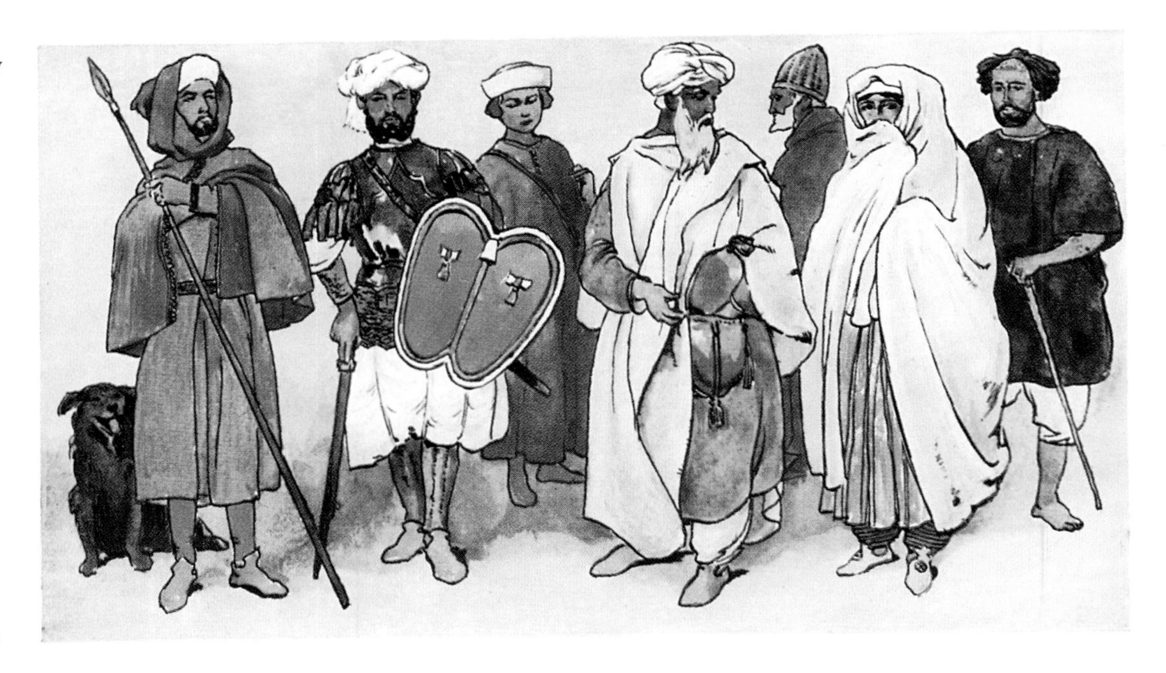

12 13 14 15 16 17 18

FRANCE
1500–1575

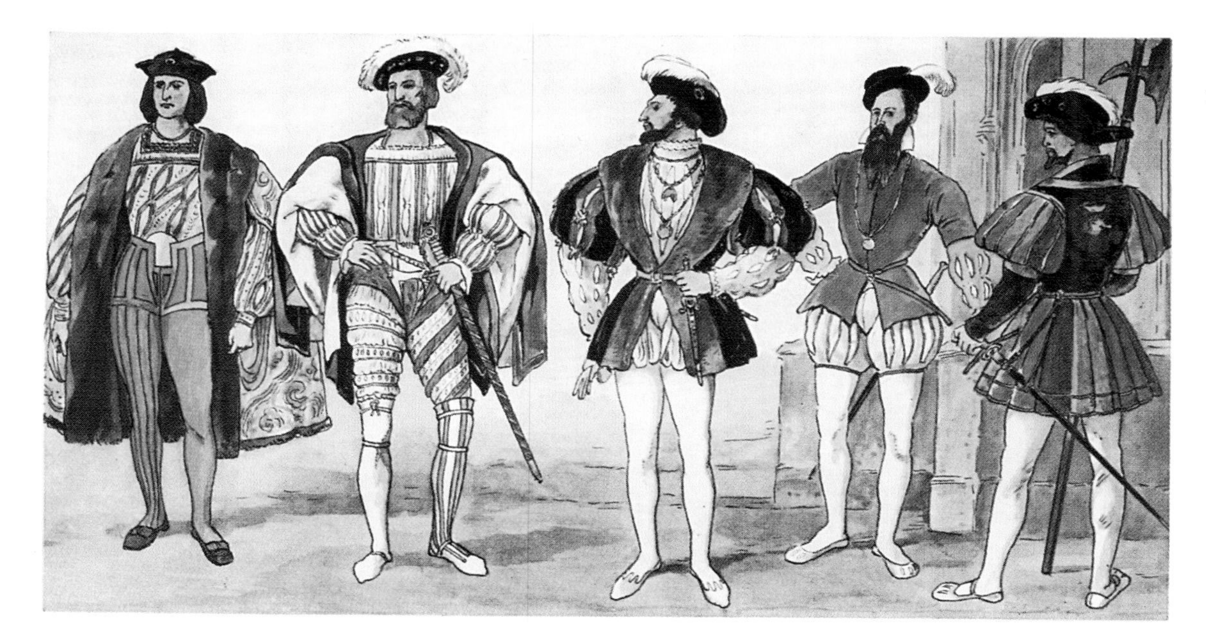

Francis I. and his Court
1515–1550

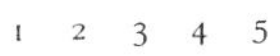

1 2 3 4 5

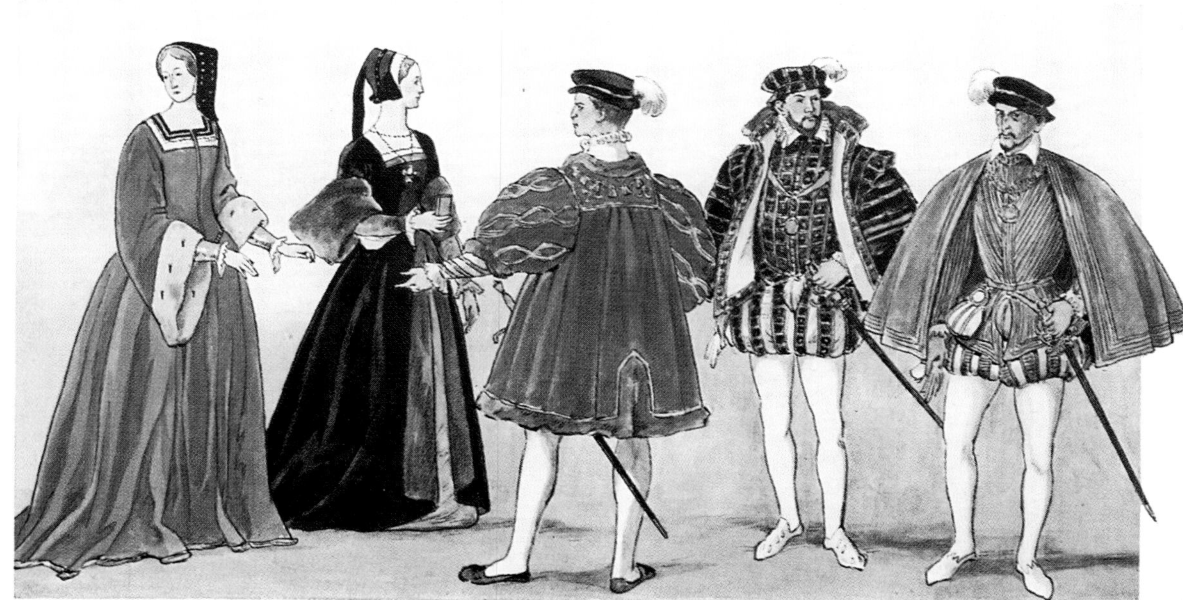

Francis I. and his Court
about 1540–1560

6 7 8 9 10

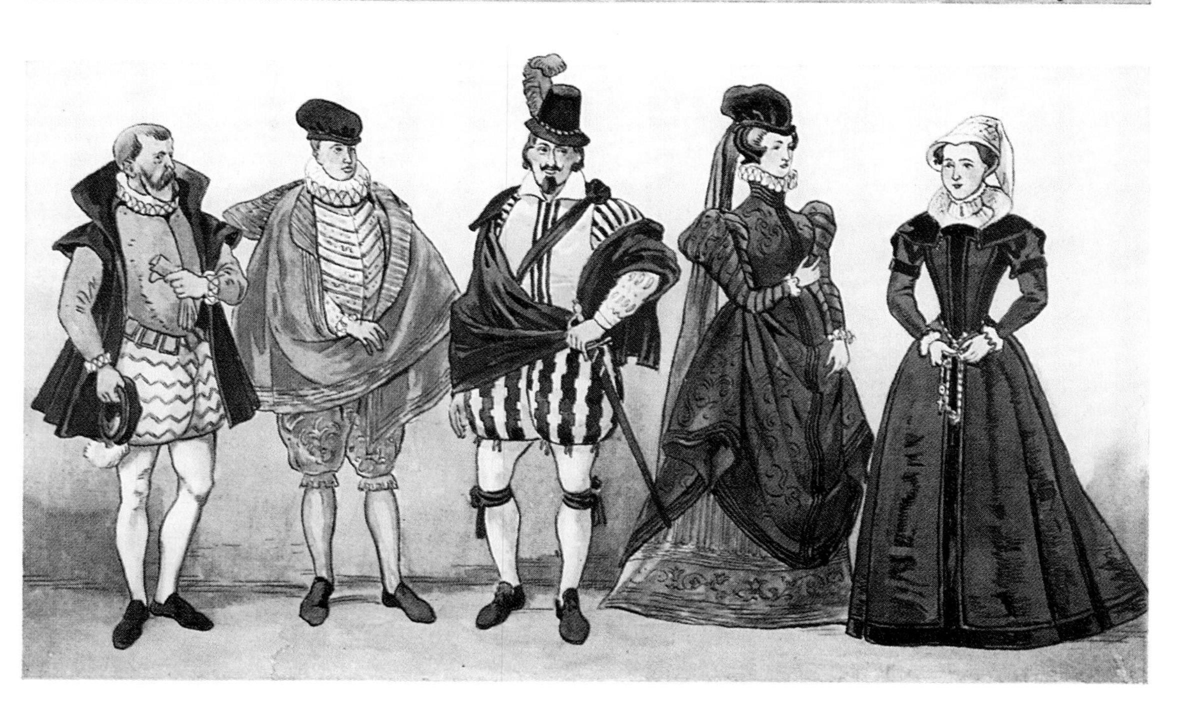

Spanish Fashion
at the French Court

11 12 13 14 15

FRANCE
1560–1590
Spanish Fashion

Charles IX. and his Court
1560–1574

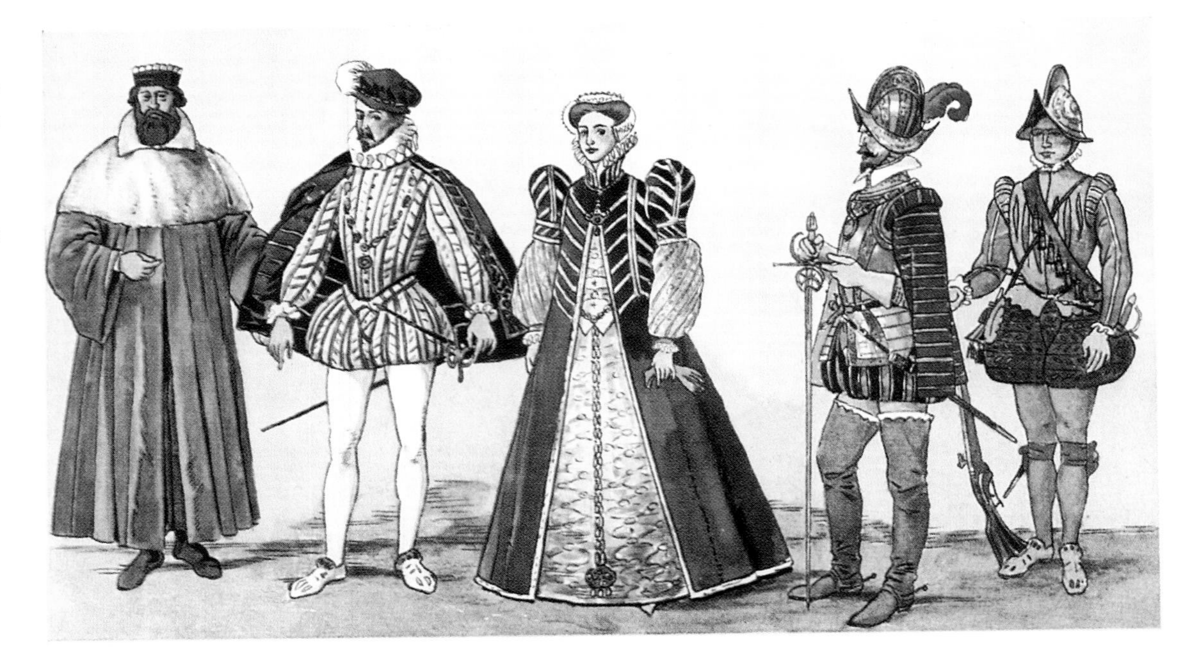

1 2 3 4 5

Soldiers and Citizens
1560–1580

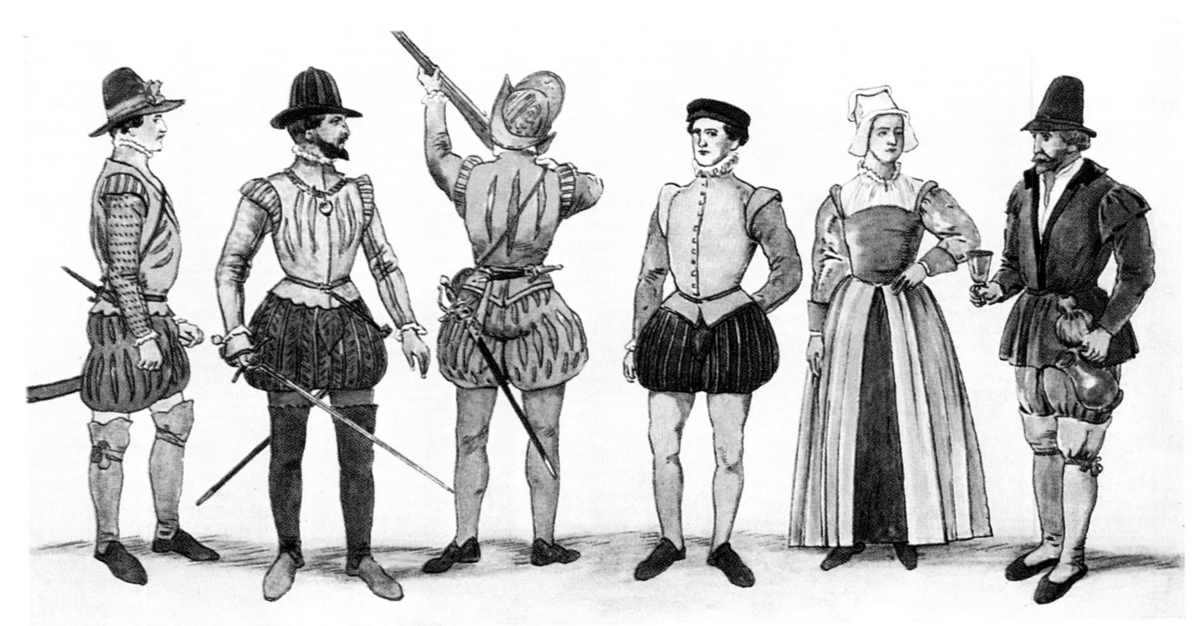

6 7 8 9 10 11

Citizens and Peasants
1580–1590

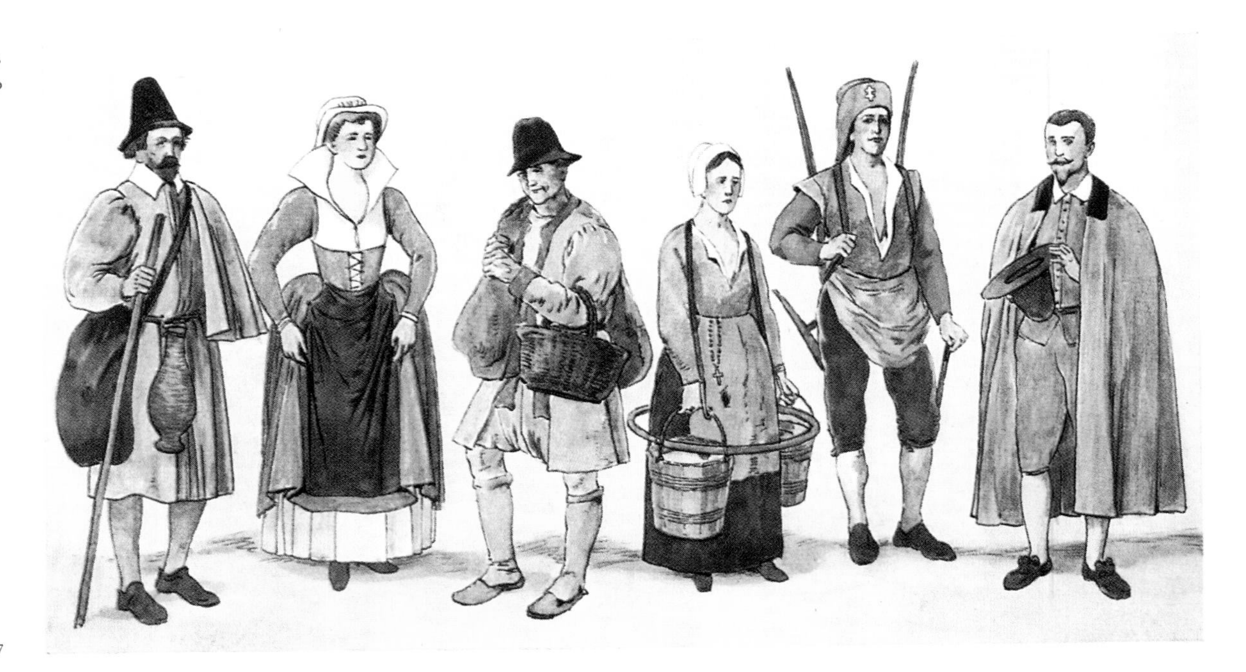

12 13 14 15 16 17

FRANCE

1575–1590
Spanish Fashion

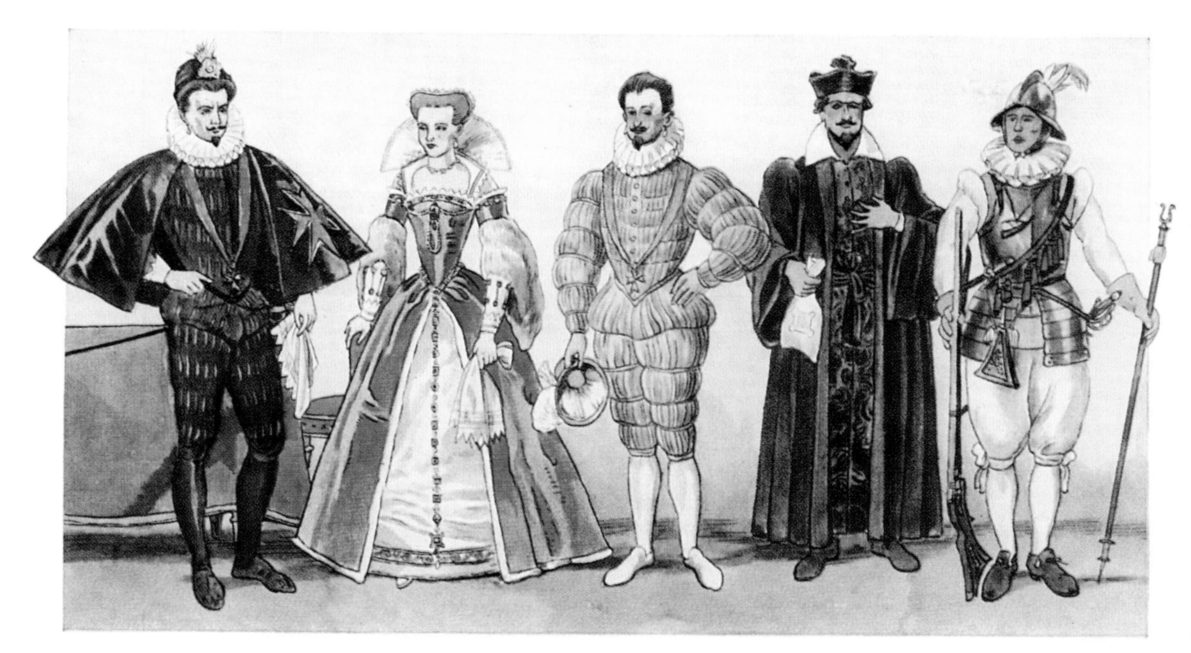

Henry III. and his Court
Huguenots

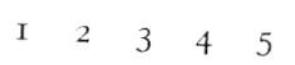

1 2 3 4 5

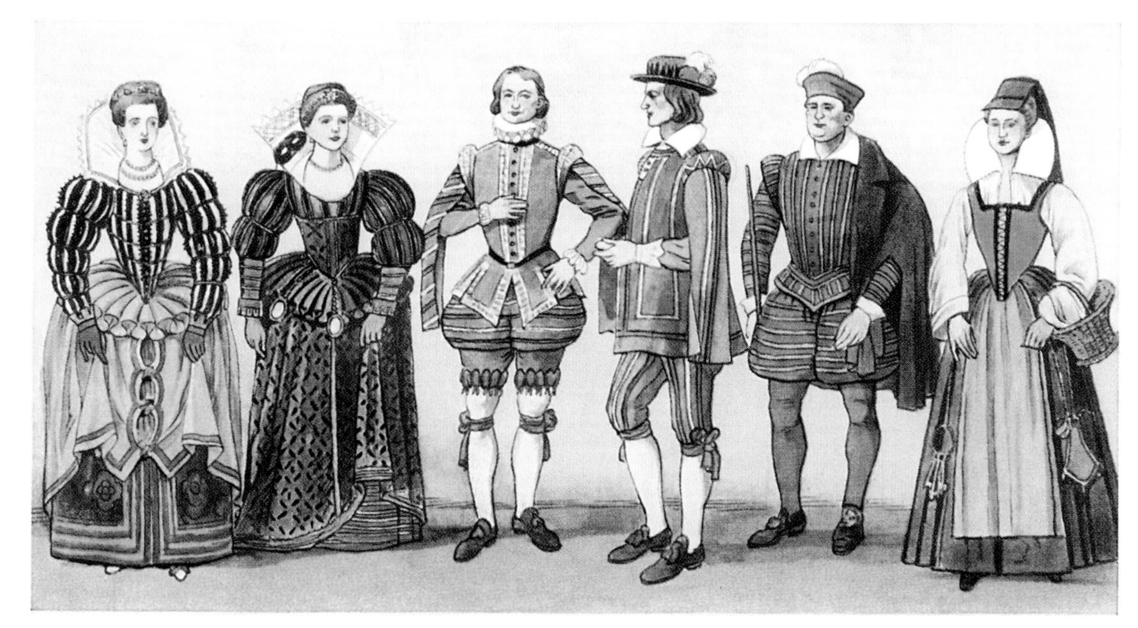

Noble Women, Pages

6 7 8 9 10 11

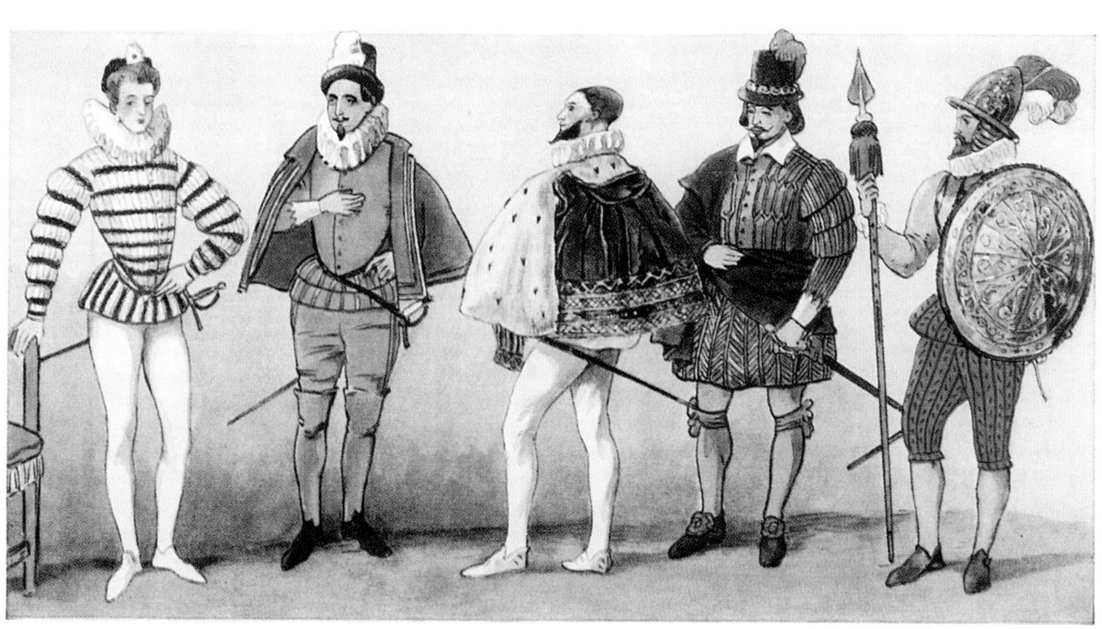

Courtiers, Bodyguard

12 13 14 15 16

ITALY
1590–1610

Respectable Women and Courtesans

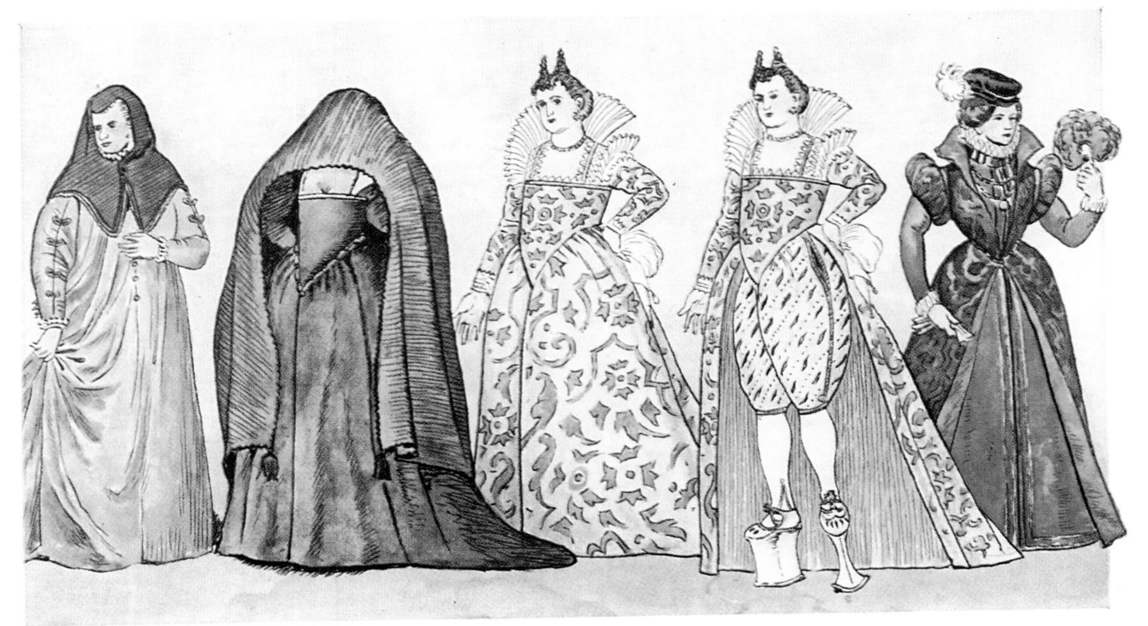

1 2 3 4 5

Venice and Ferrara

1590–1610

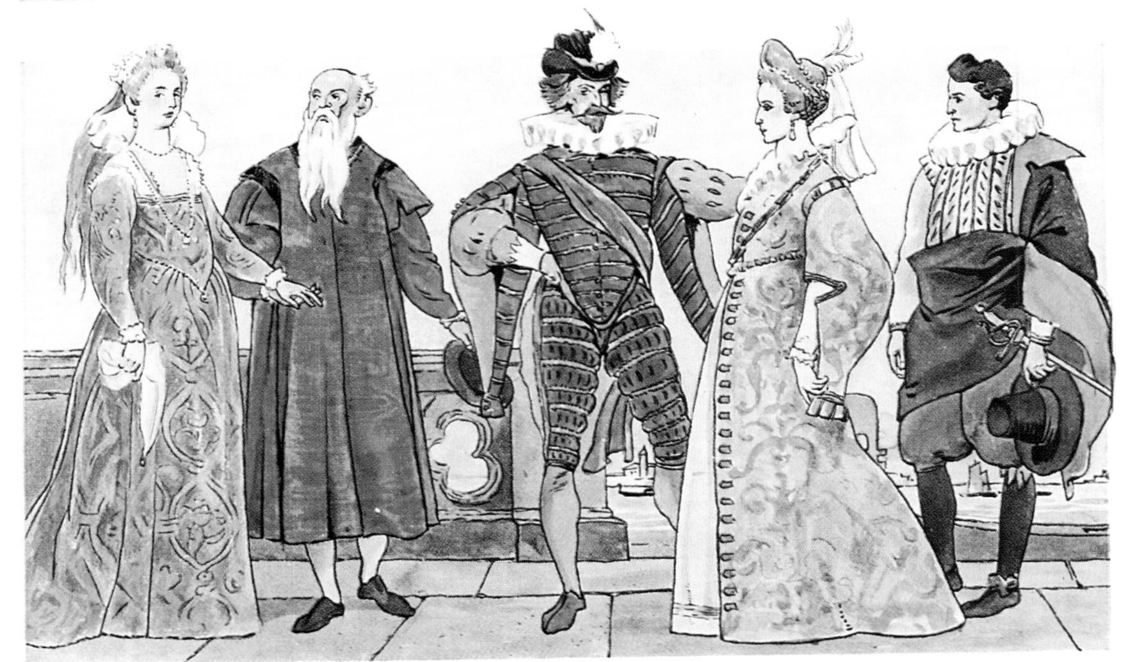

6 7 8 9 10

Milan 1604

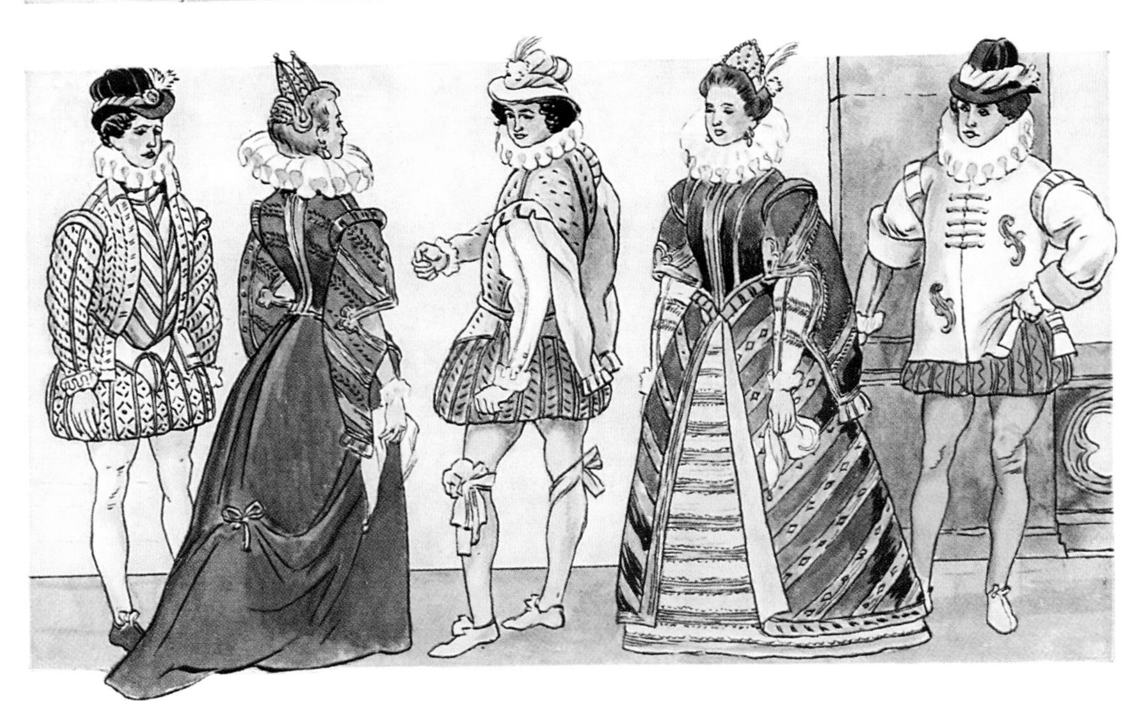

11 12 13 14 15

FRANCE
1600–1640

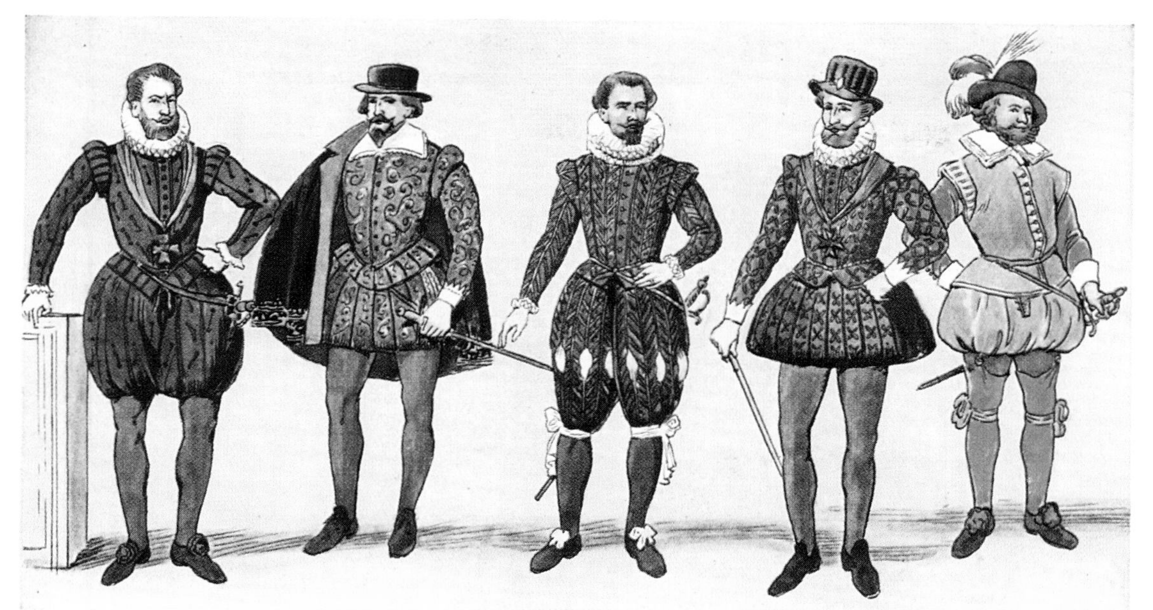

Henry IV. and his Court

1 2 3 4 5

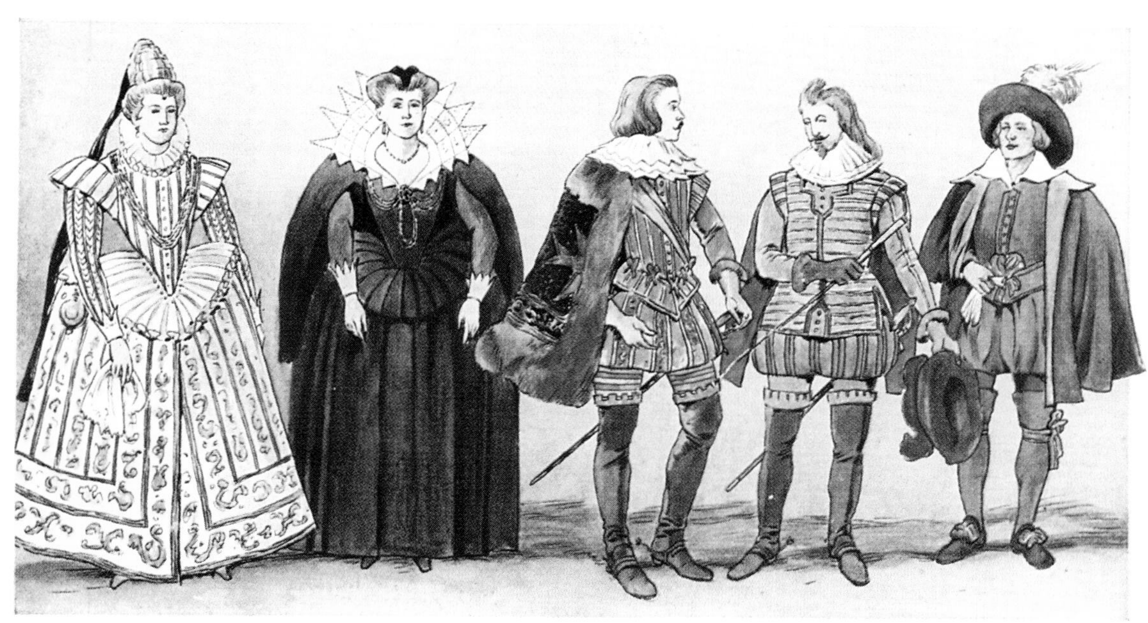

Henry IV. and Louis XIII.

6 7 8 9 10

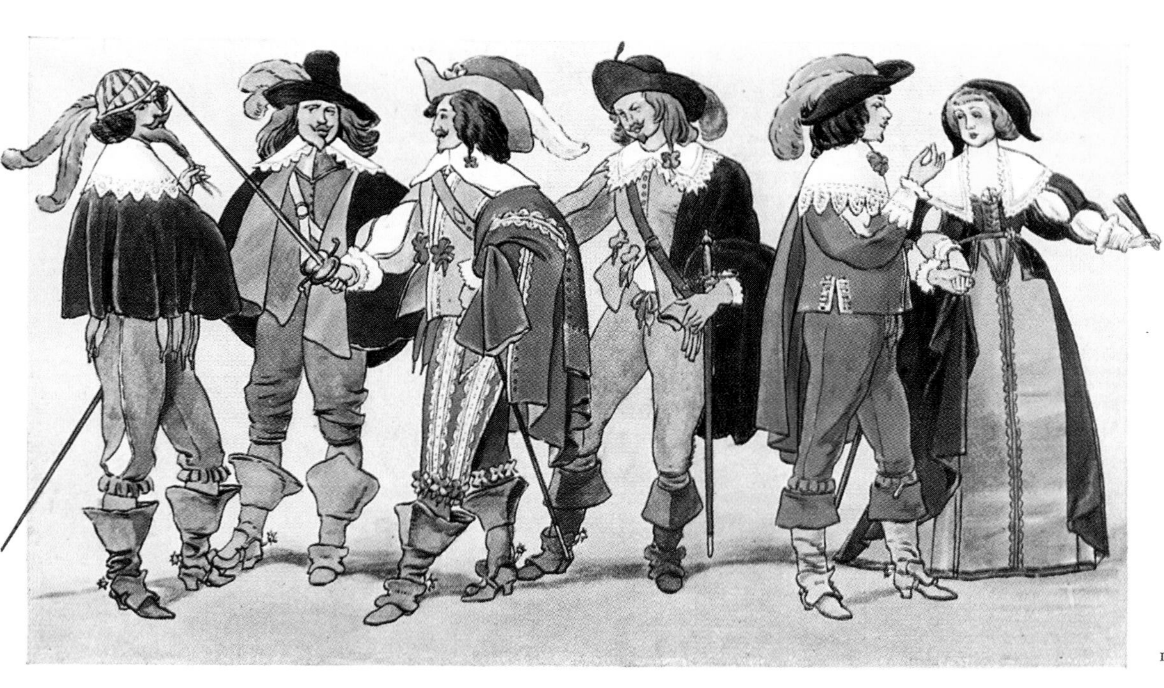

«Messieurs à la mode»
1630–1640

11 12 13 14 15 16

SPAIN
16th and 17th Centuries

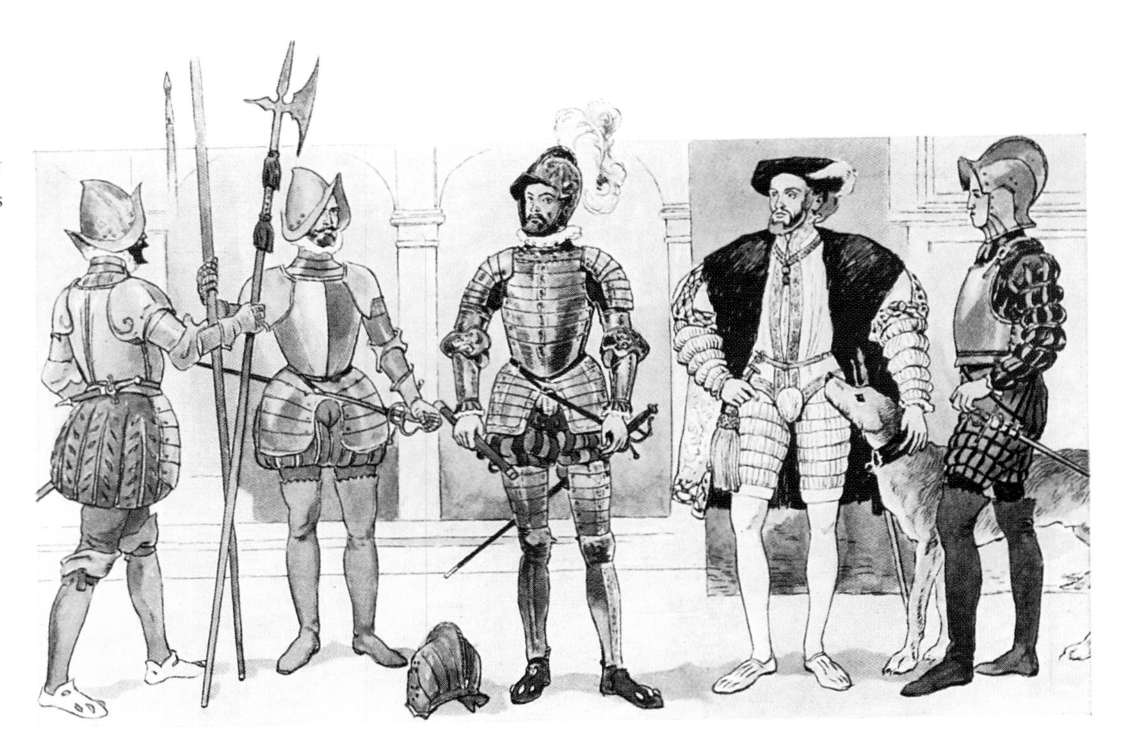

1 2 3 4 5

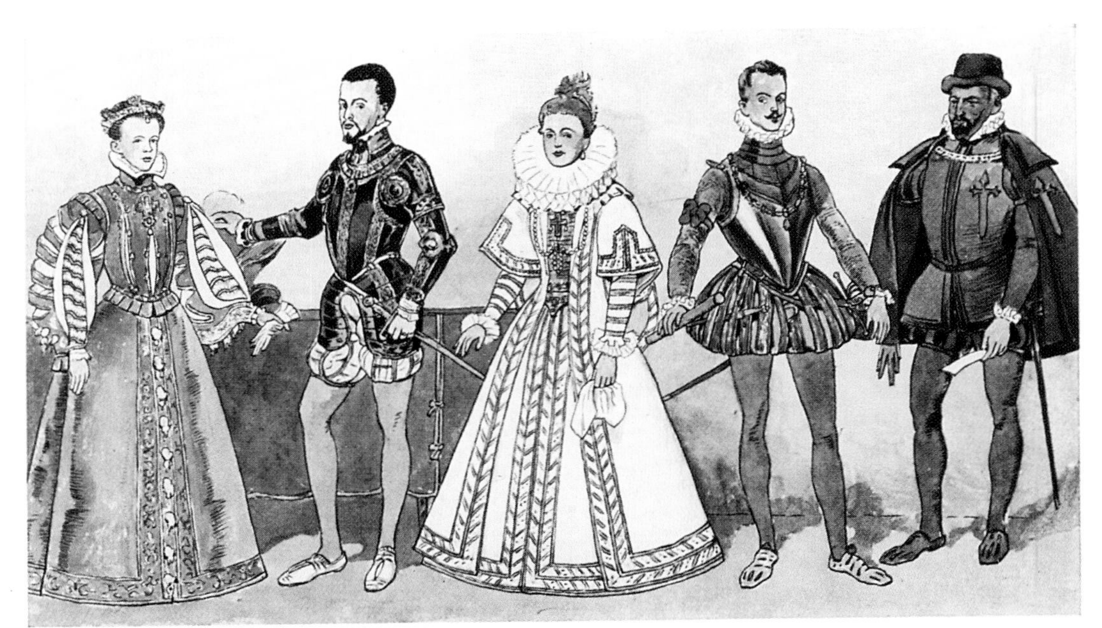

6 7 8 9 10

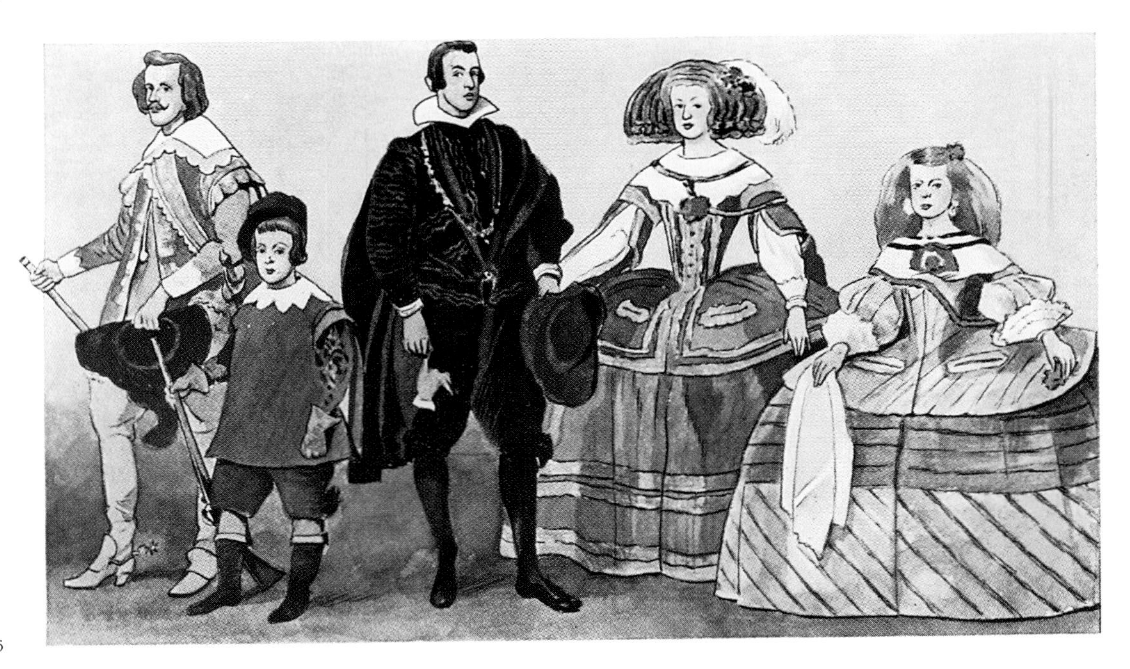

11 12 13 14 15

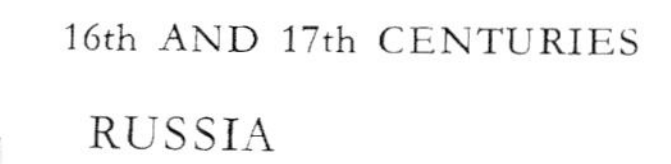

RUSSIA

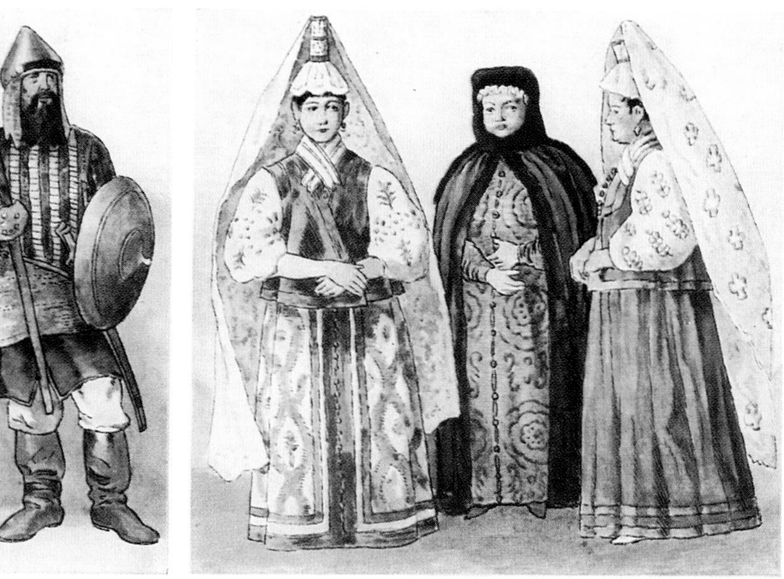

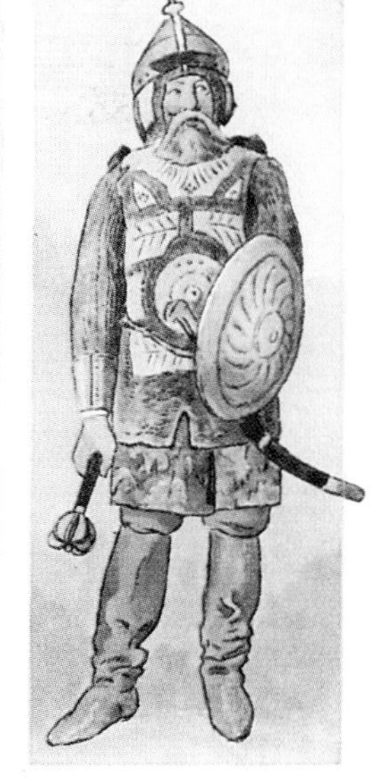

Boyard Women, Warriors

1 2 3 4 5

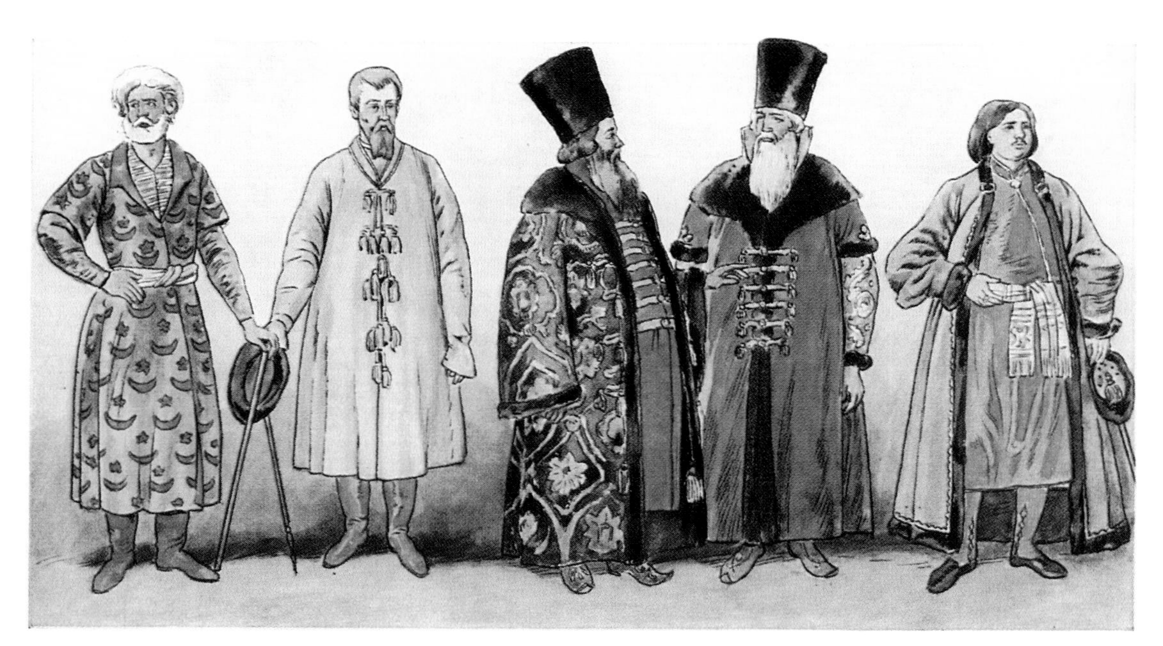

Boyards

6 7 8 9 10

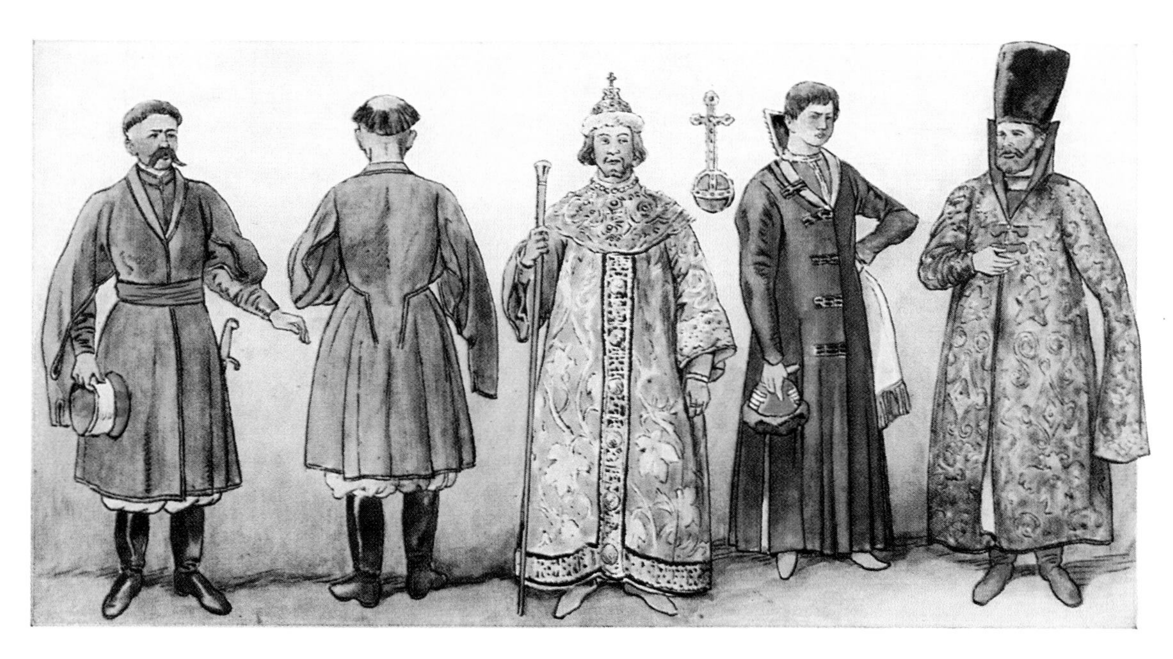

Tsar and Boyards

11 12 13 14 15

POLAND, HUNGARY, UKRAINE

Poland

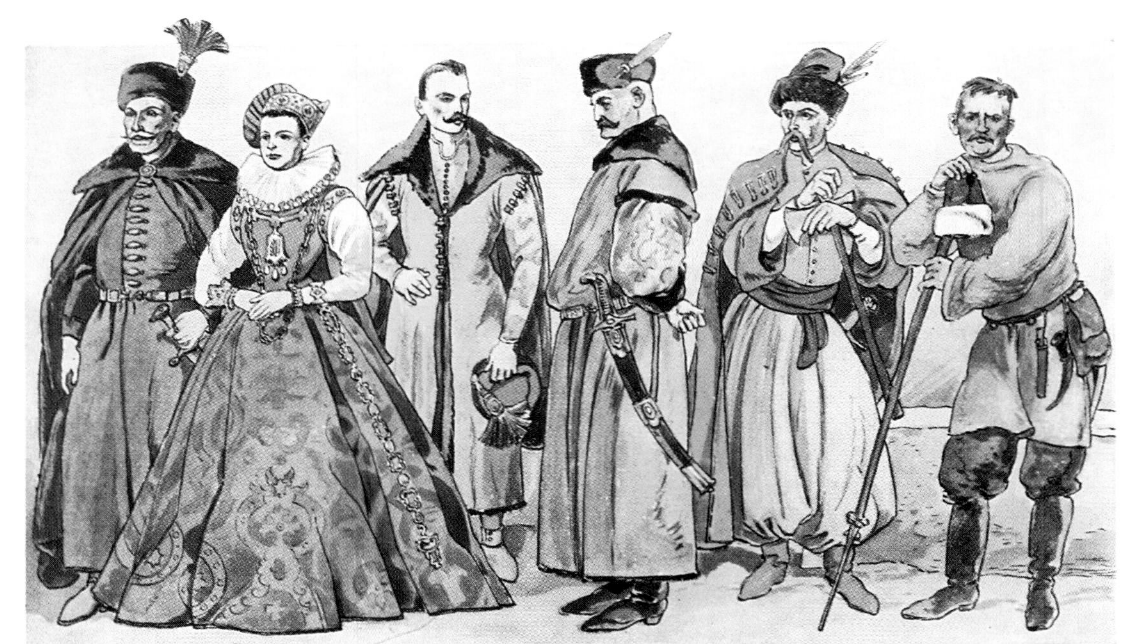

1 2 3 4 5 6

Poland

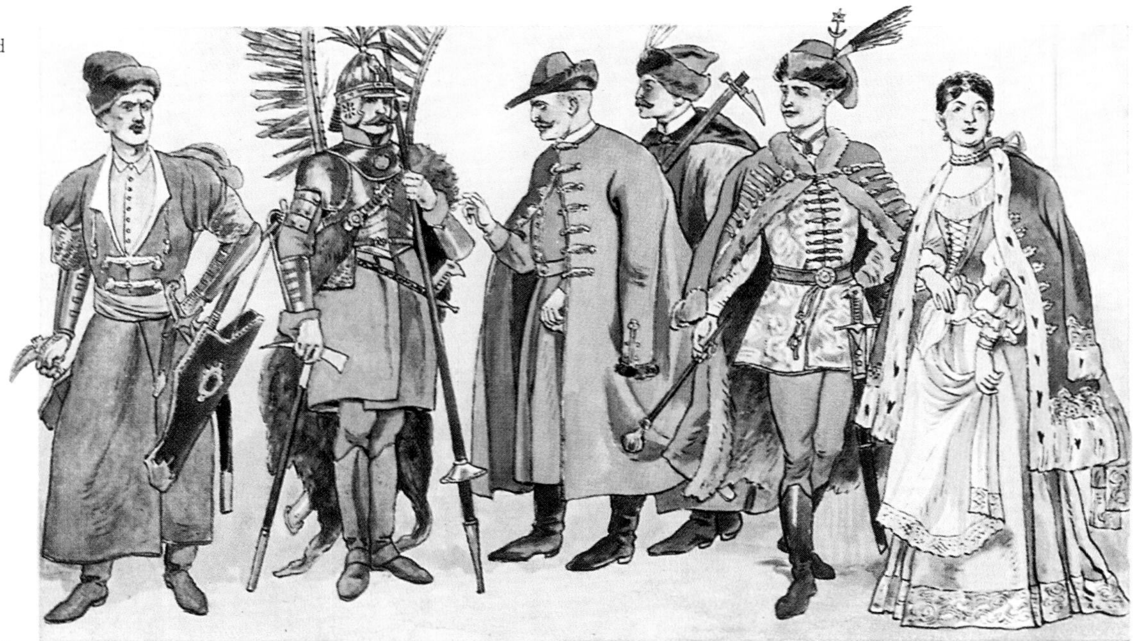

7 8 9 10 11 12

Hungary and Ukraine

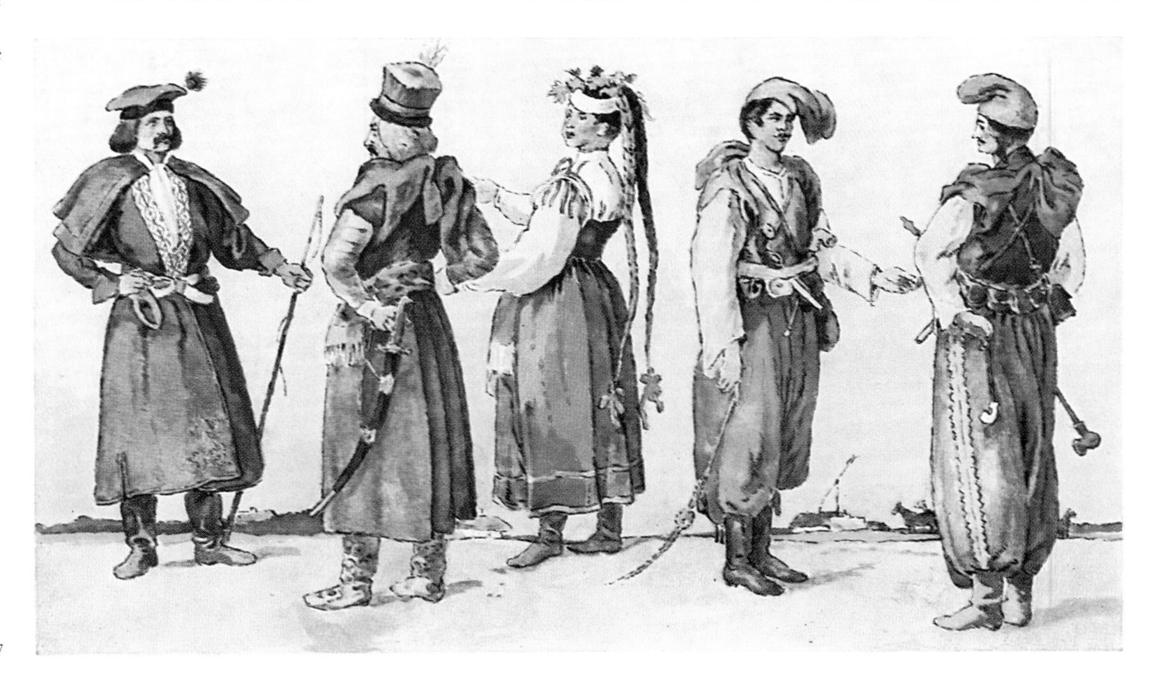

13 14 15 16 17

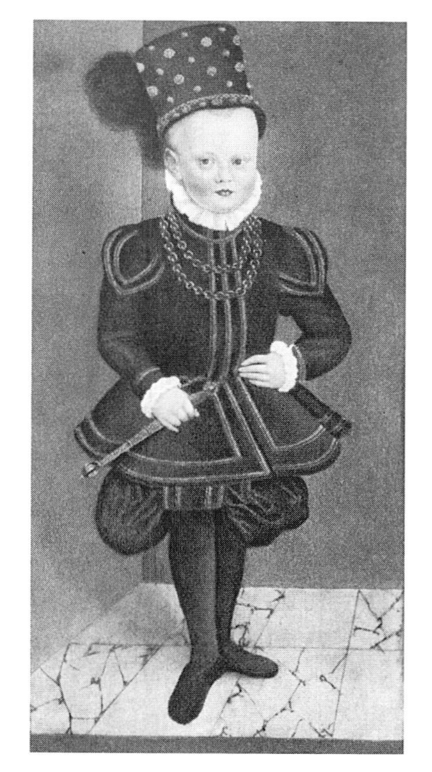

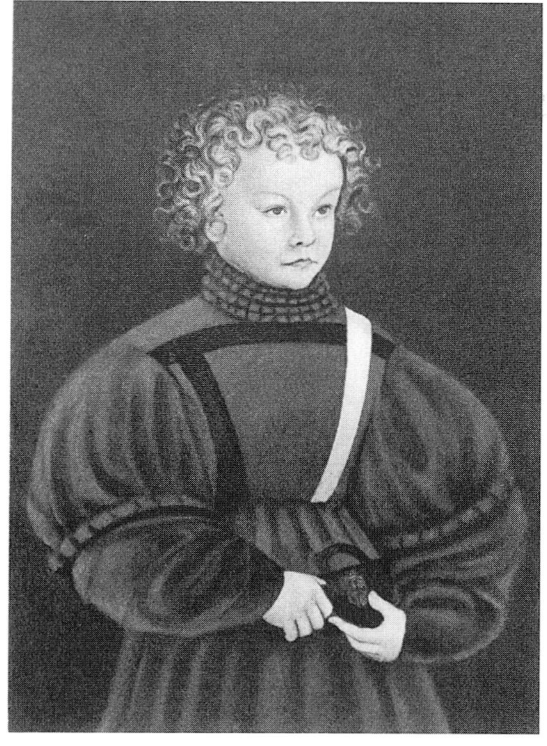

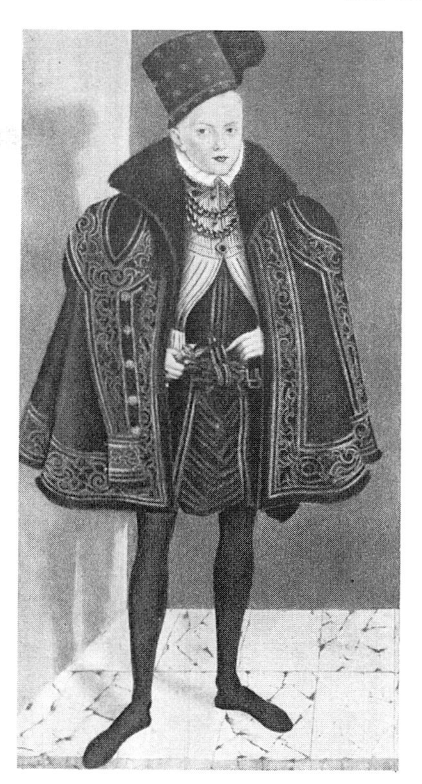

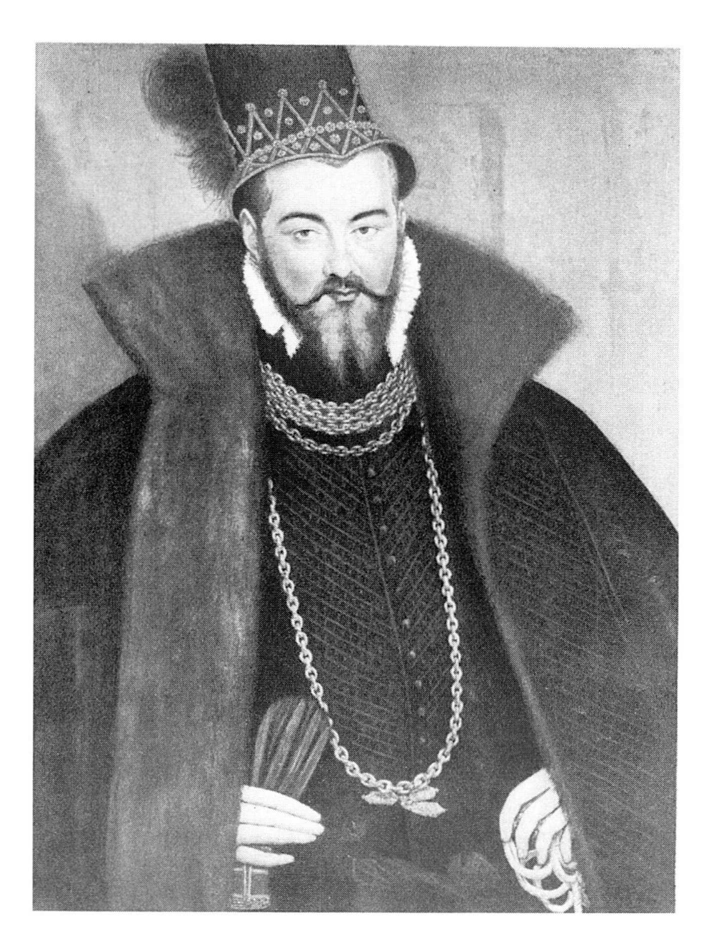

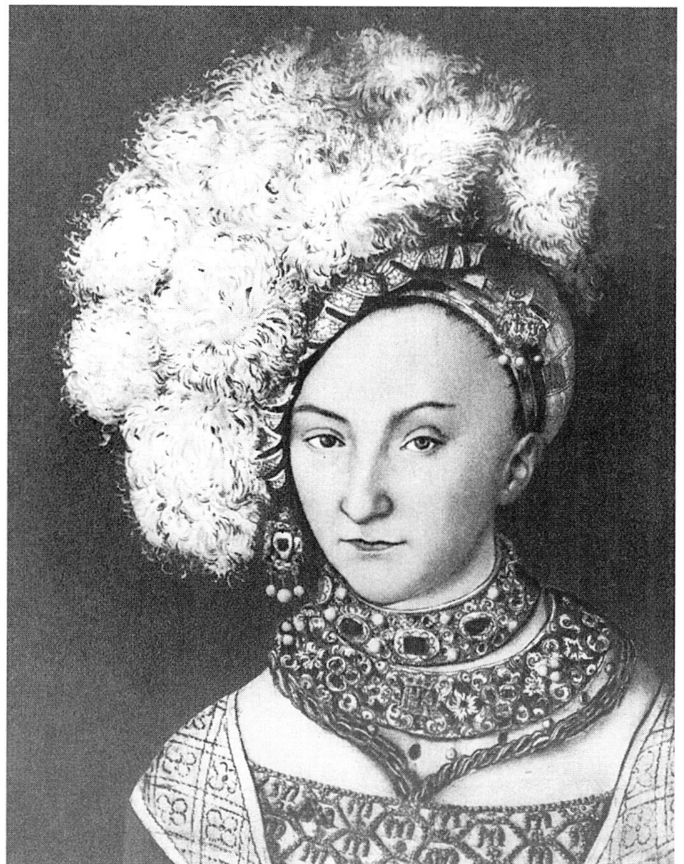

Reformation and Spanish Fashion 1514–1564

Costume worn at the Court of Saxony

GERMANY
about 1560–1580
(Spanish Fashion)

Citizens' and Craftsmen's Wives
from Dantzig, Cologne and Lübeck

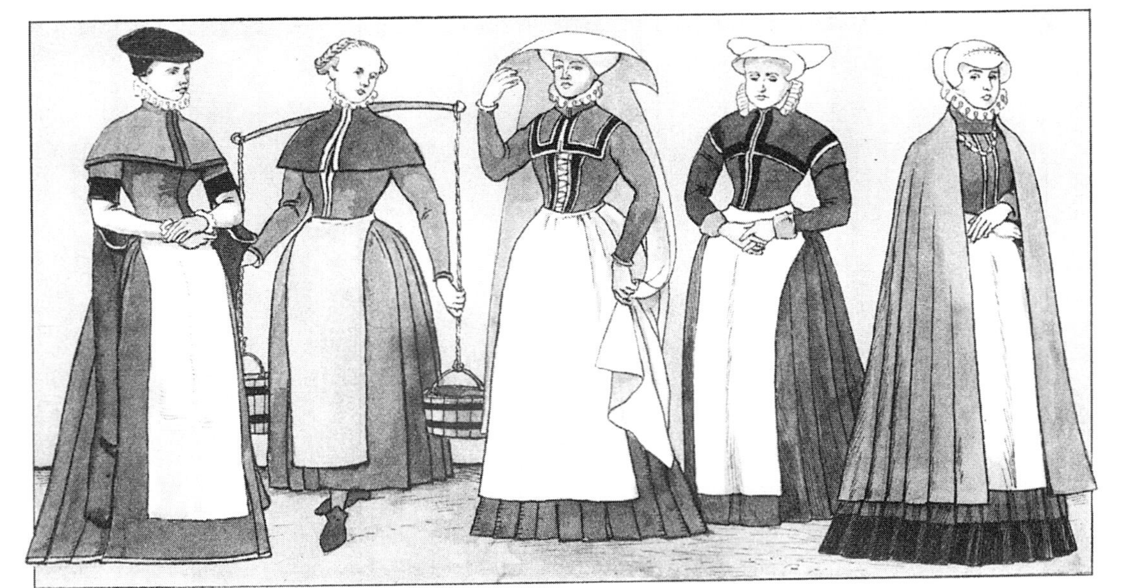

1 2 3 4 5

Citizens' and Craftsmen's Wives
from Nuremberg and Augsburg

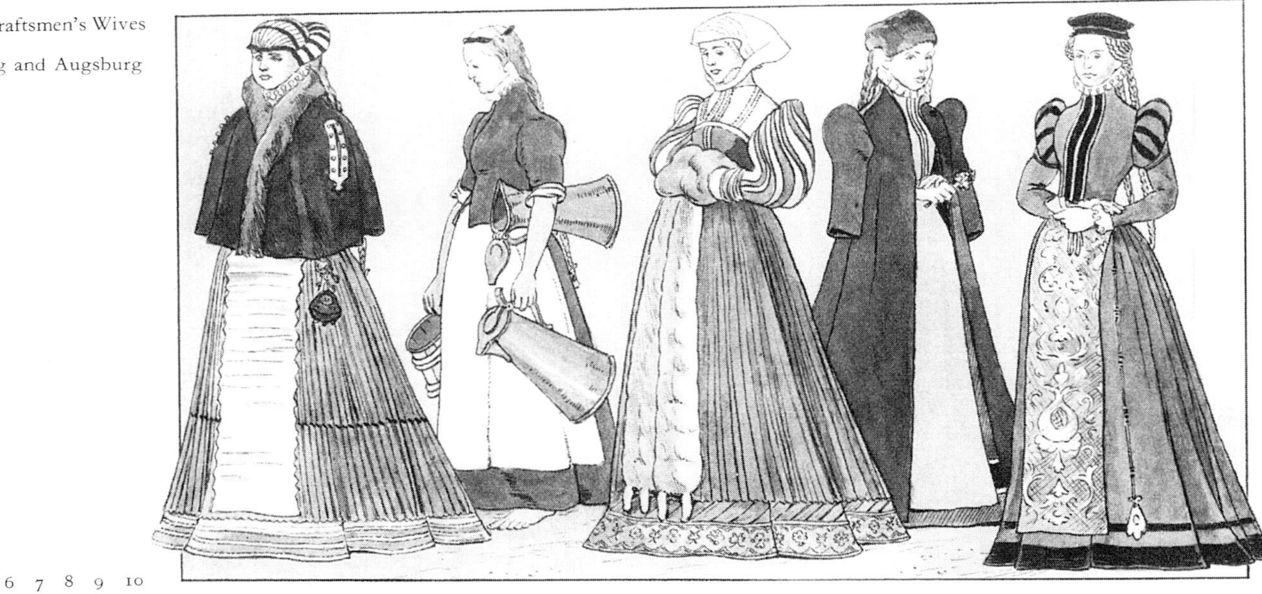

6 7 8 9 10

Men's Costume

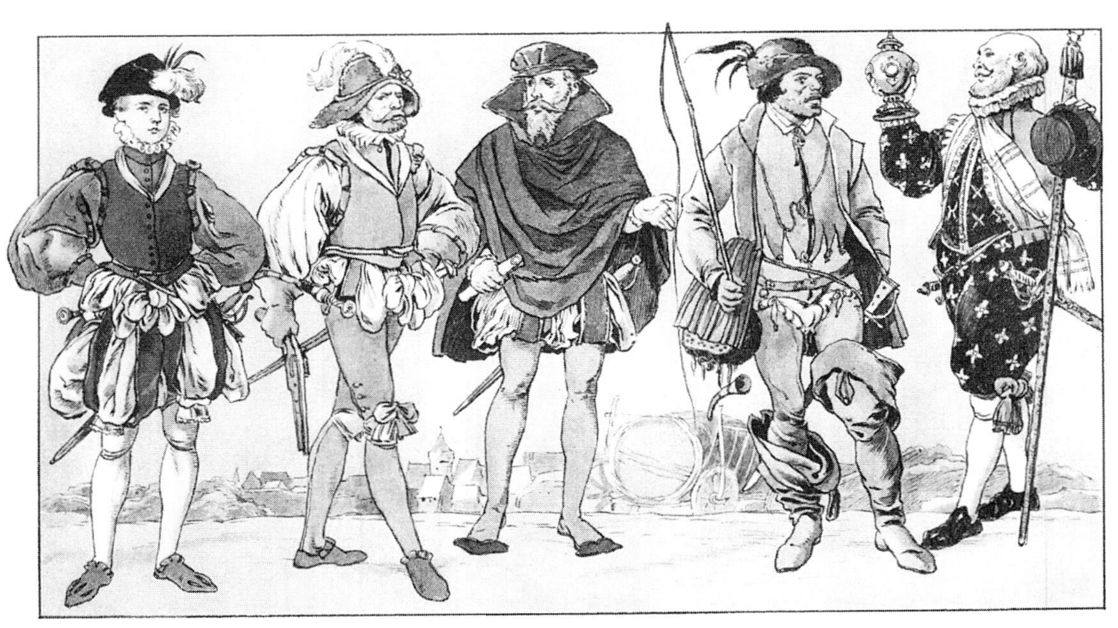

11 12 13 14 15

EUROPE
1550–1590

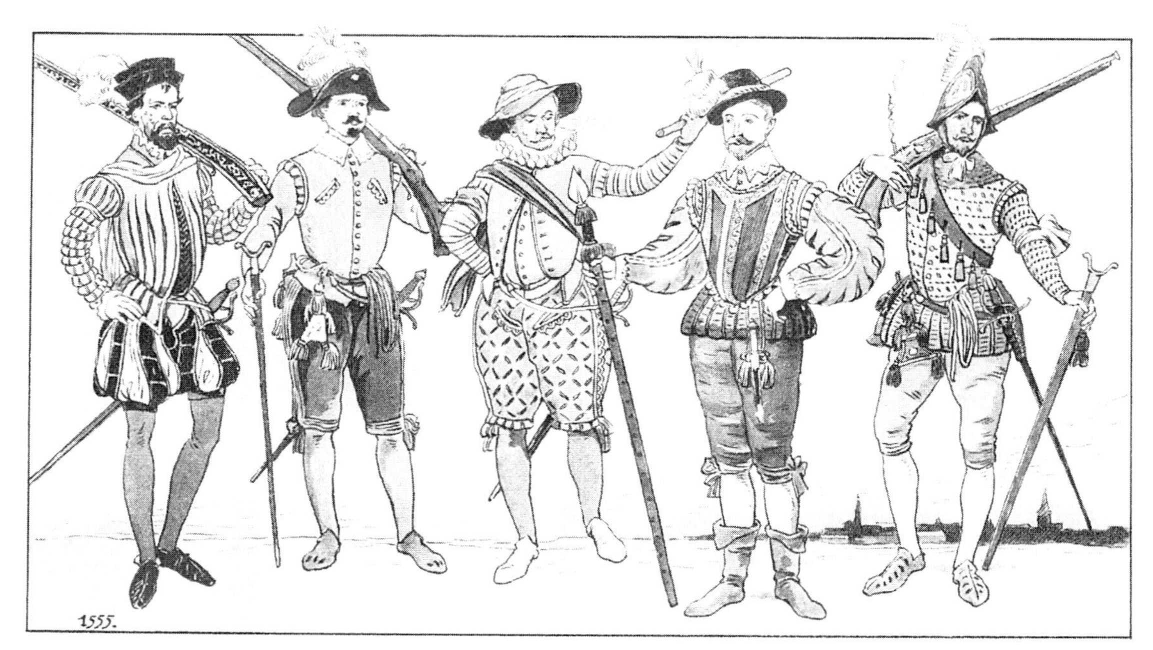

Spanish Soldiers
1555 and 1590

1 2 3 4 5

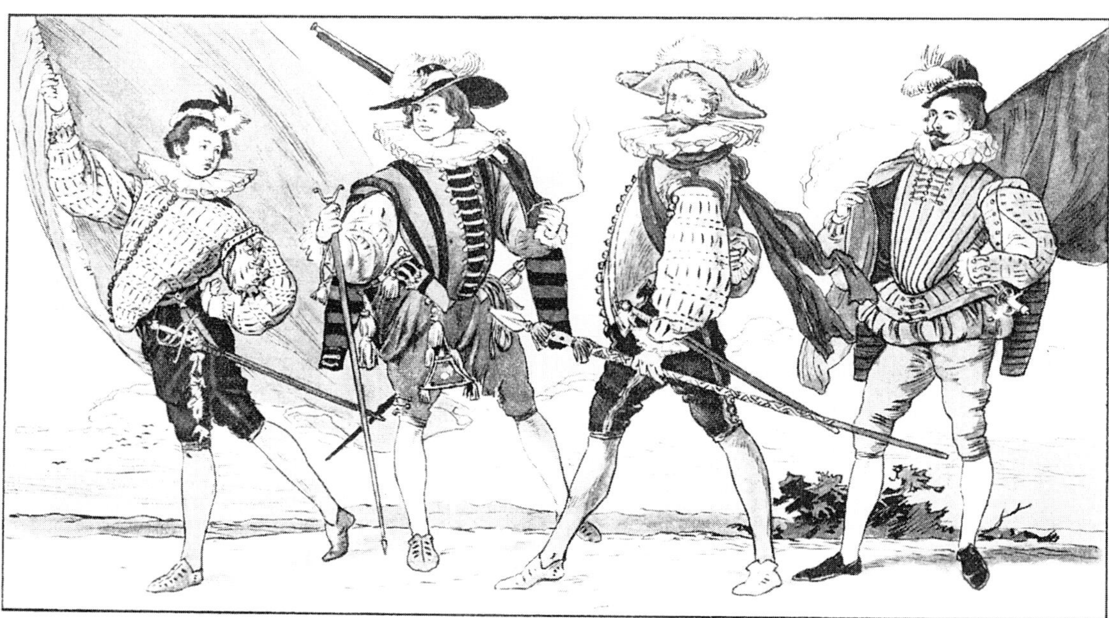

Spanish Soldiers
in the Netherlands 1585

6 7 8 9

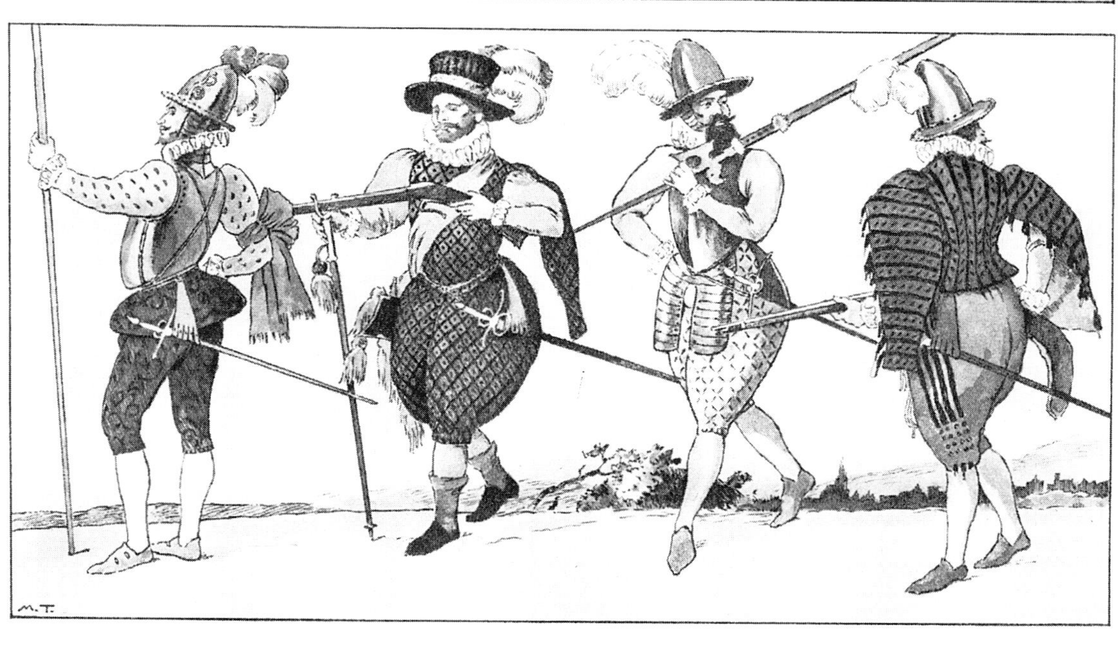

French Soldiers about 1581

10 11 12 13

GERMANY
Head-dress 1550–1595
(Spanish Fashion)

Small Cap (Toque)

Small Spanish Hats

Stiff Ruffs

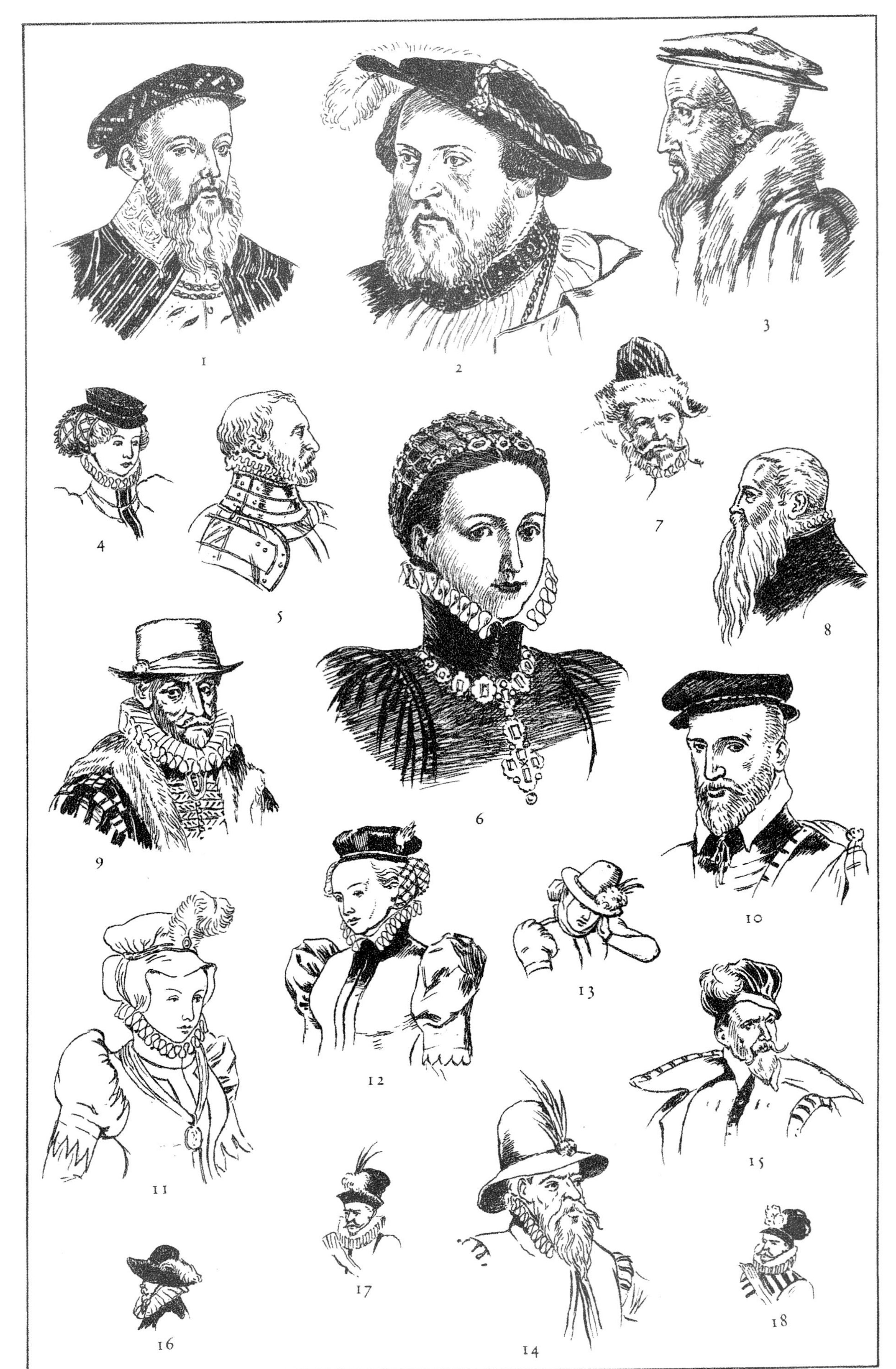

GERMANY AND FRANCE

Thirty Years' War

Immagination haar
Patient bart
Responsion huth
Indifferent huth schnur
5 Legation feder
6 Varsat Kroß
7 Accordant kamsohl
8 Male content wammes
9 Alamodo hosen
10 Difident schenckel
11 Reputation hosen binder
12 Necessitet schuh
13 Respect rosen
14 occasion stiefel
15 Resonant sporen
16 Accomodat gurtel
17 Poenitent degen
18 Diligent mantel
19 Inter medys handschuh
20 Stultissimus gang und geberden

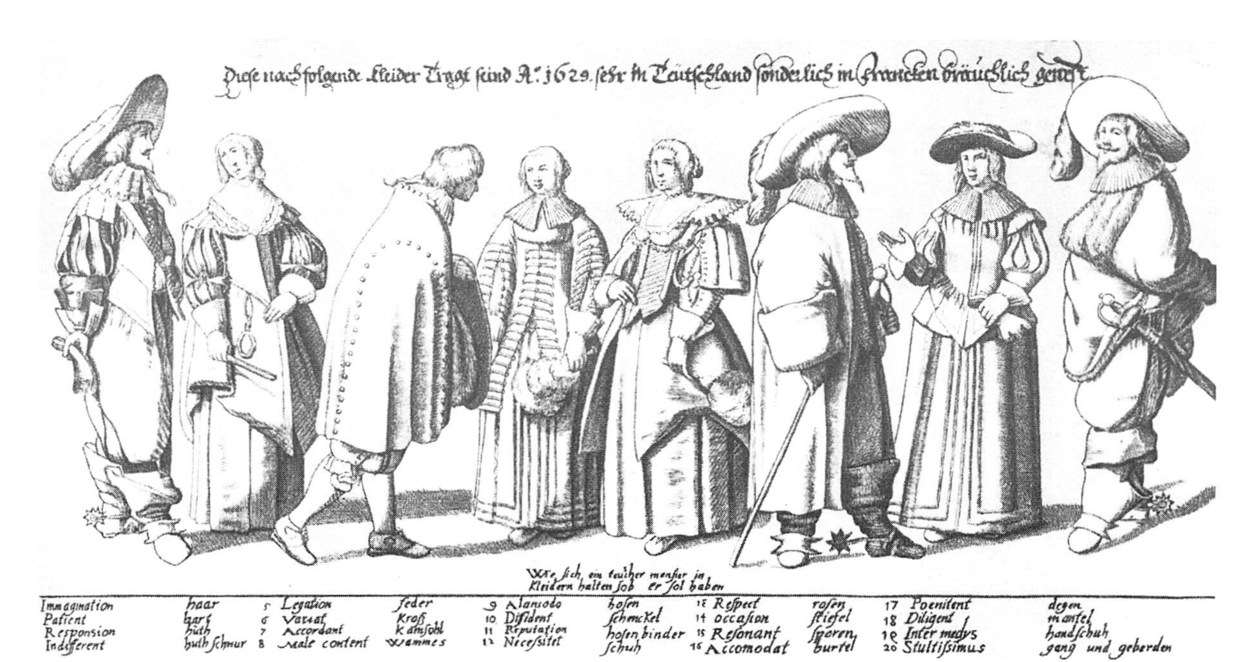

"Alla modo" Costume 1629

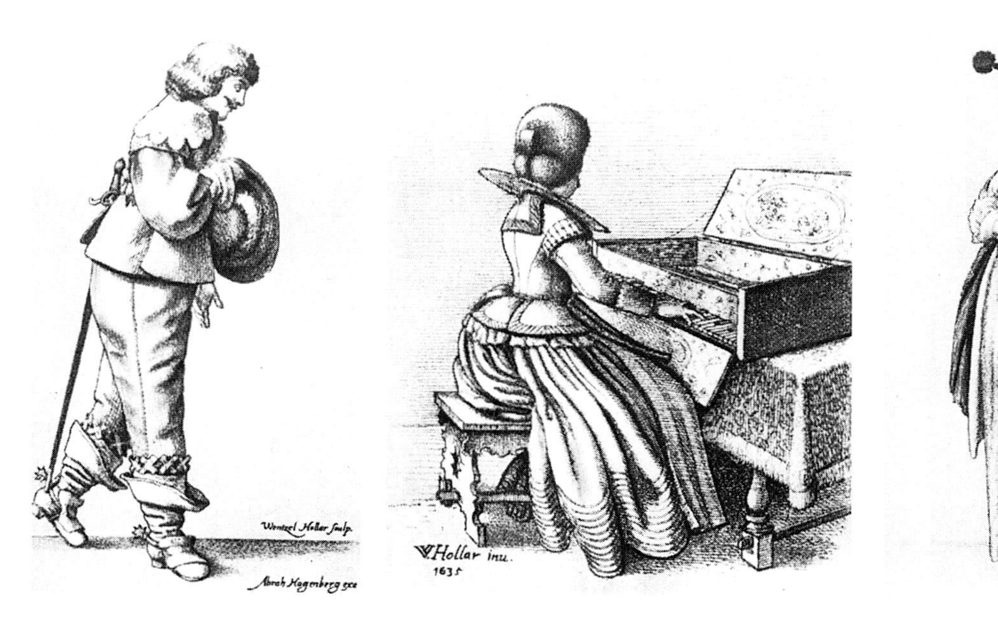

Courtier, Women

Monsieurisch Alla modo, vnd Damische Bisarrie.

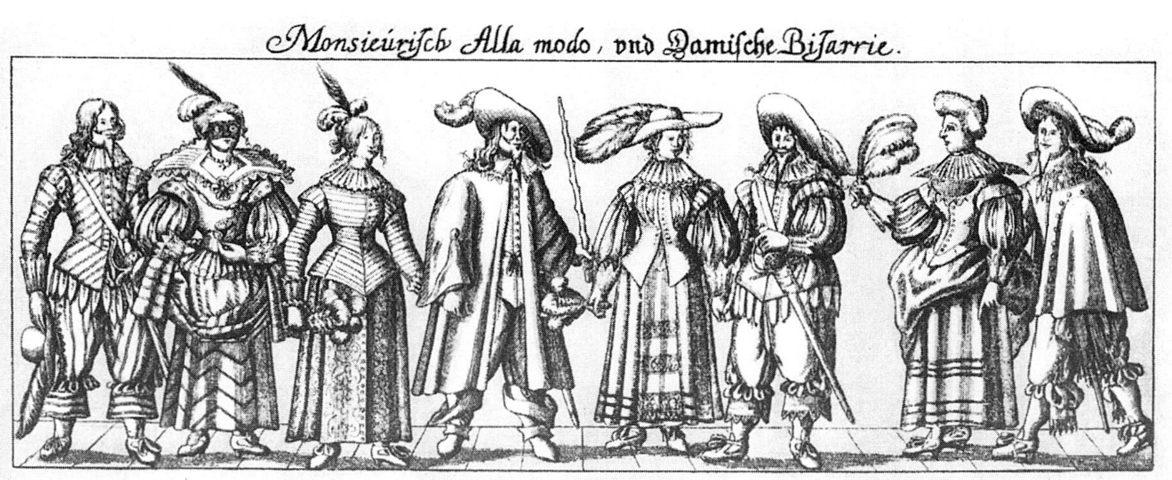

"Alla modo" Costume

ENGLAND
Time of Elizabeth and
Mary Queen of Scots
1550–1605

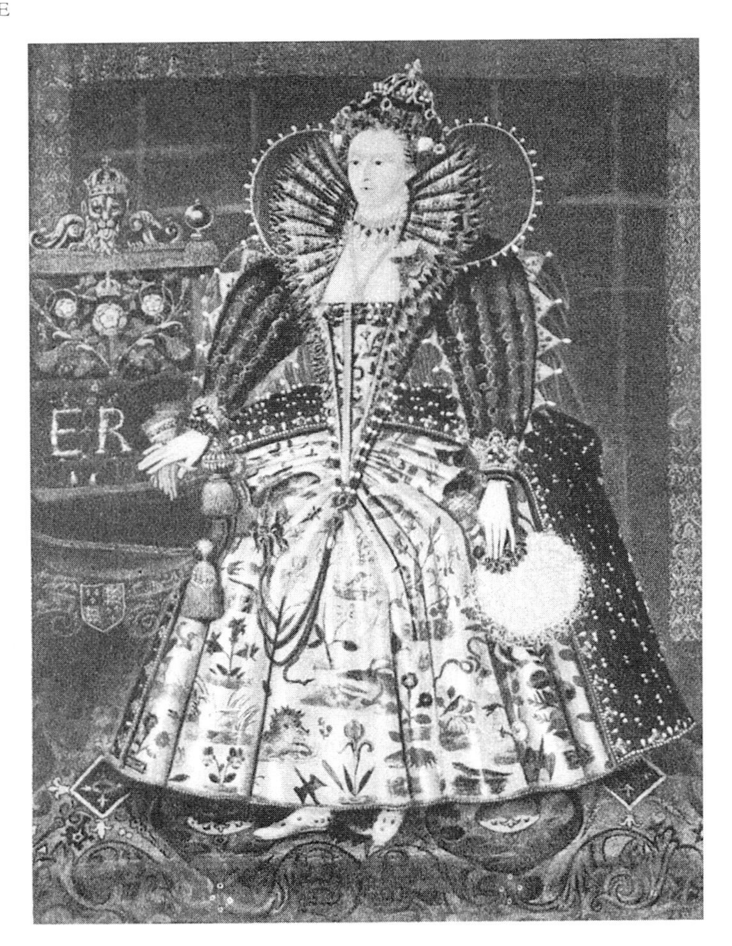

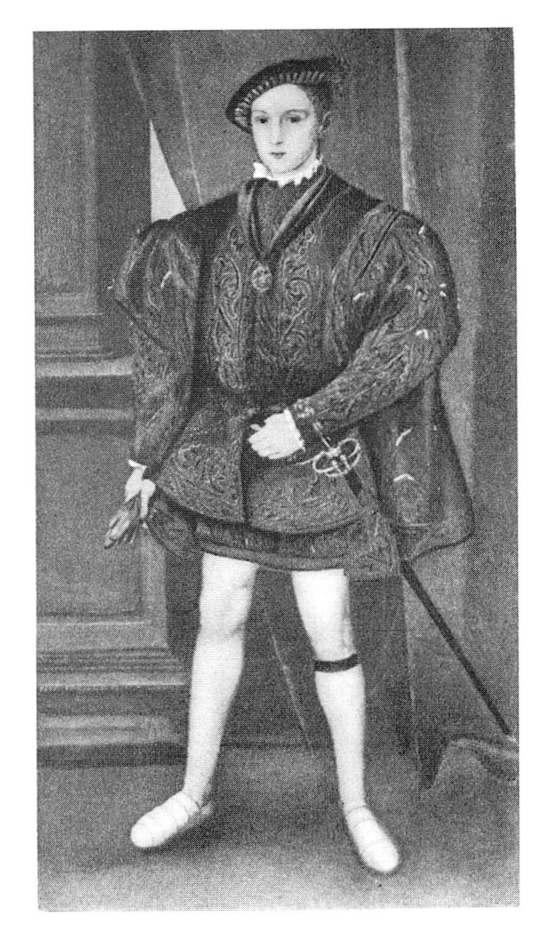

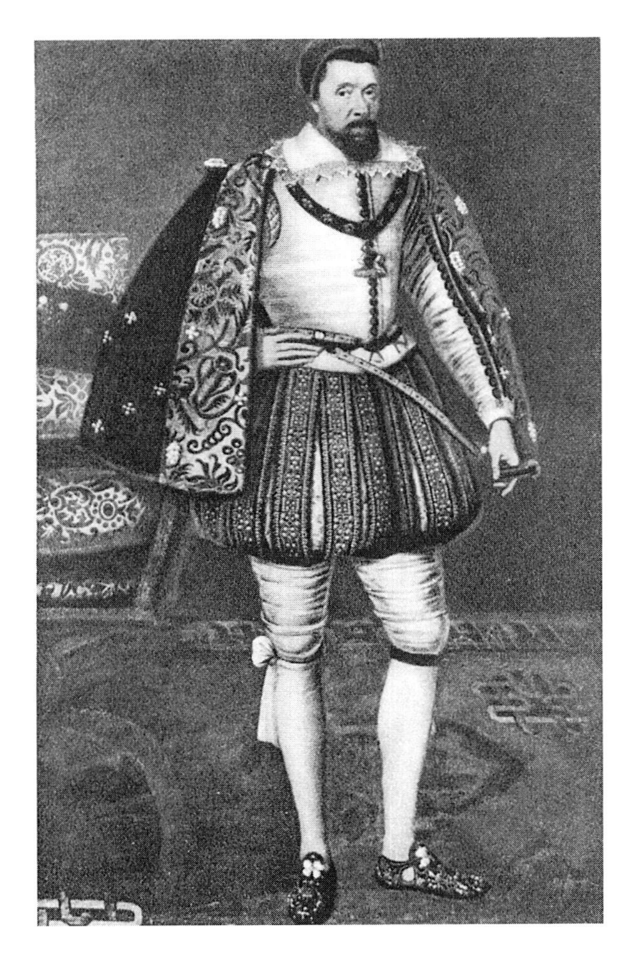

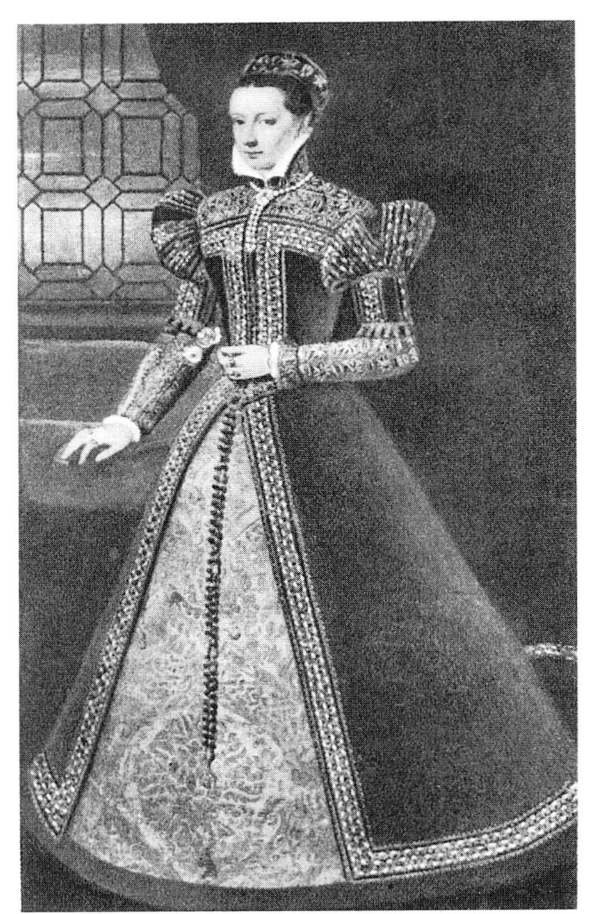

SPAIN
Time of Philip IV.
1630–1660

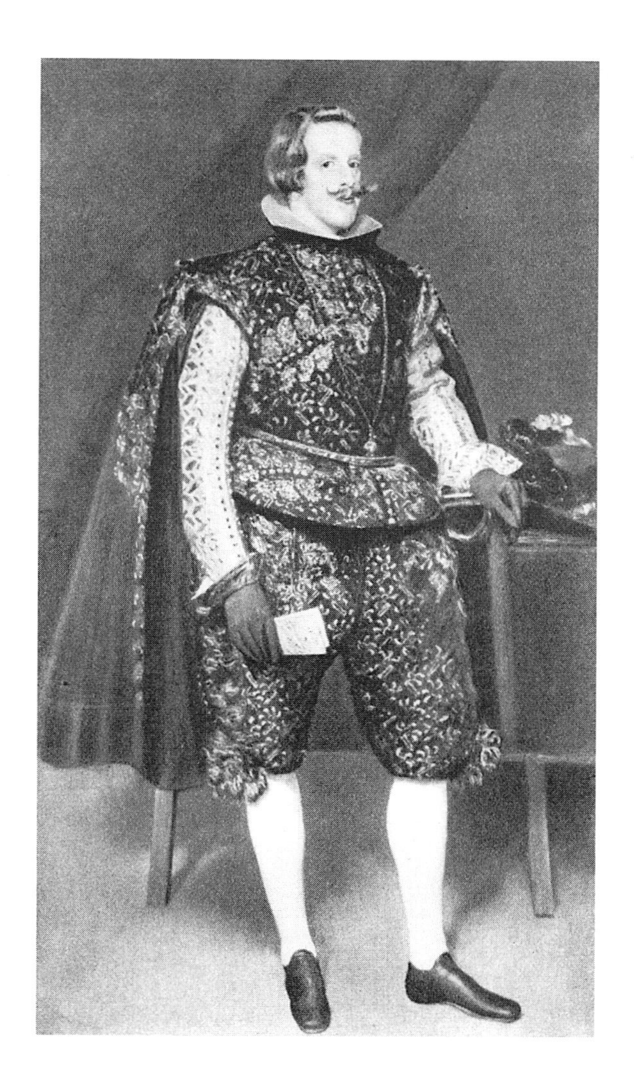

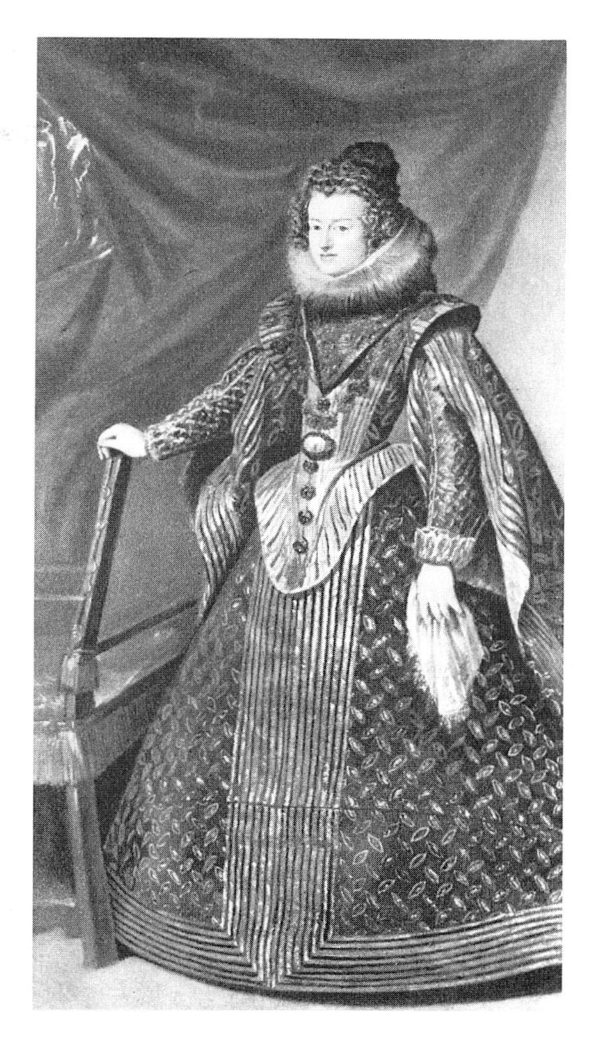

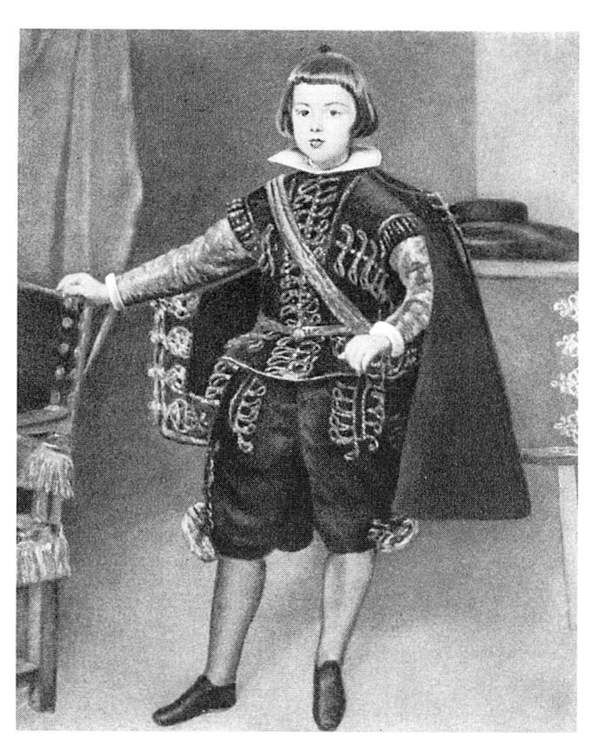

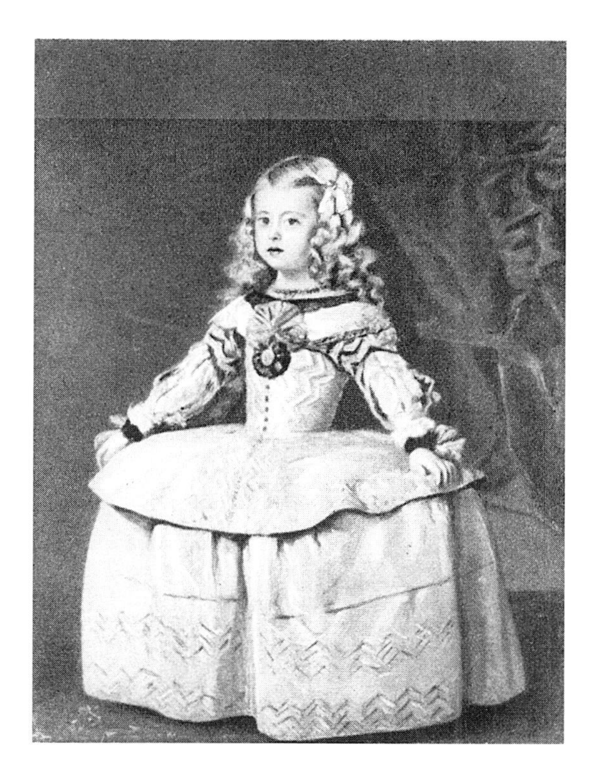

TURKEY

Turkey about 1575

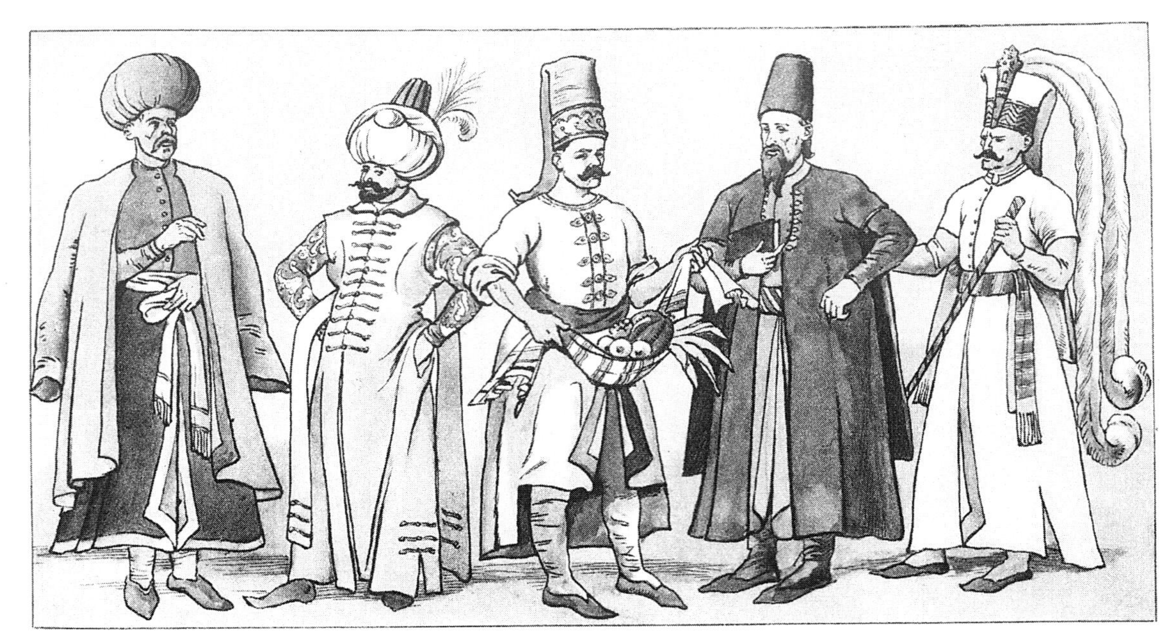

1 2 3 4 5

Turkey about 1575

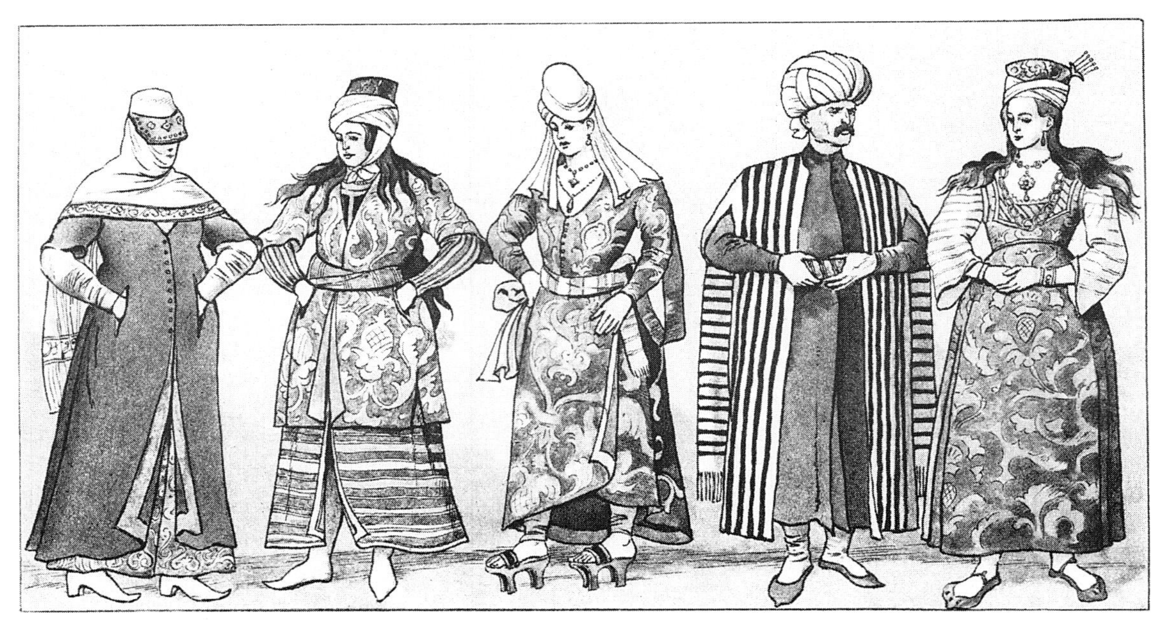

6 7 8 9 10

Women of the Seraglio, Dervish, etc.

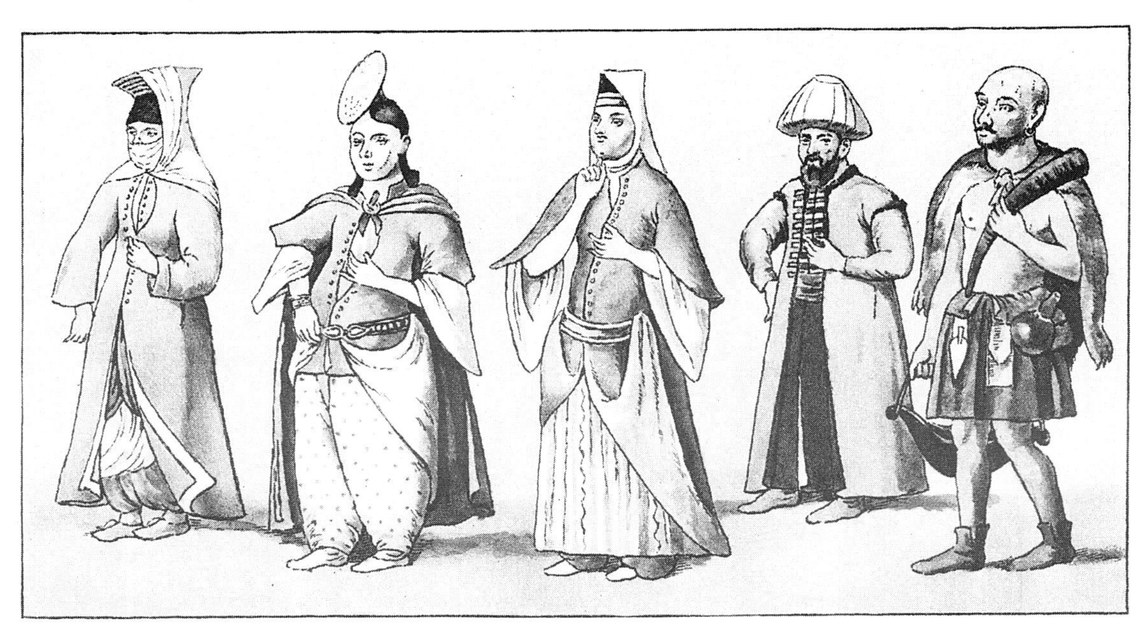

11 12 13 14 15

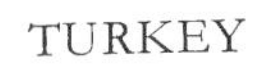

TURKEY

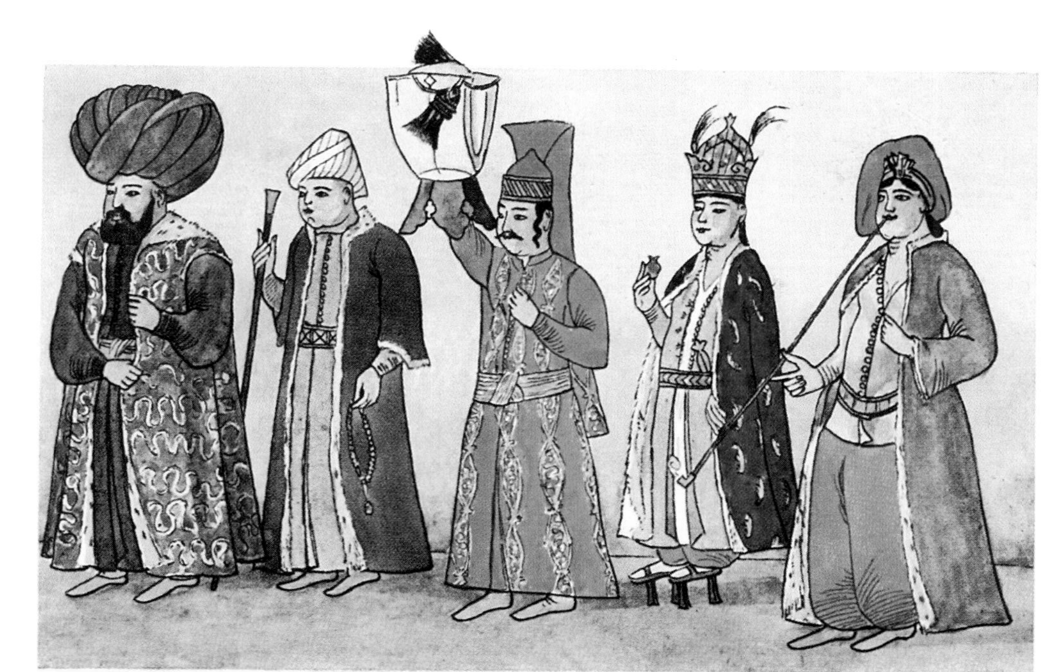

Officials, etc.

1 2 3 4 5

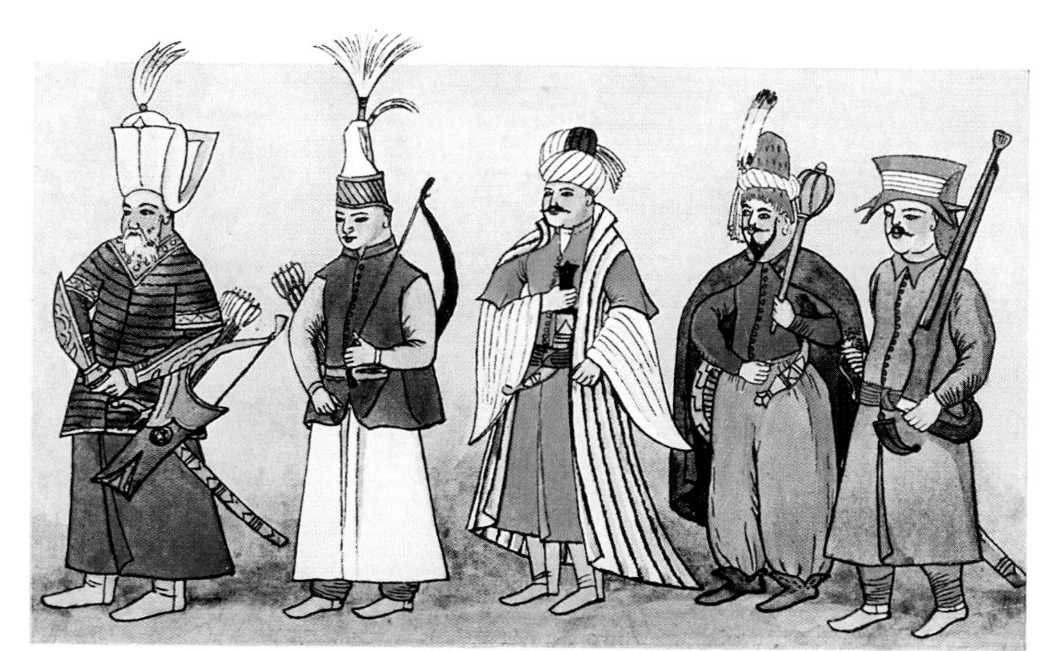

Officers and Soldiers

6 7 8 9 10

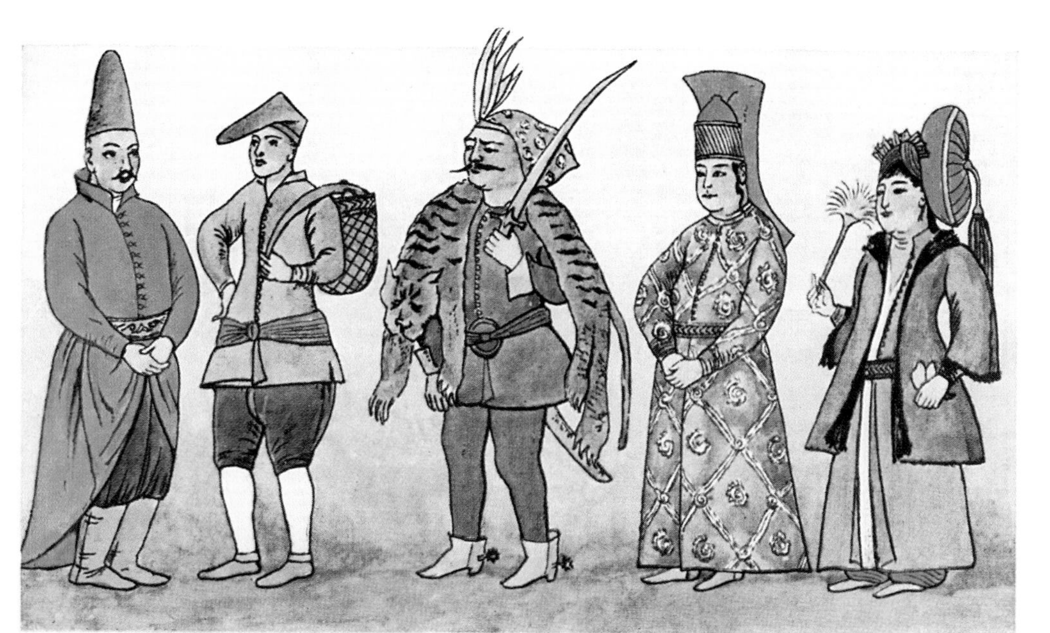

Sultan's Retinue

11 12 13 14 15

EUROPE

Military Costume during the Thirty Years' War 1600–1650

Musketeers and Pikemen 1600–1615

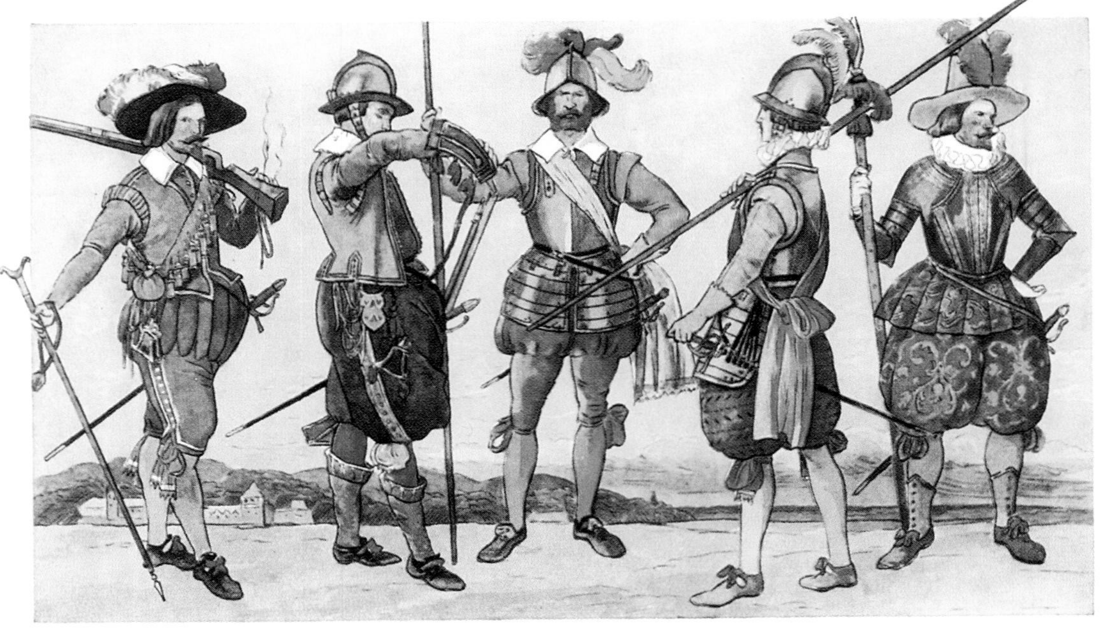

1 2 3 4 5

Commanders about 1630–1635

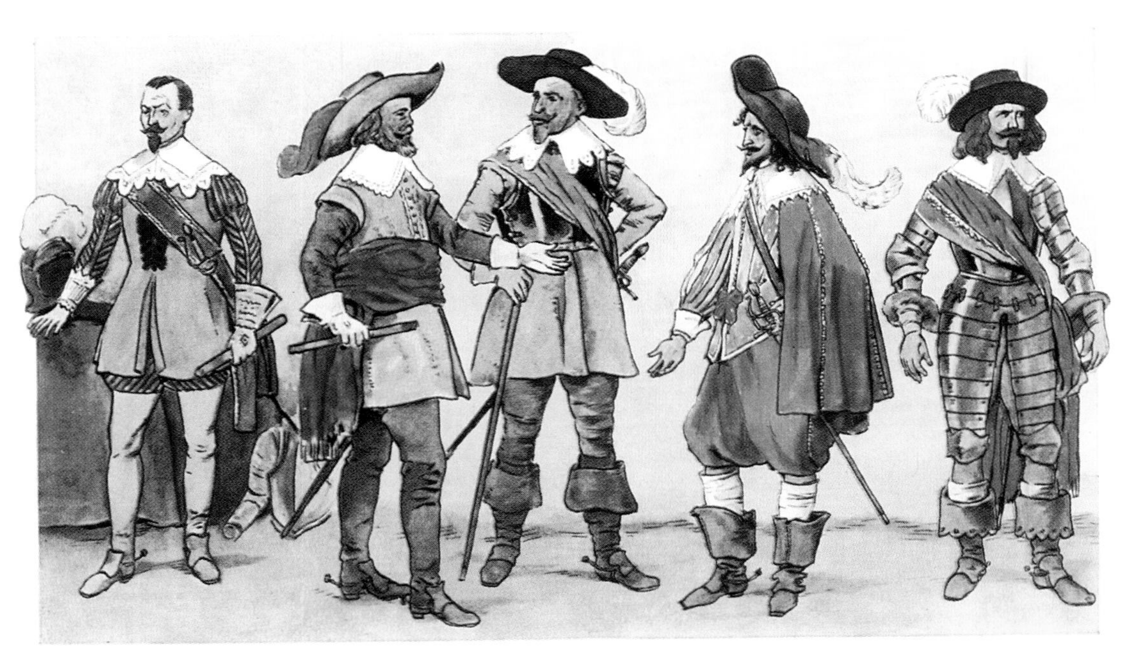

6 7 8 9 10

Soldiers and Officers 1635–1650

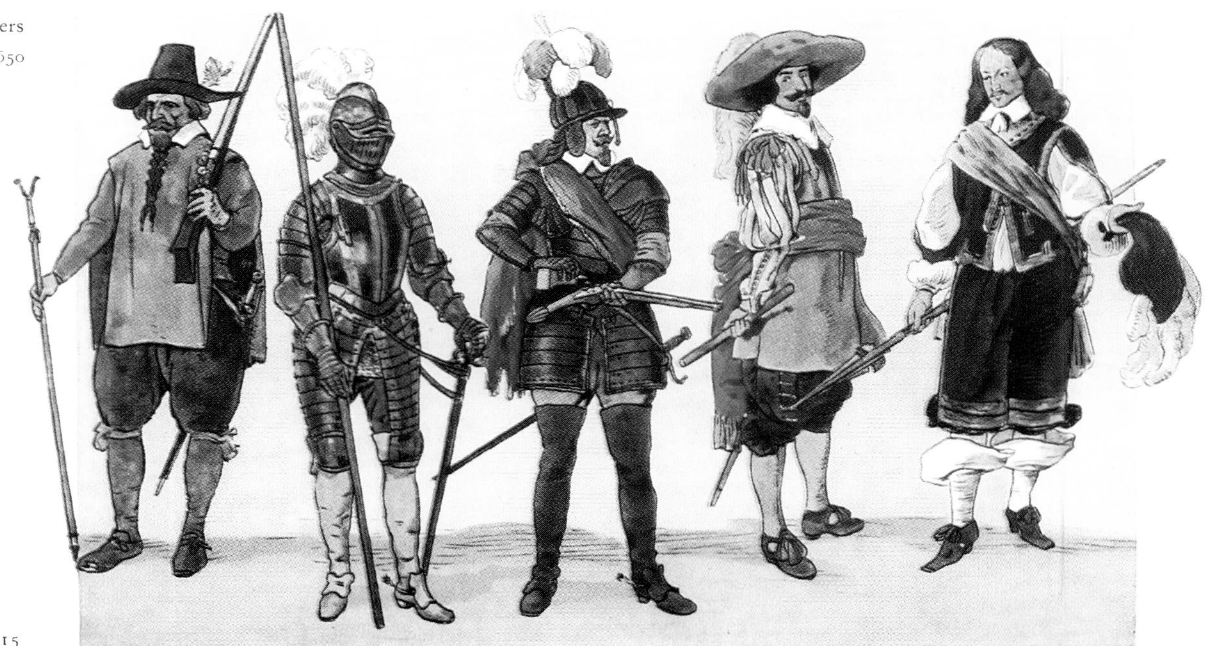

11 12 13 14 15

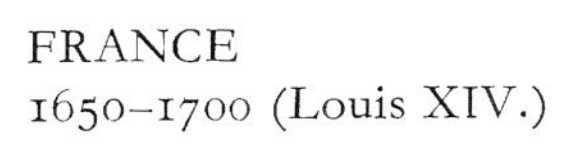

FRANCE
1650–1700 (Louis XIV.)

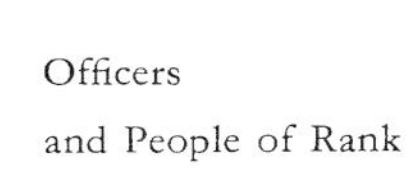

Officers
and People of Rank

1 2 3 4 5 6

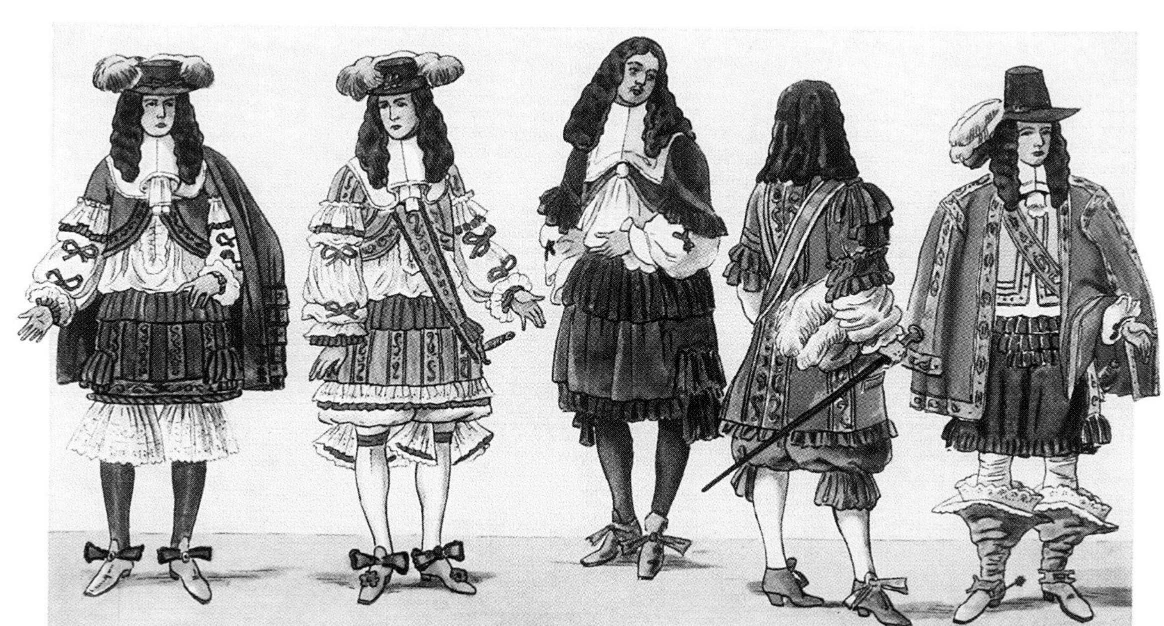

Louis XIV.
and People of Rank

7 8 9 10 11

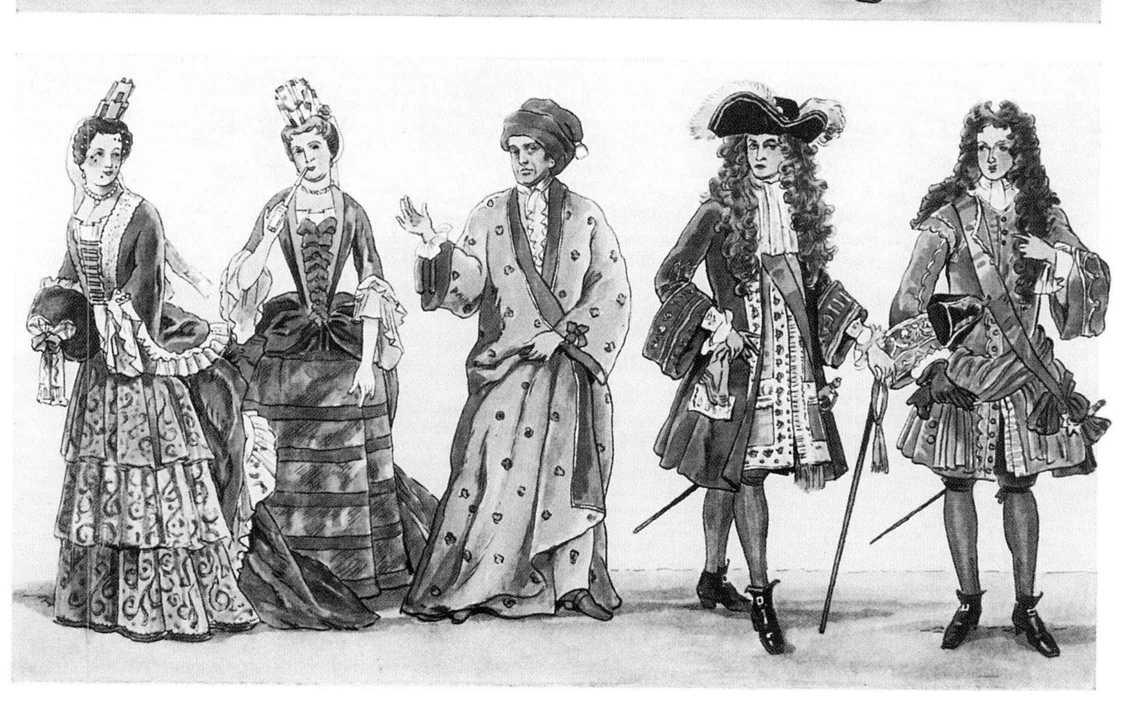

12 13 14 15 16

FRANCE
Theatre and Dancers

Italian Comedy about 1715

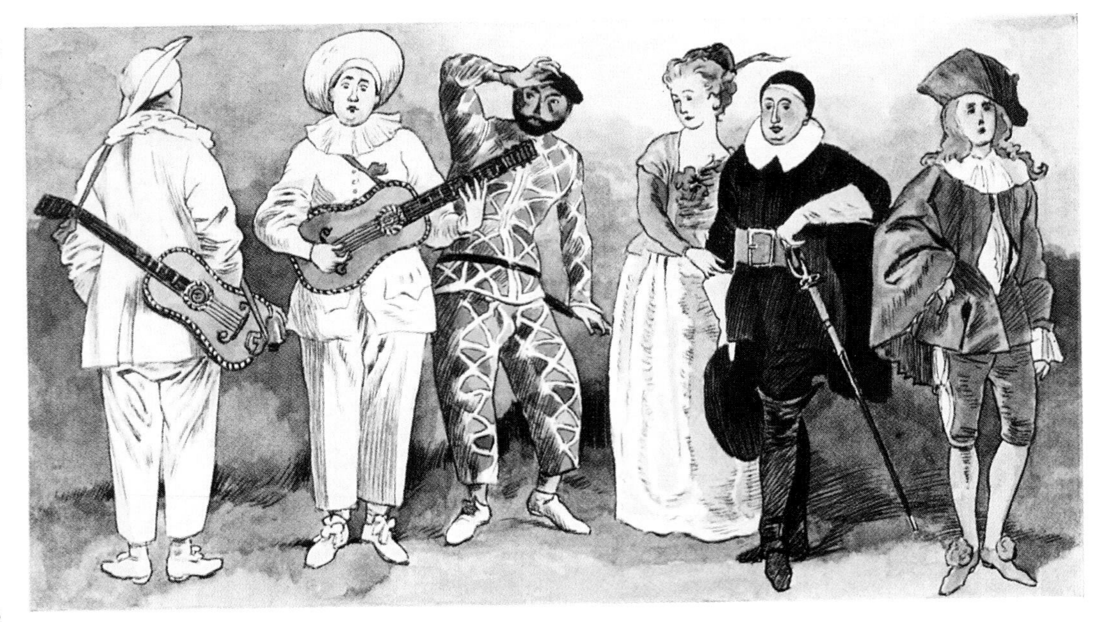

1 2 3 4 5 6

Dancers about 1725

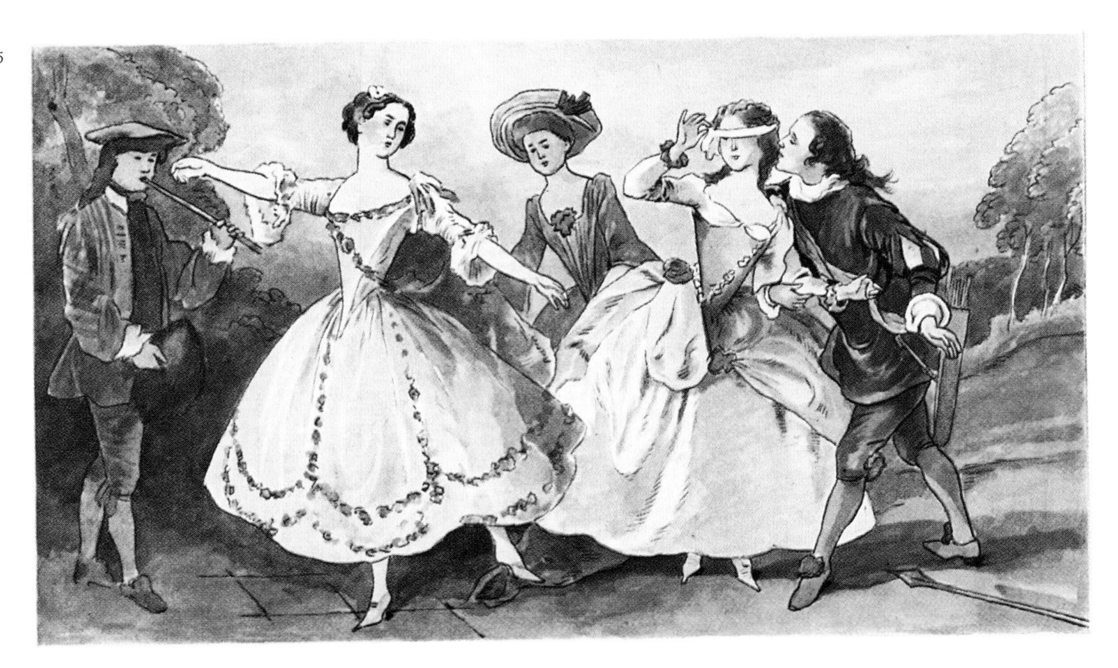

7 8 9 10 11

Dancers about 1730

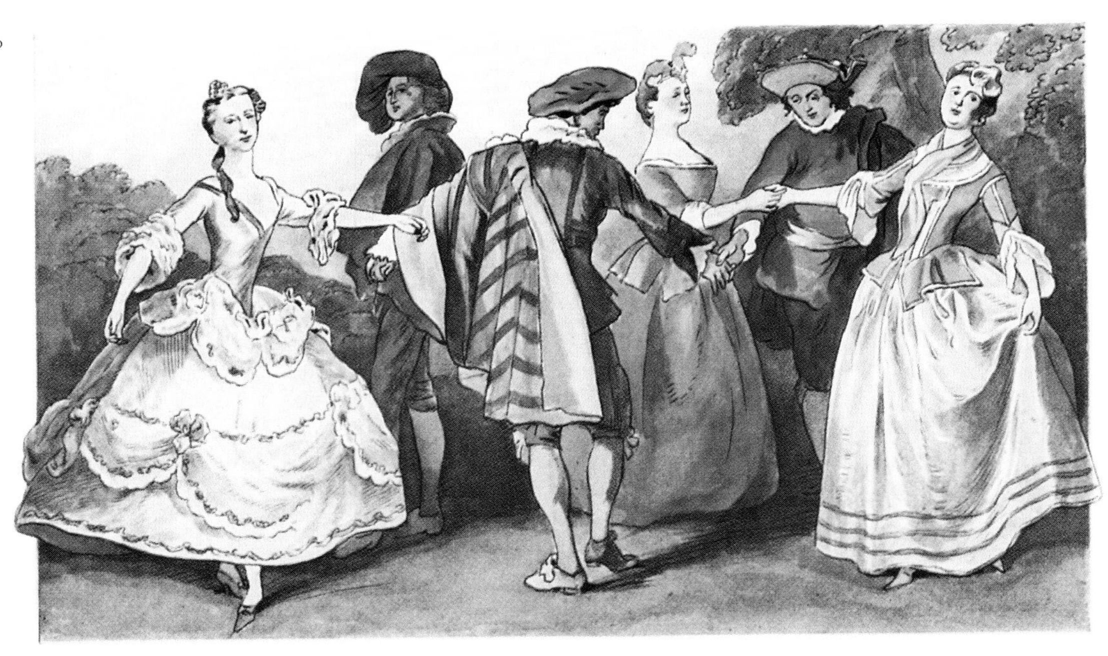

12 13 14 15 16 17

GERMANY
Citizen's Costume
1625–1675
Nuremberg, Augsburg, Cologne

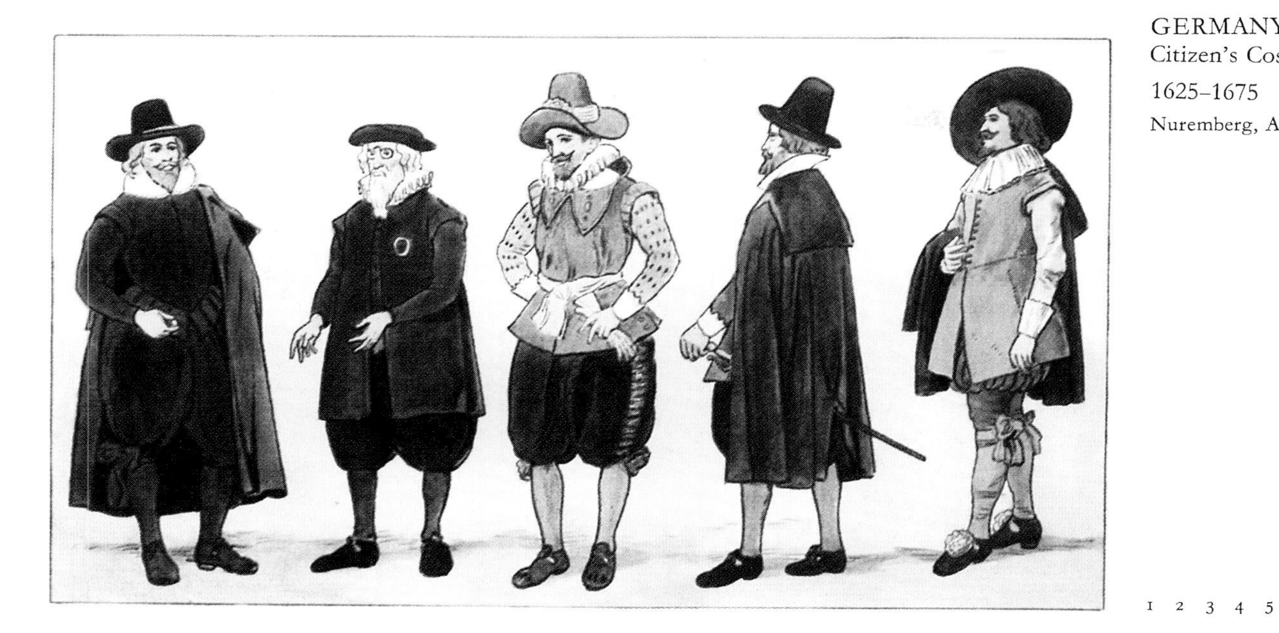

1 2 3 4 5

The "Rhinegrave"
Breeches in Germany, etc.

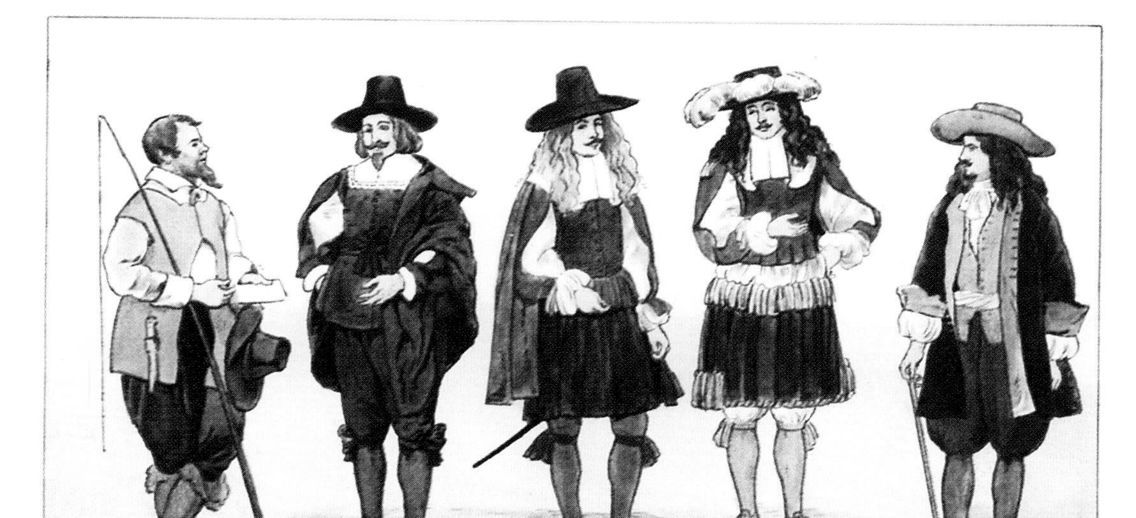

6 7 8 9 10

Augsburg and Strasburg
Women's Costume about 1640

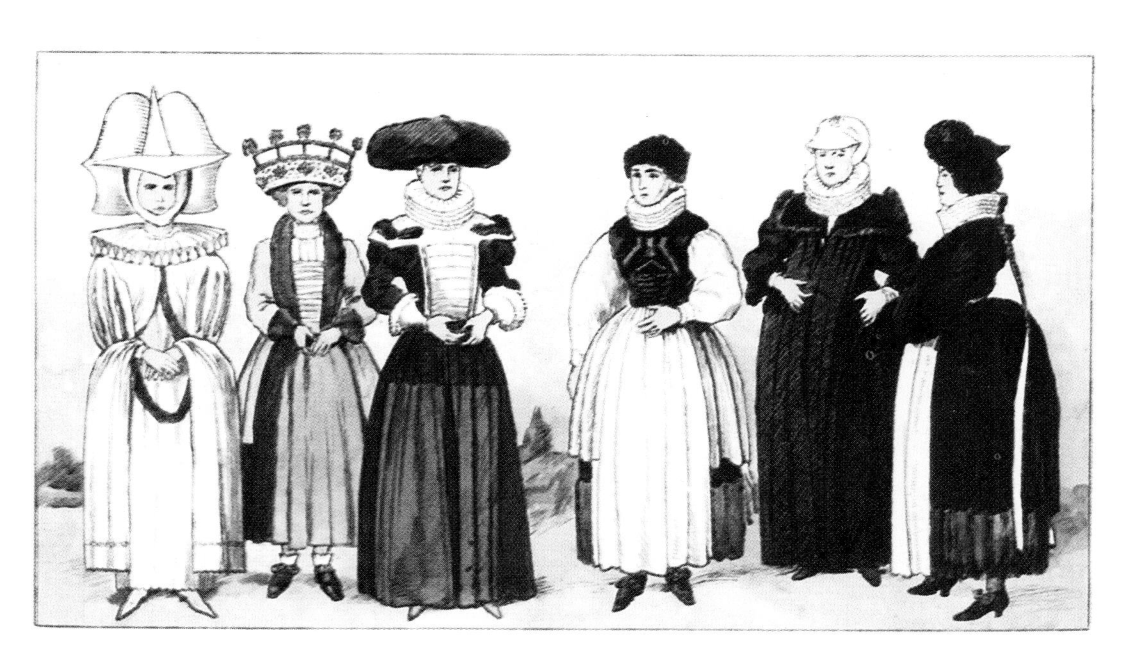

11 12 13 14 15 16

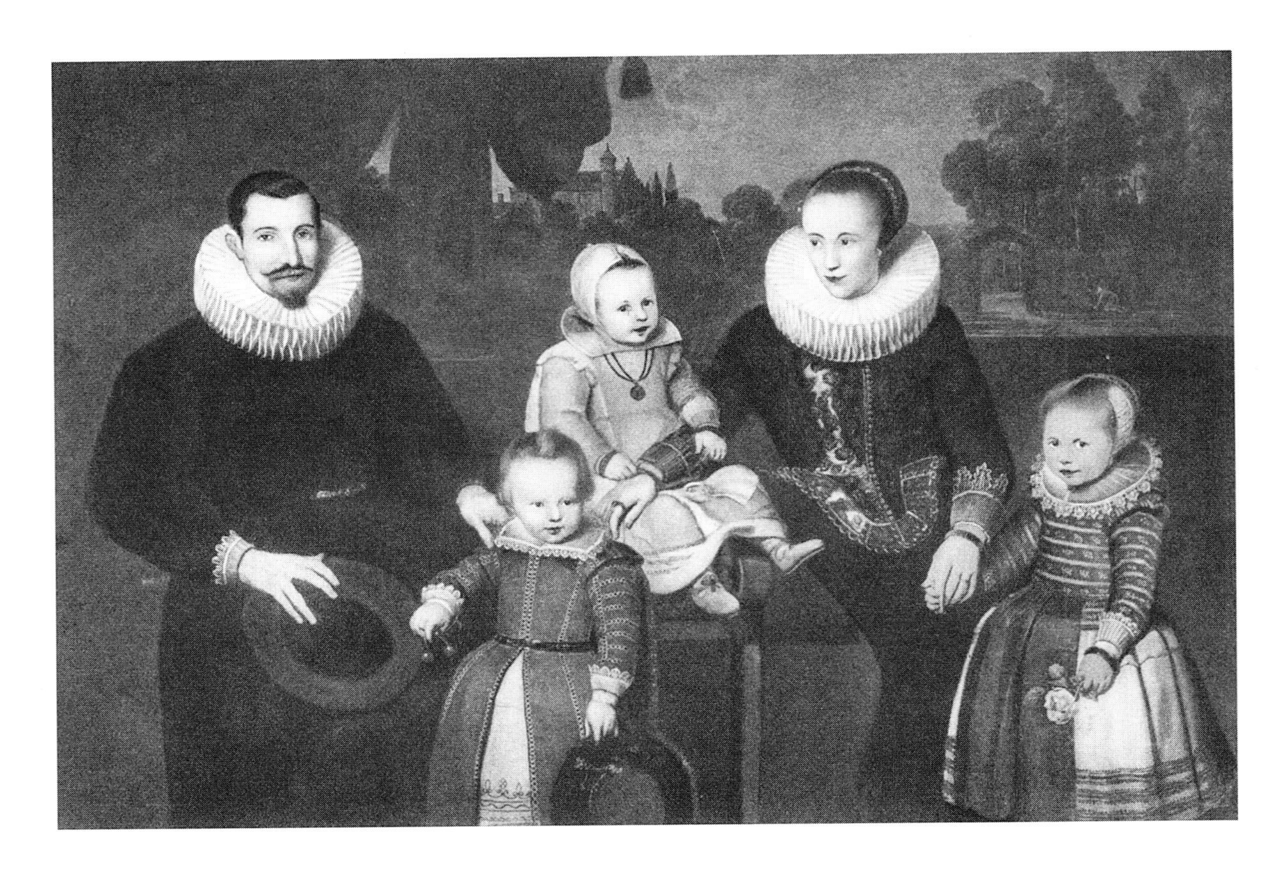

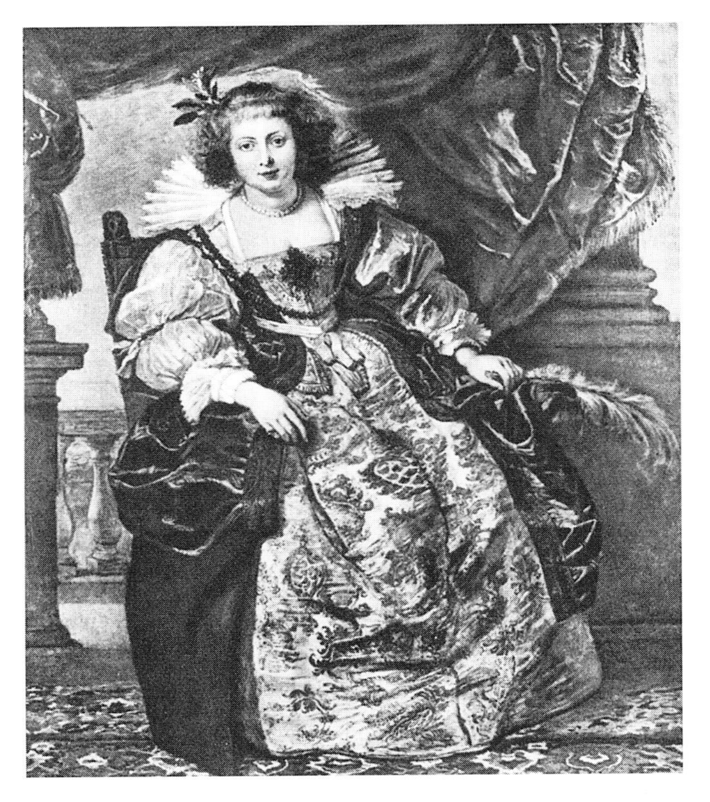

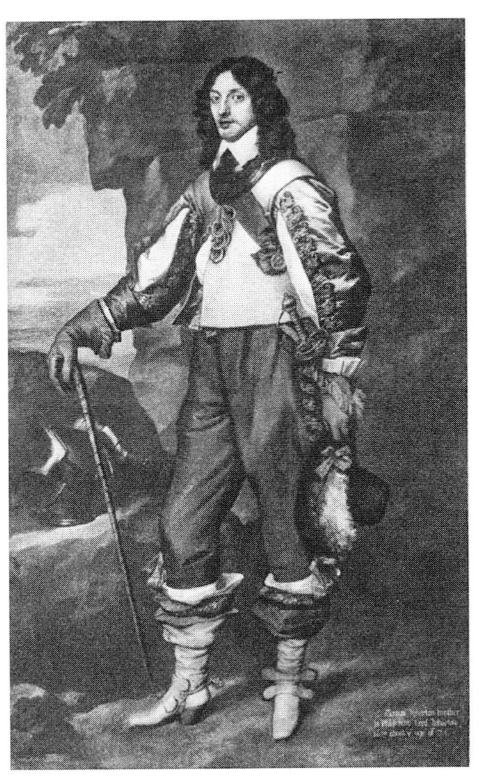

NETHERLANDS AND ENGLAND

NETHERLANDS
1650–1680

Dutch Citizens' Costume

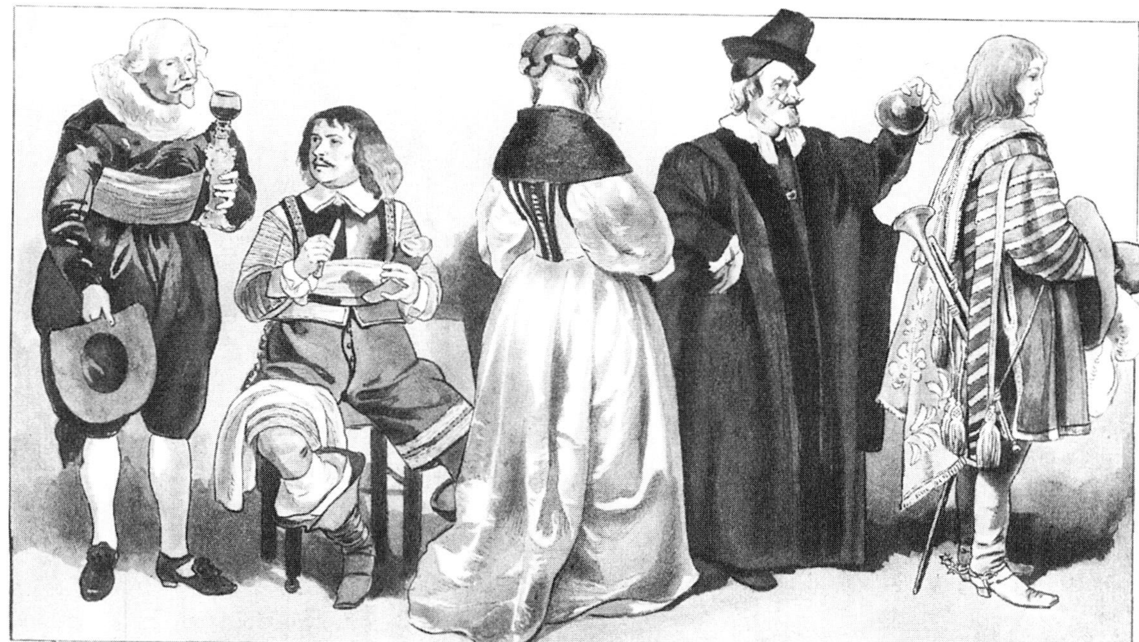

1 2 3 4 5

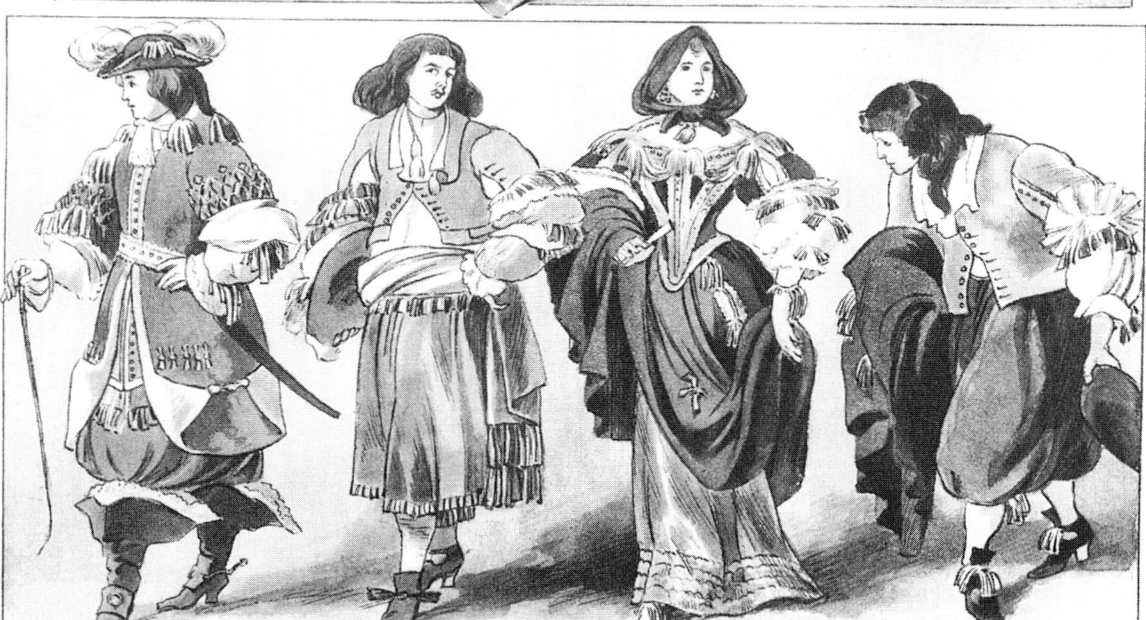

6 7 8 9

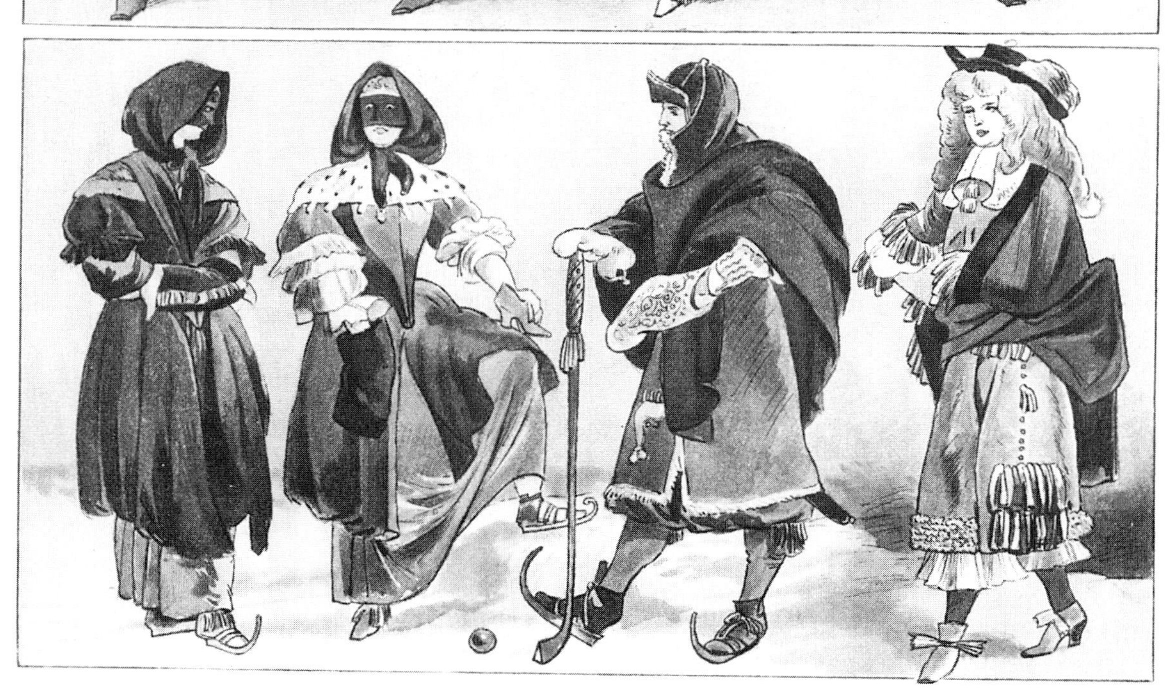

10 11 12 13

NETHERLANDS
Head-dresses,
Hair Styles;
Collars and Ruffs

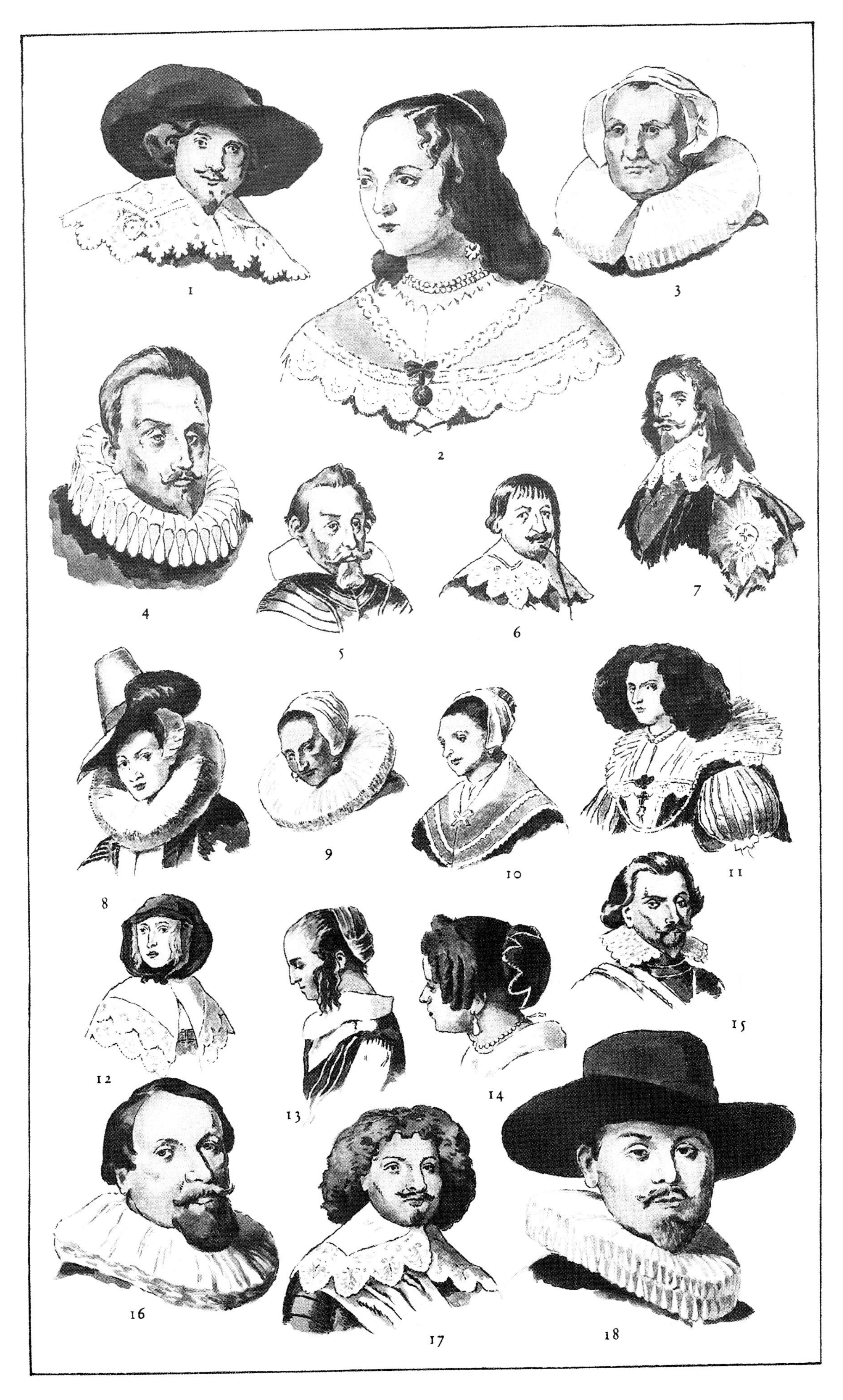

ENGLAND
about 1640

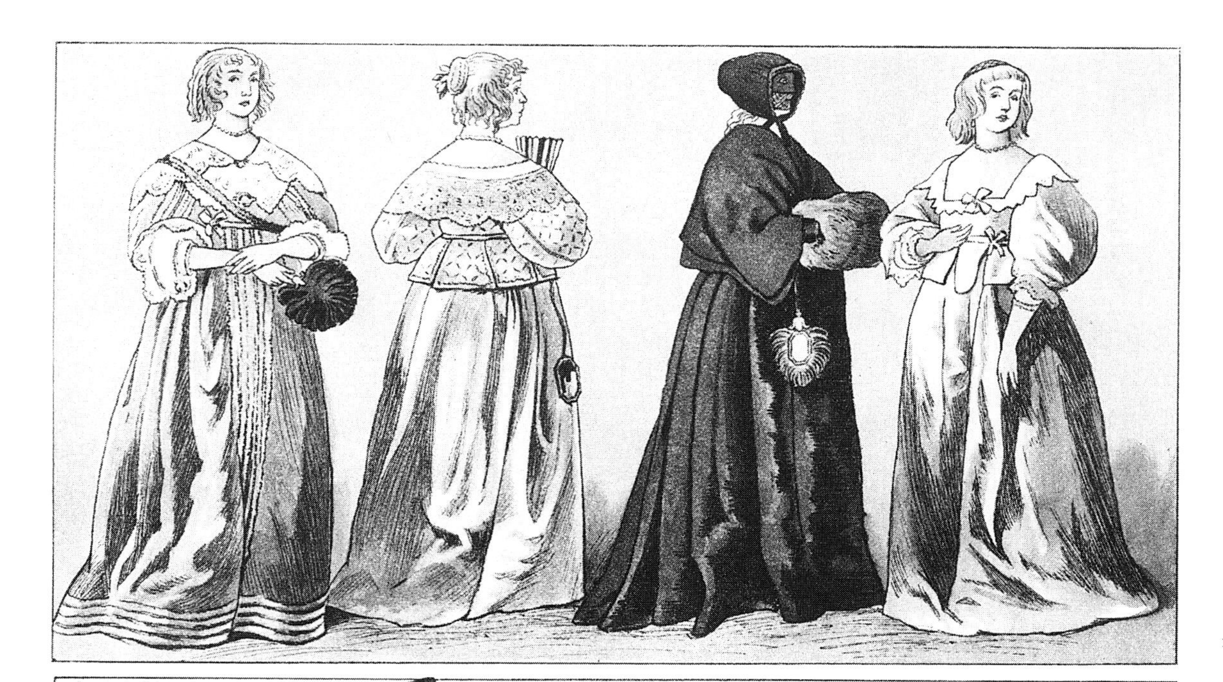

Noble Ladies

1 2 3 4

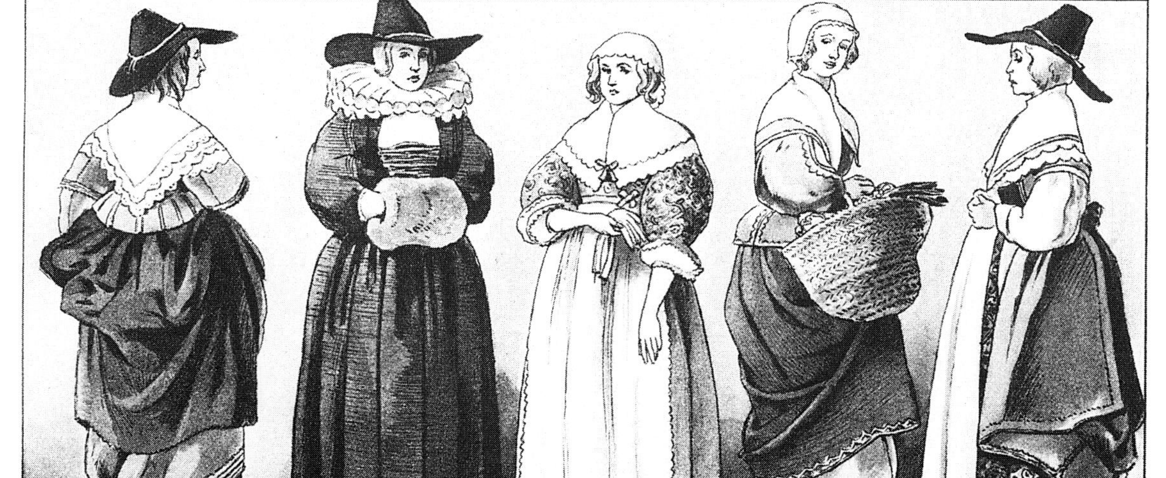

Citizens' and Craftsmen's Wives

5 6 7 8 9

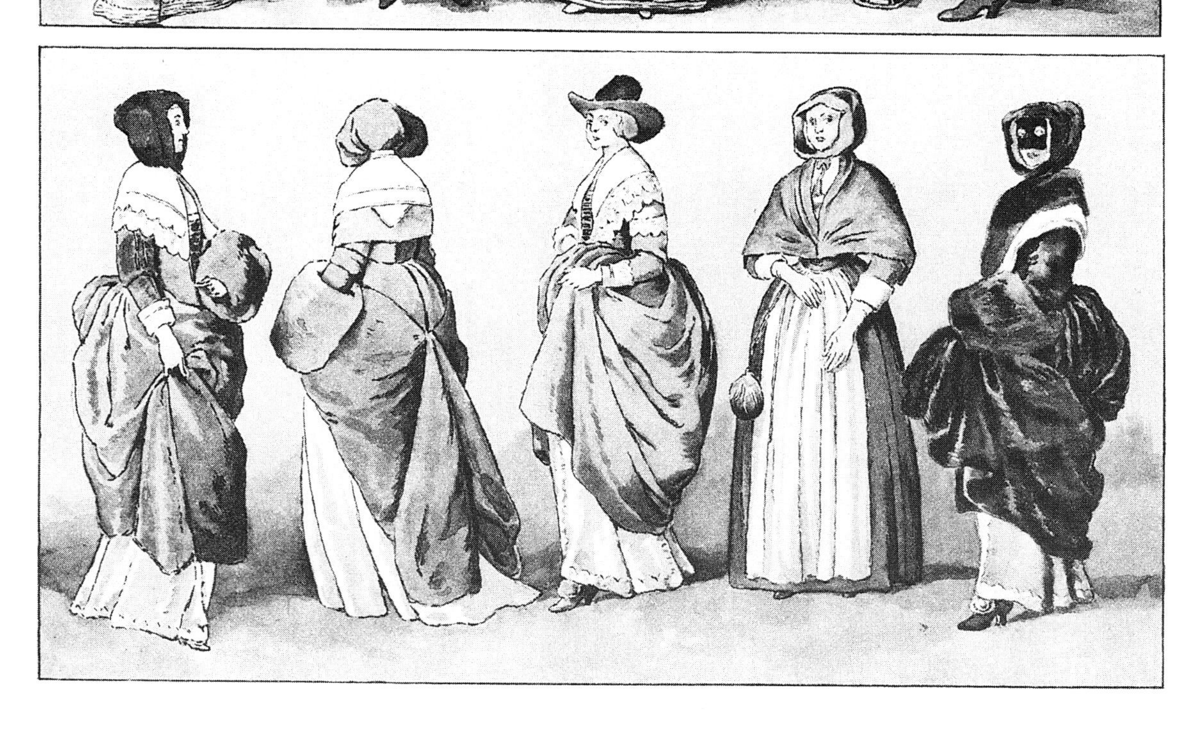

Noble Ladies

10 11 12 13 14

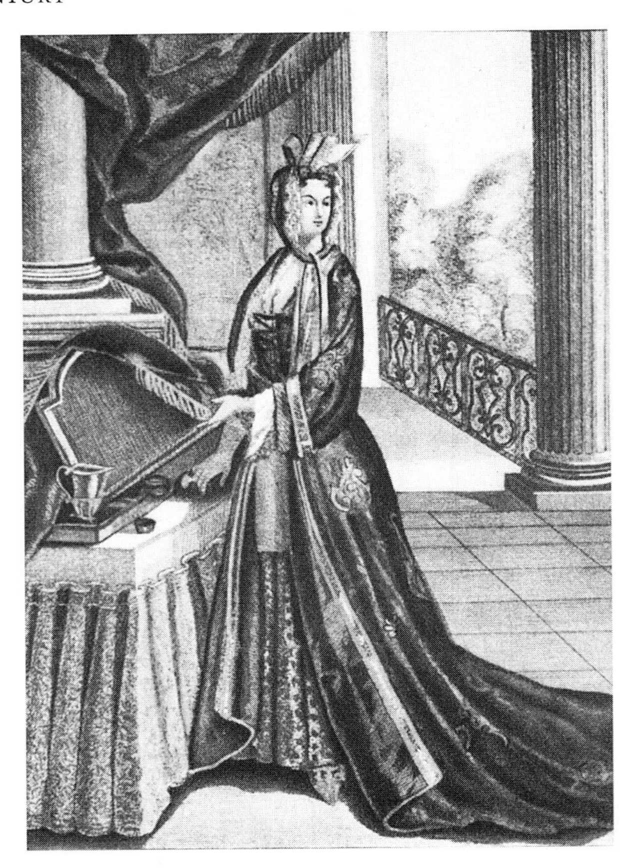

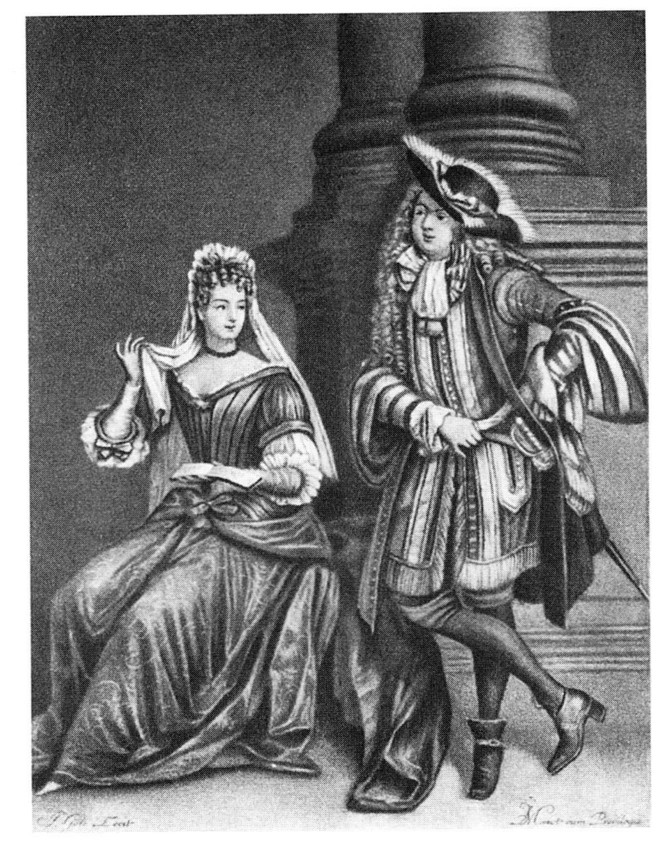

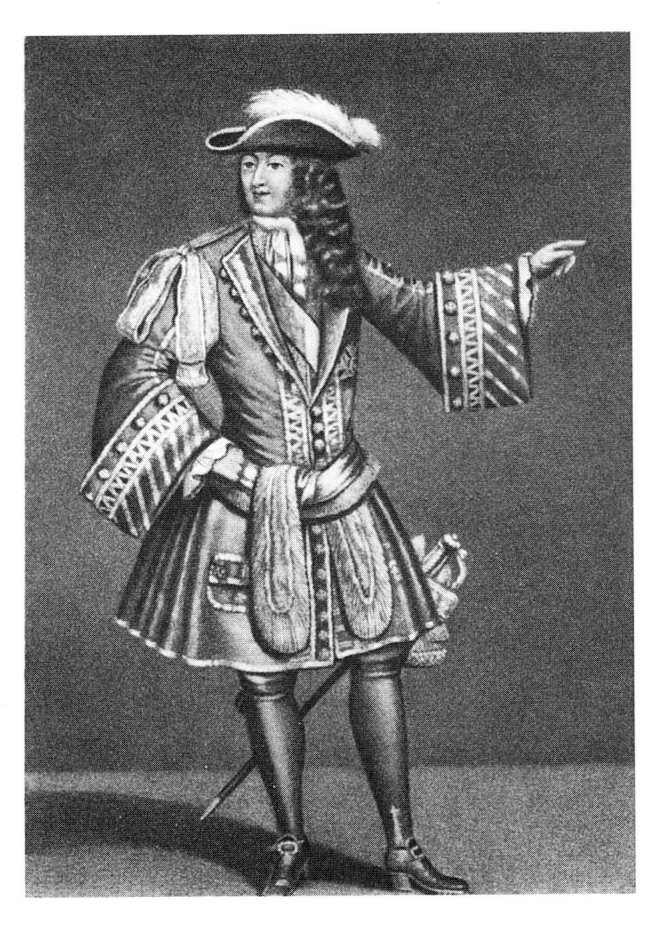

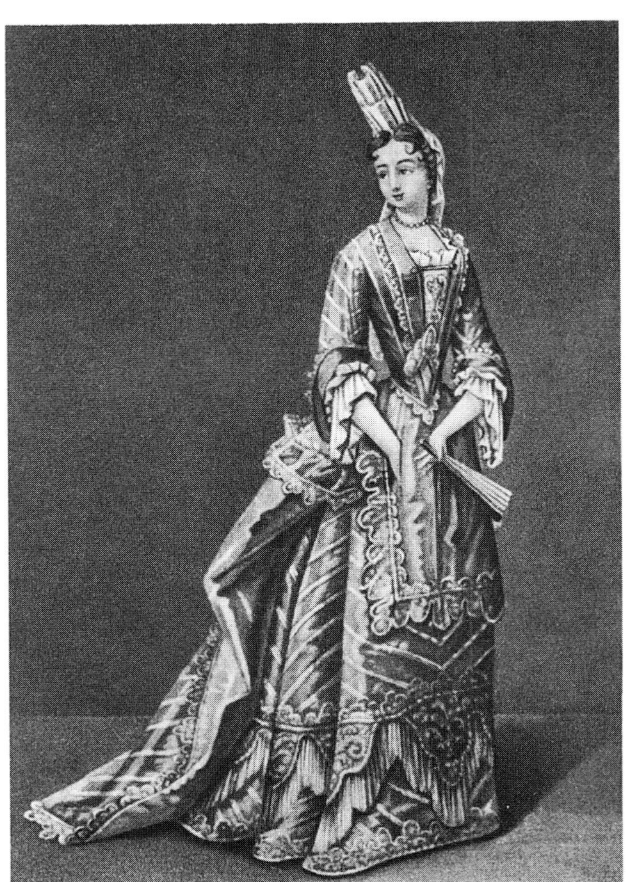

Time of Louis XIV. about 1700 (Court Dress at Versailles)

FRANCE
1695–1700

Paris Citizens' Costume

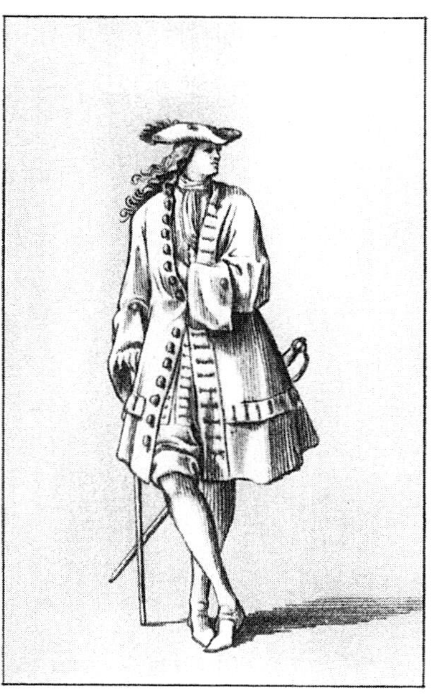
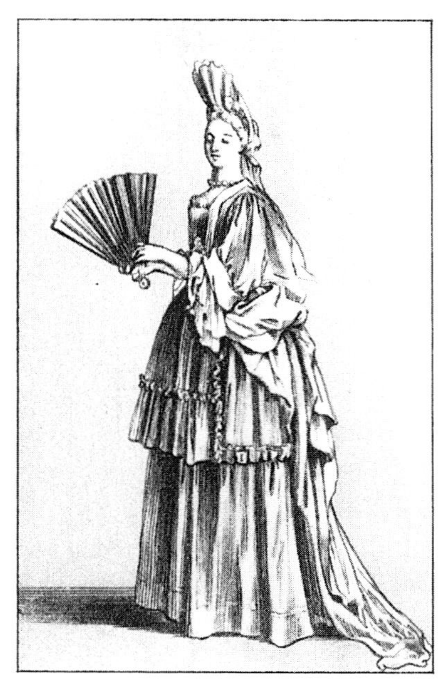
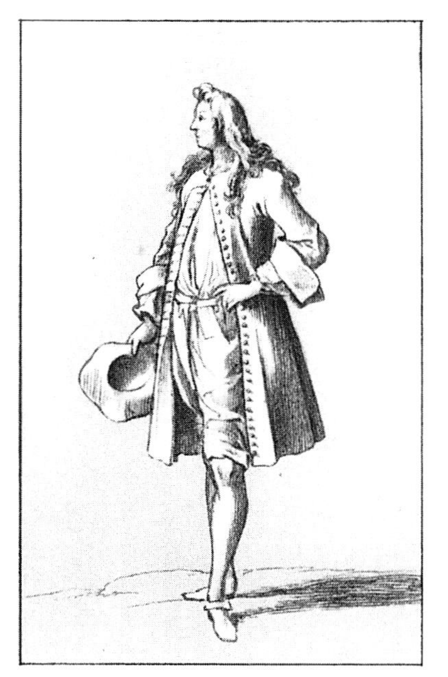
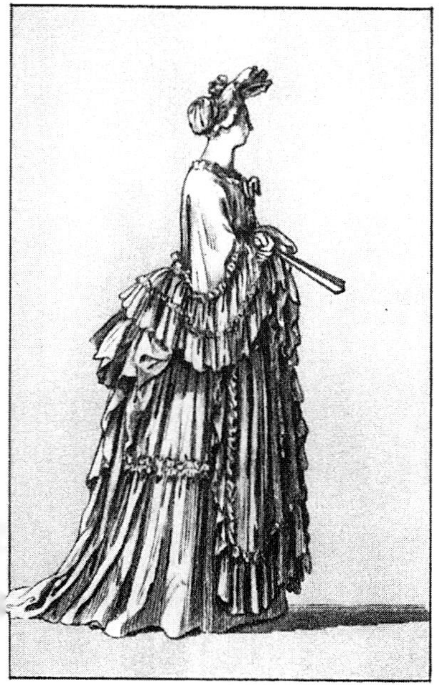
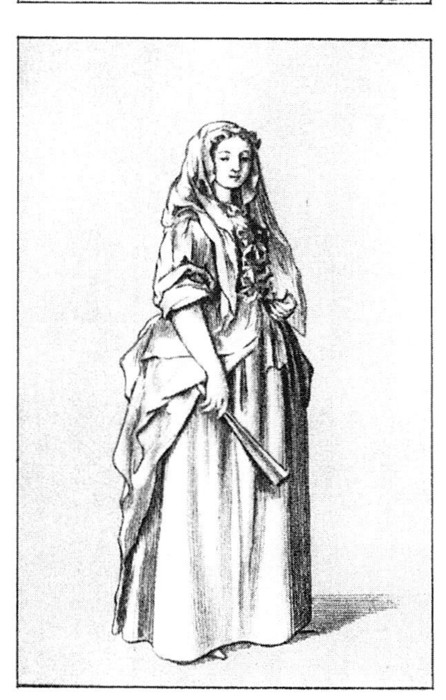
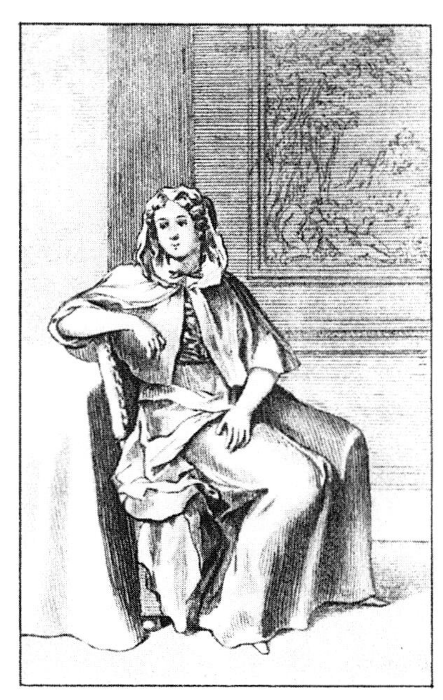
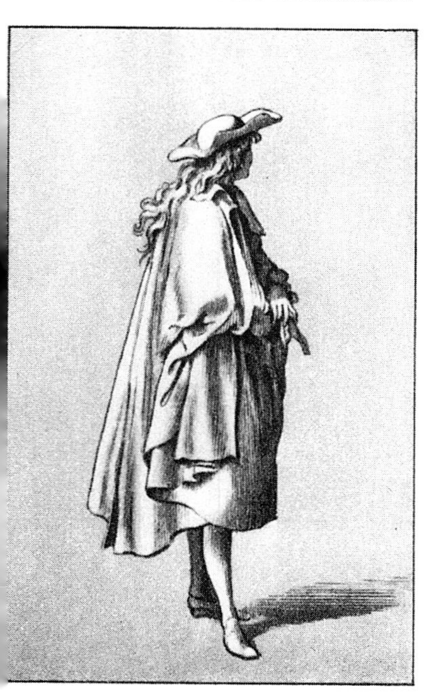
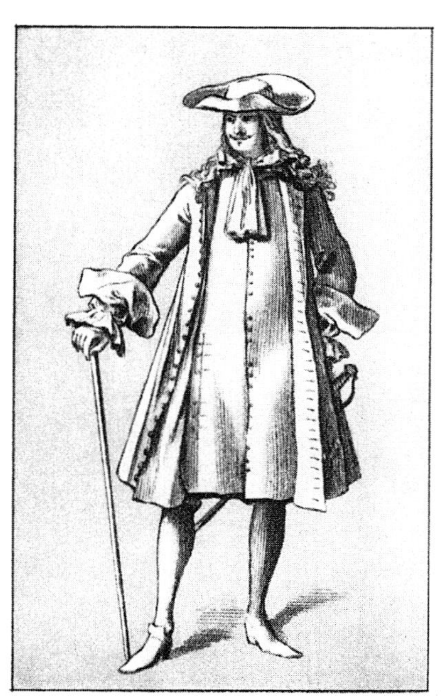
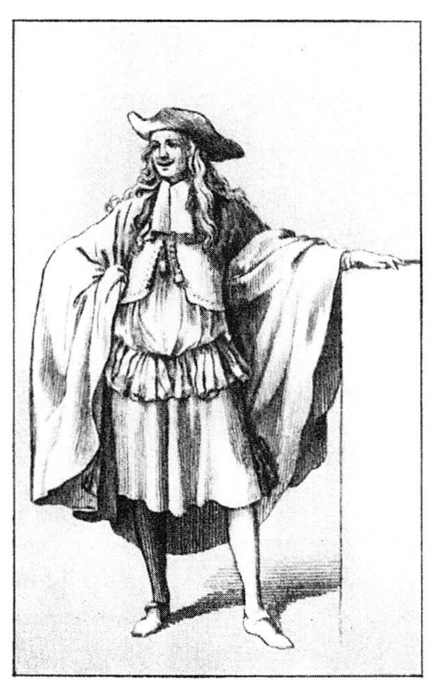

FRANCE
1715–1720

Paris Citizens

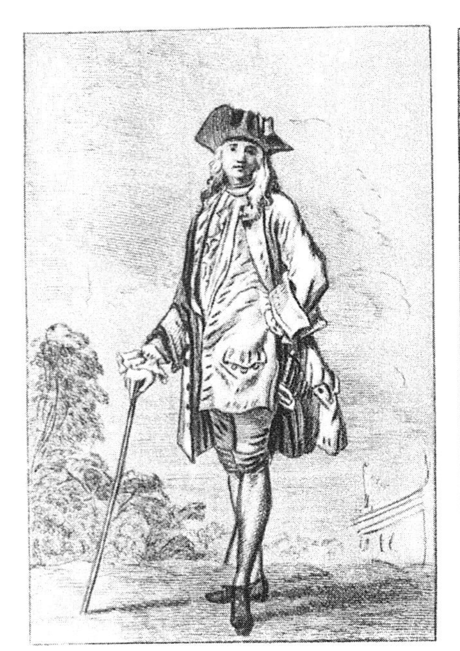
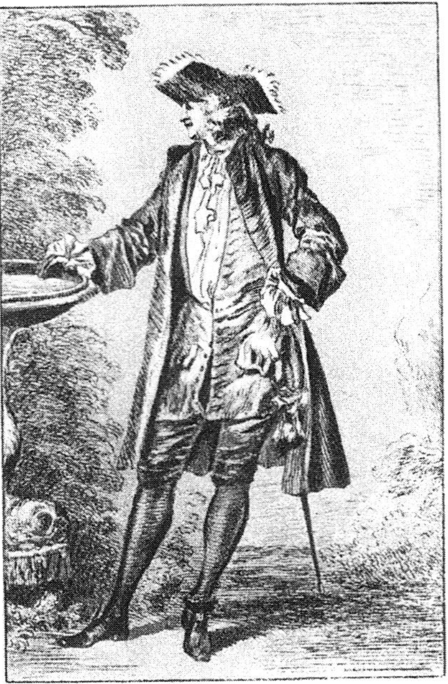
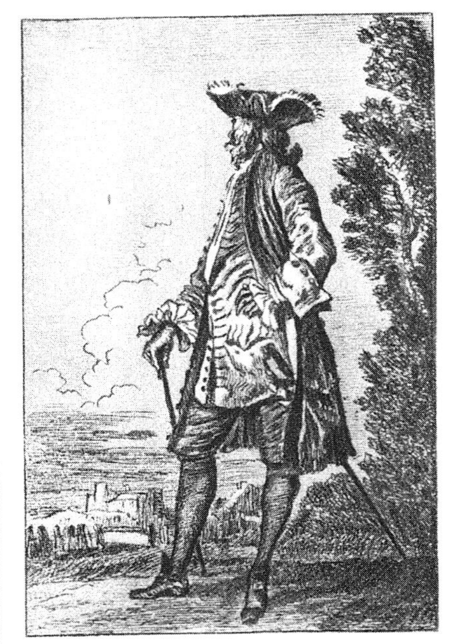
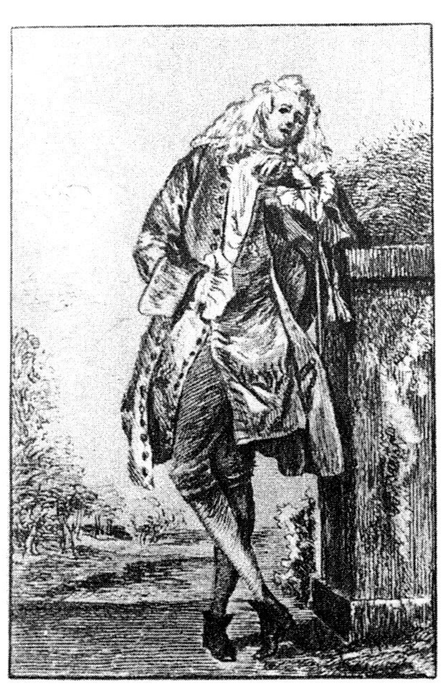
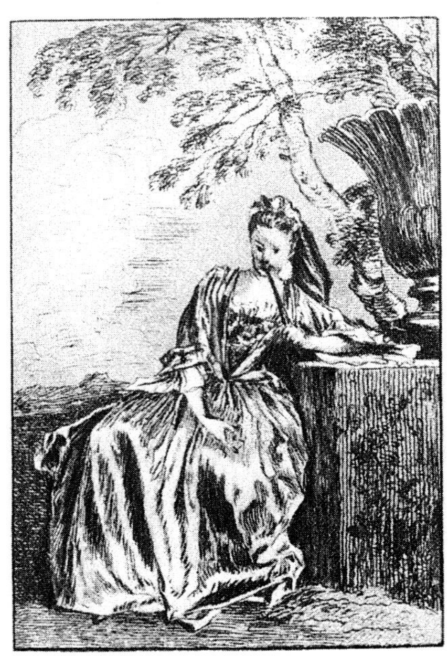
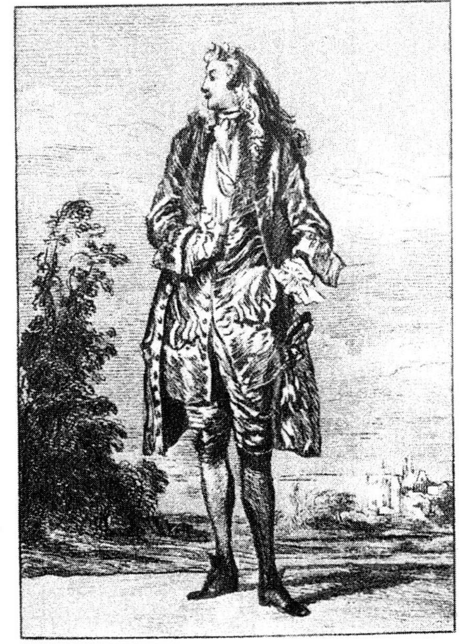
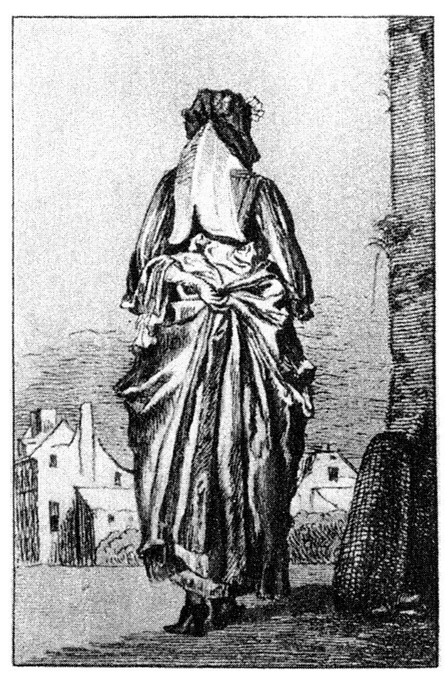
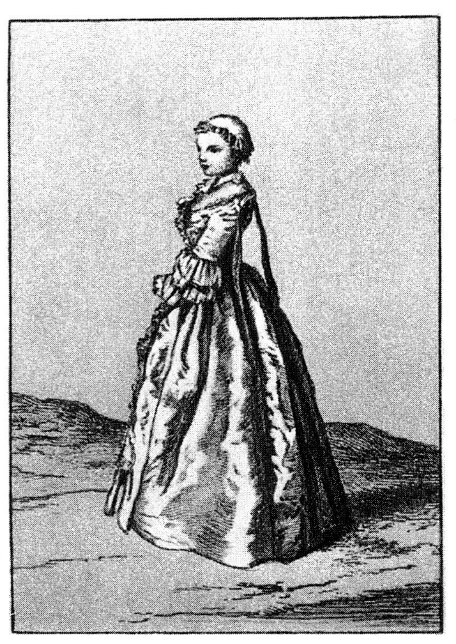
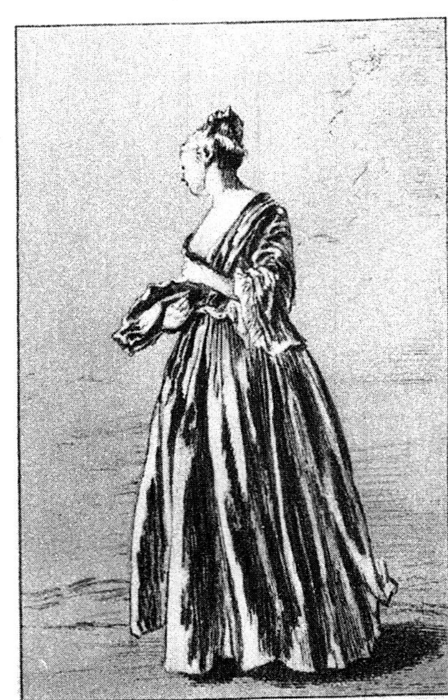

ITALIAN COMEDY
1680–1730

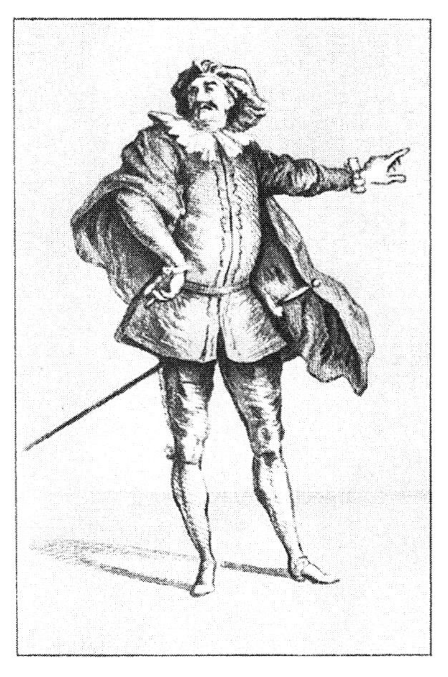
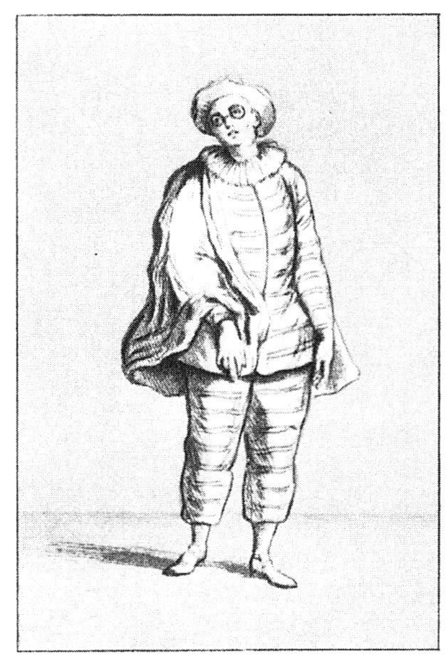
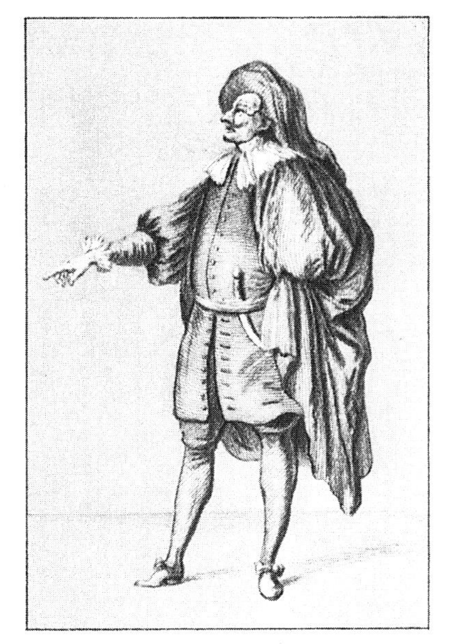
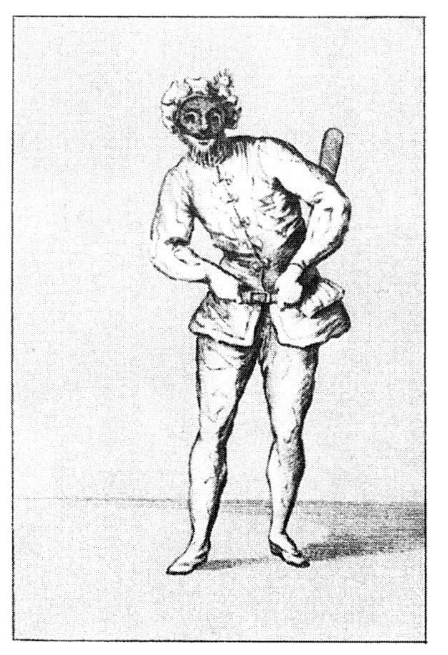
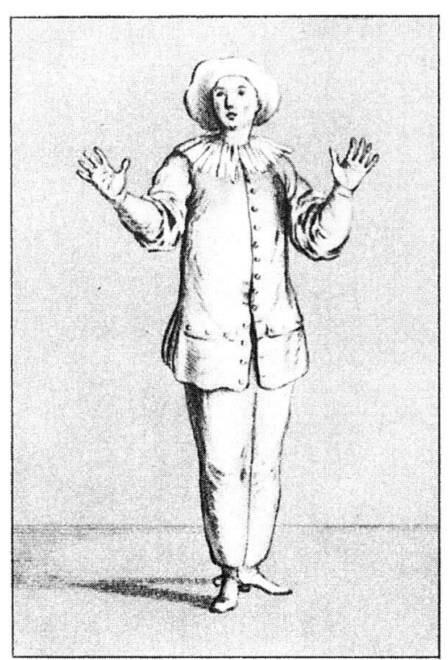
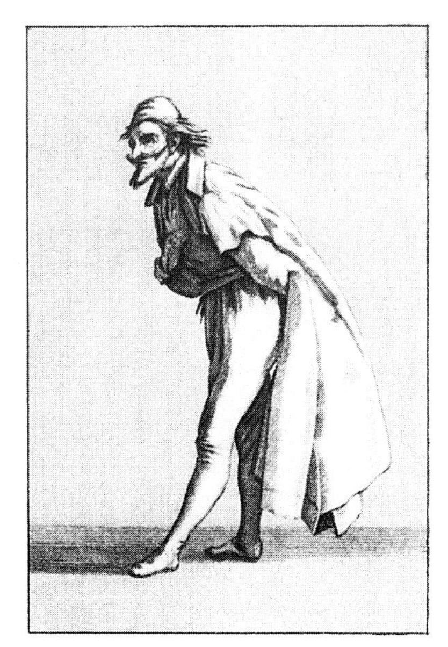
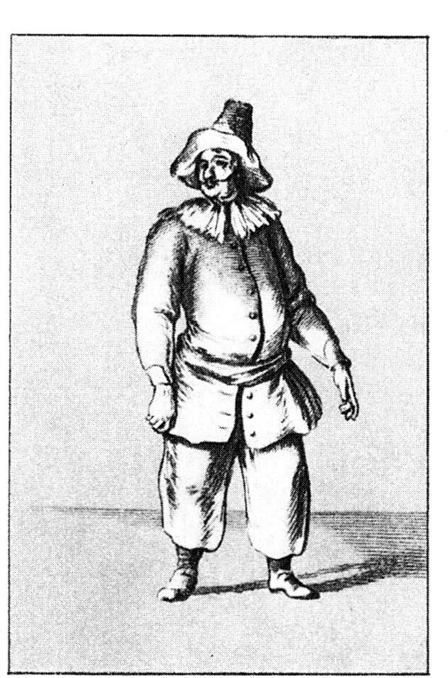
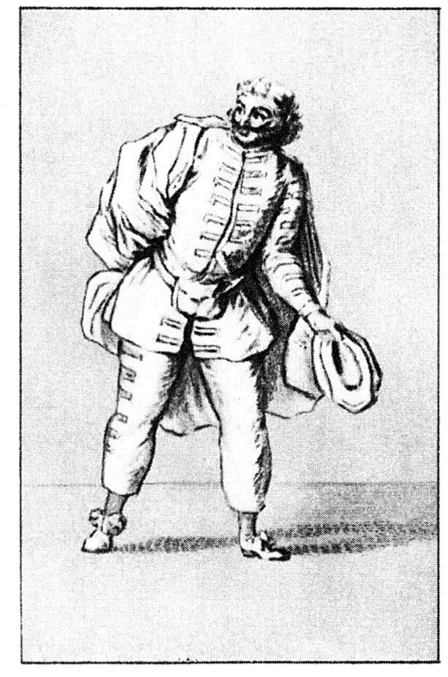
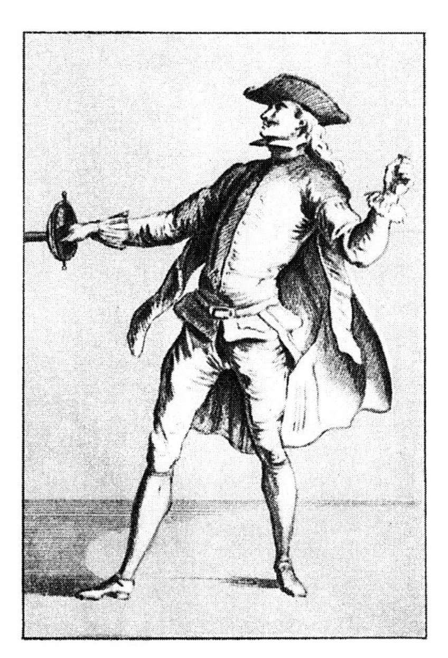

HOLLAND AND ENGLAND
1740–1750

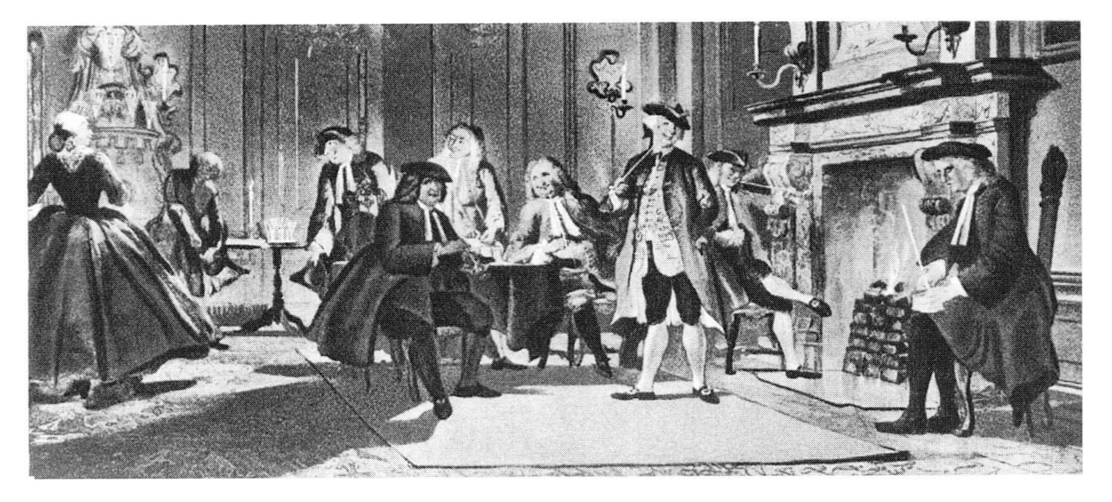

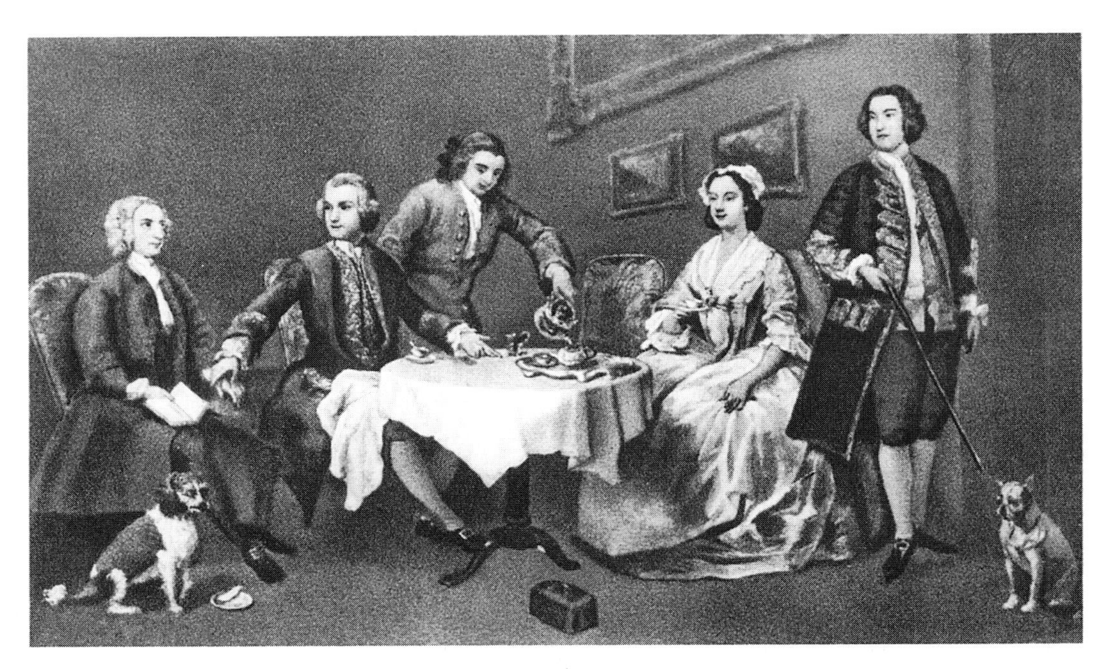

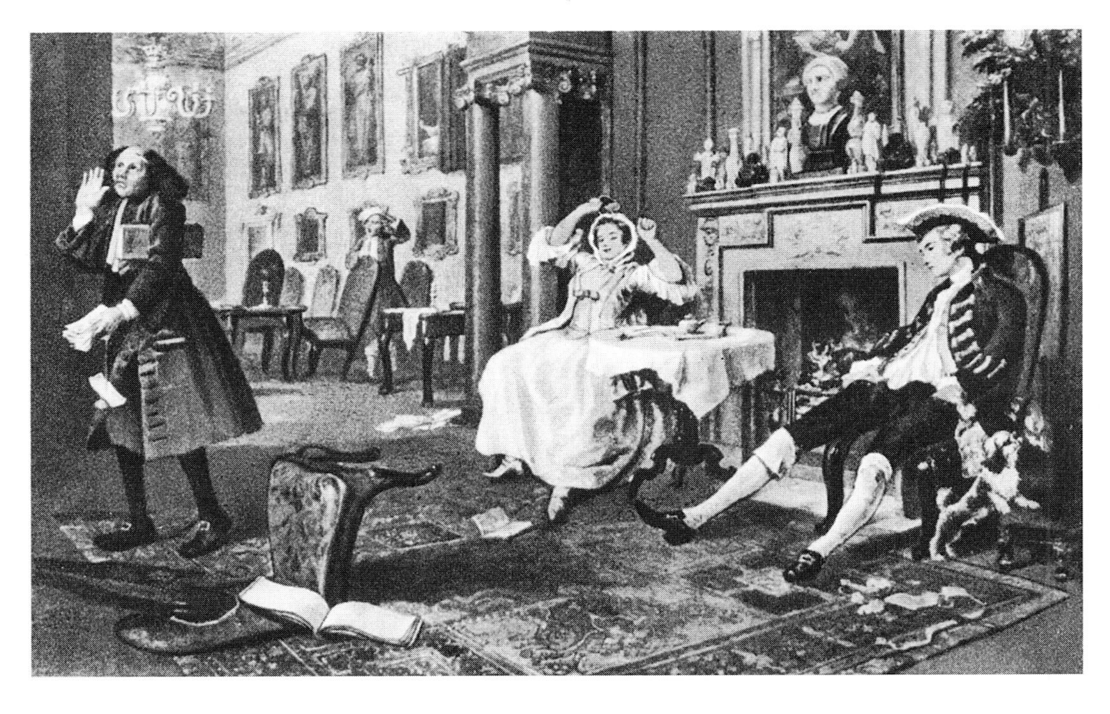

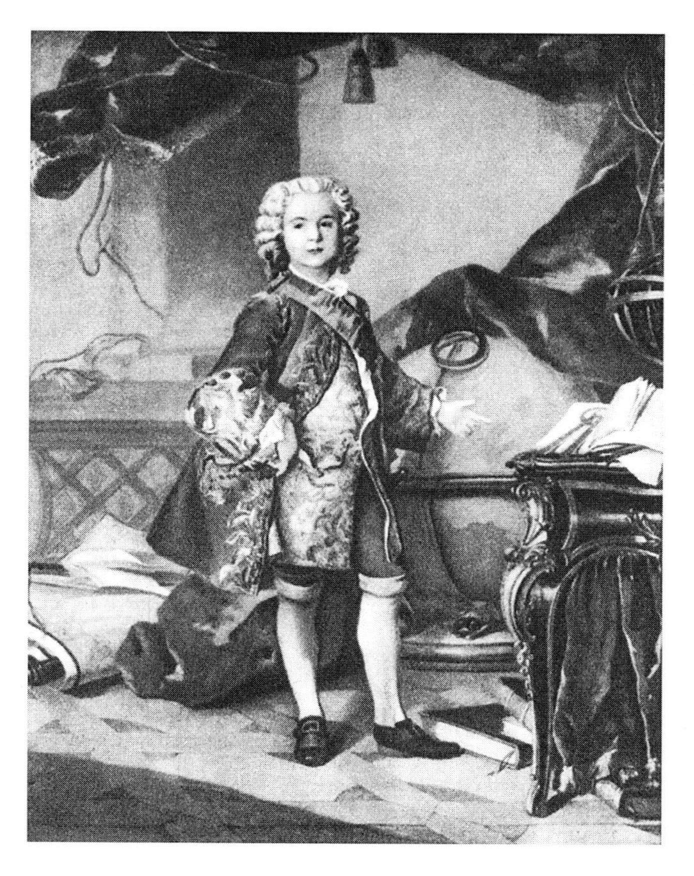

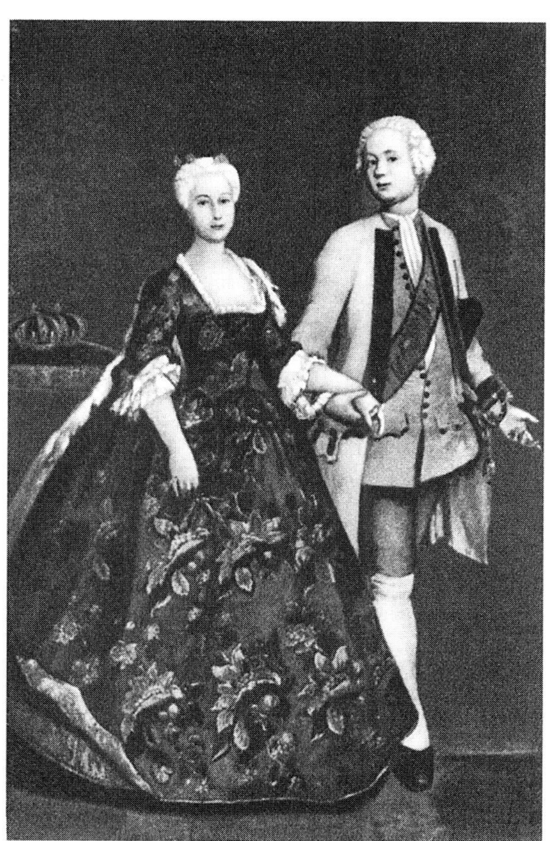

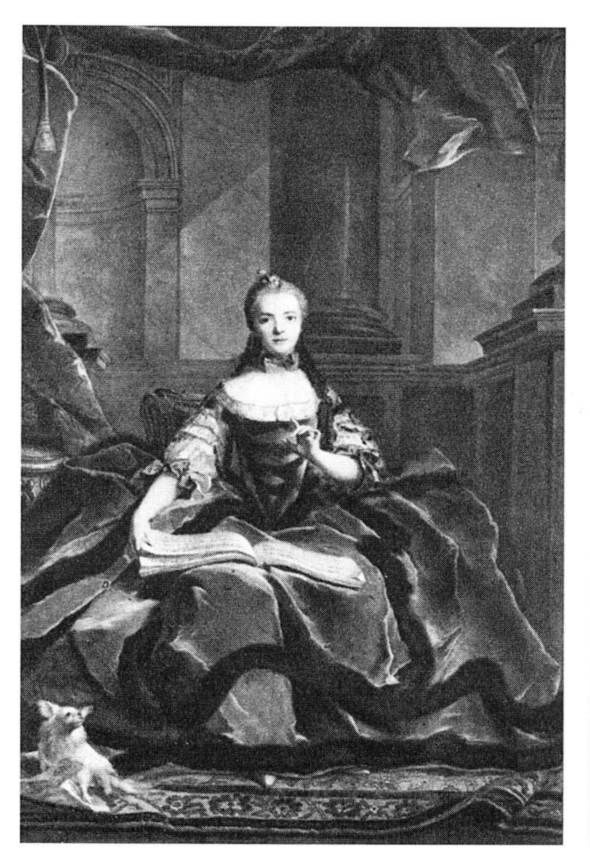

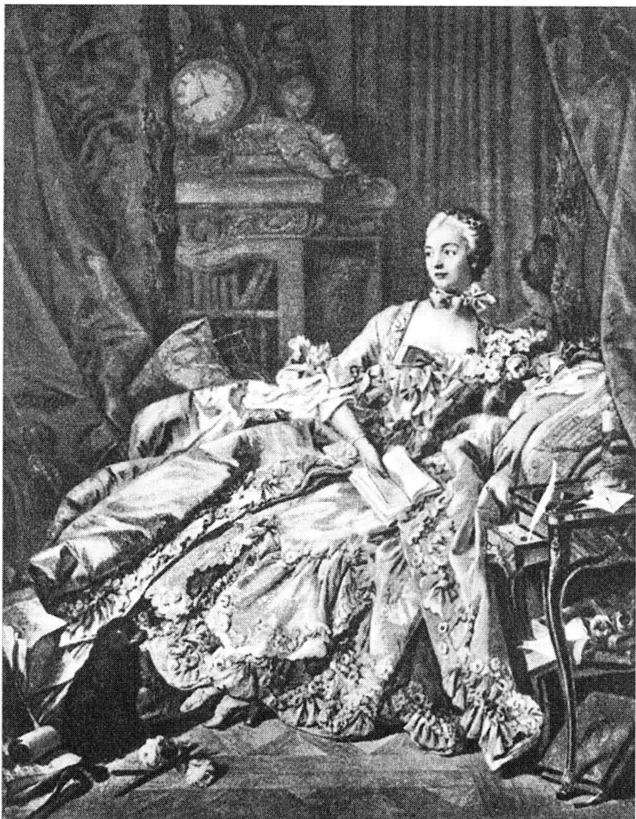

FRANCE AND GERMANY 1730–1760

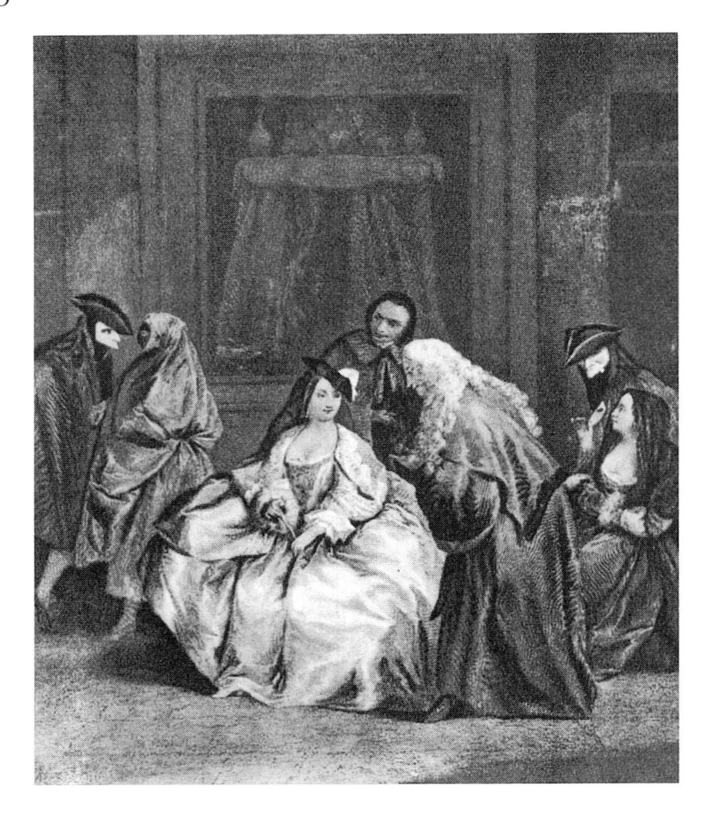

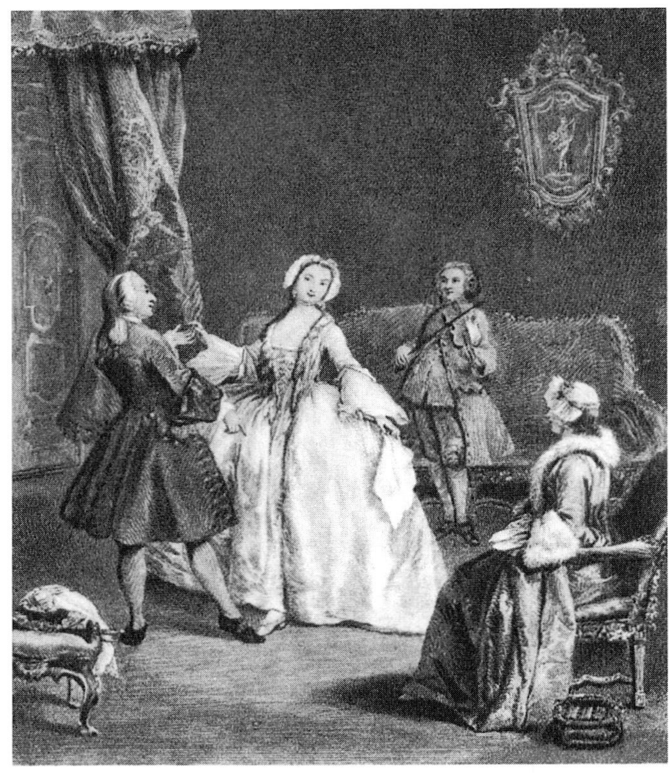

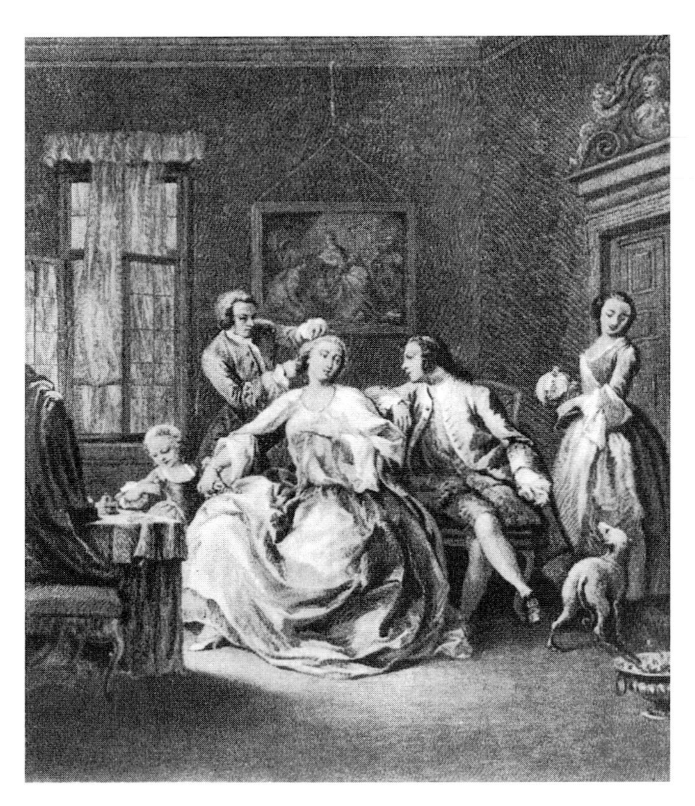

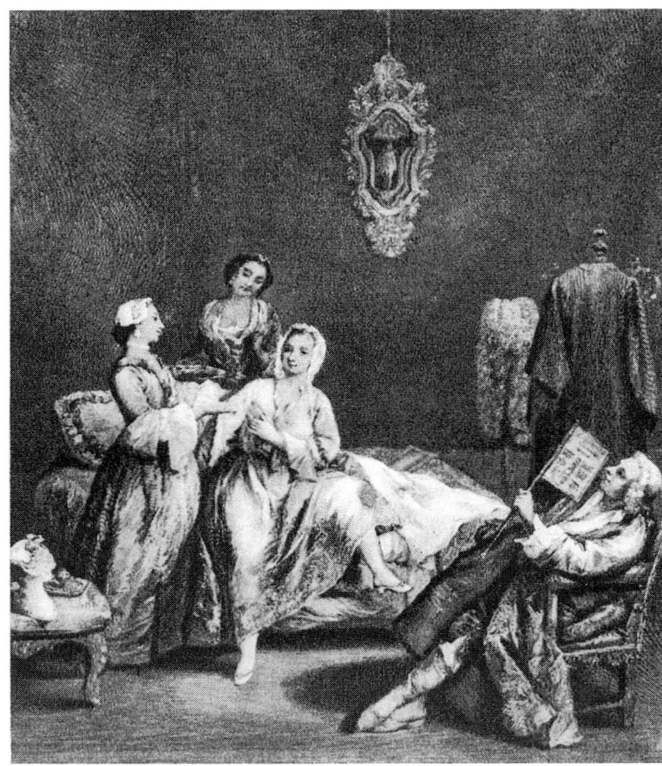

ITALY Venice about 1750

FRANCE
about 1740
Paris Street Life

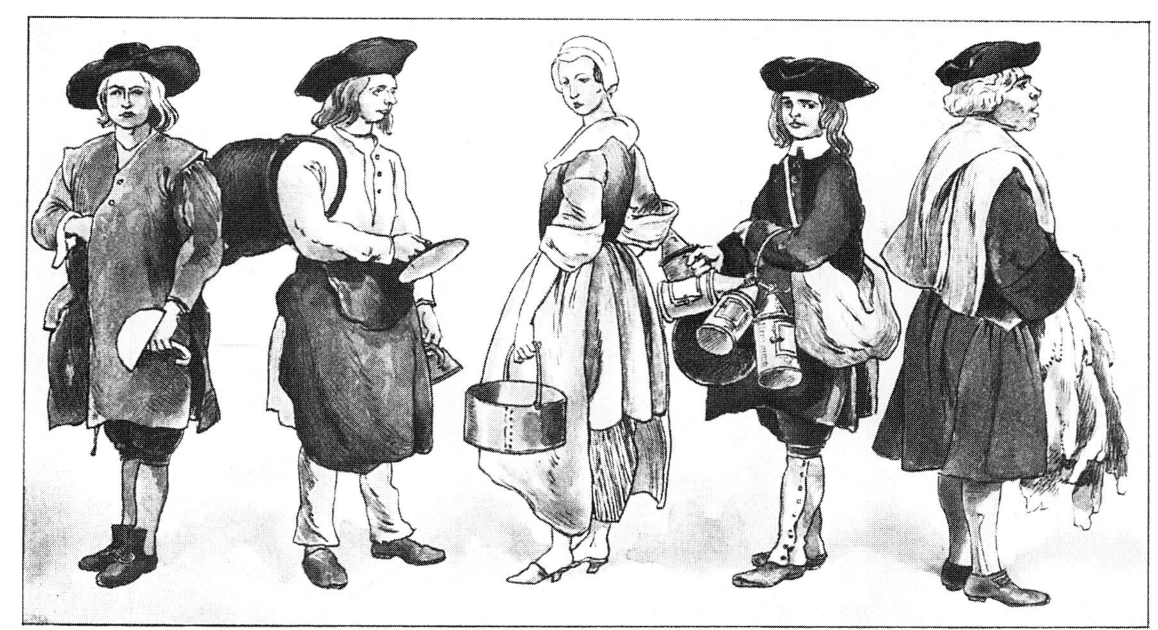

Street-criers and Tradesmen

1 2 3 4 5

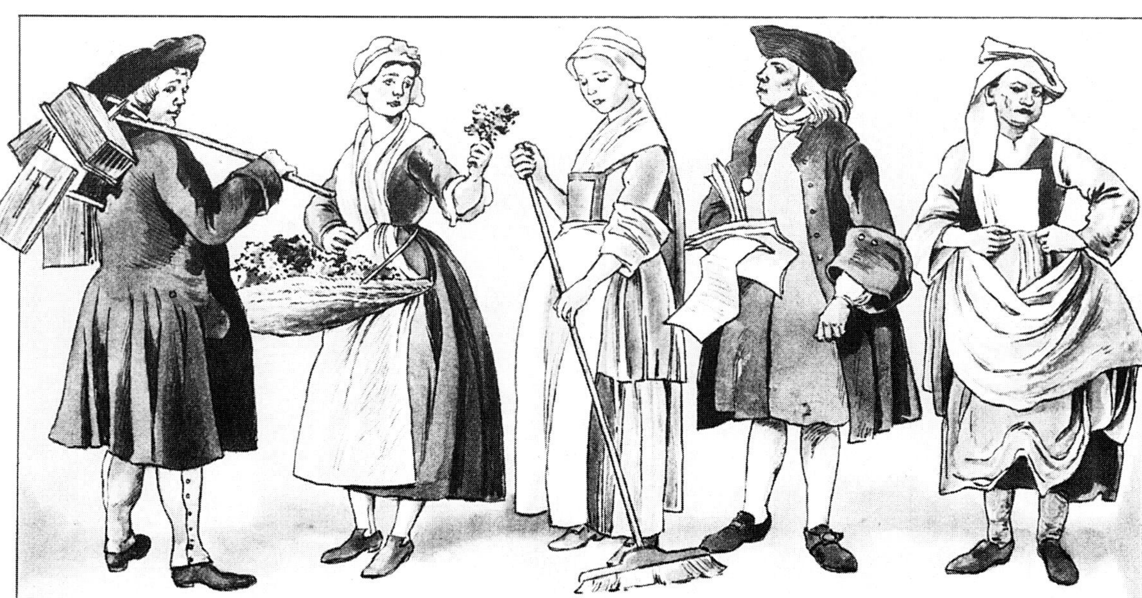

Tradesmen and Hawkers

6 7 8 9 10

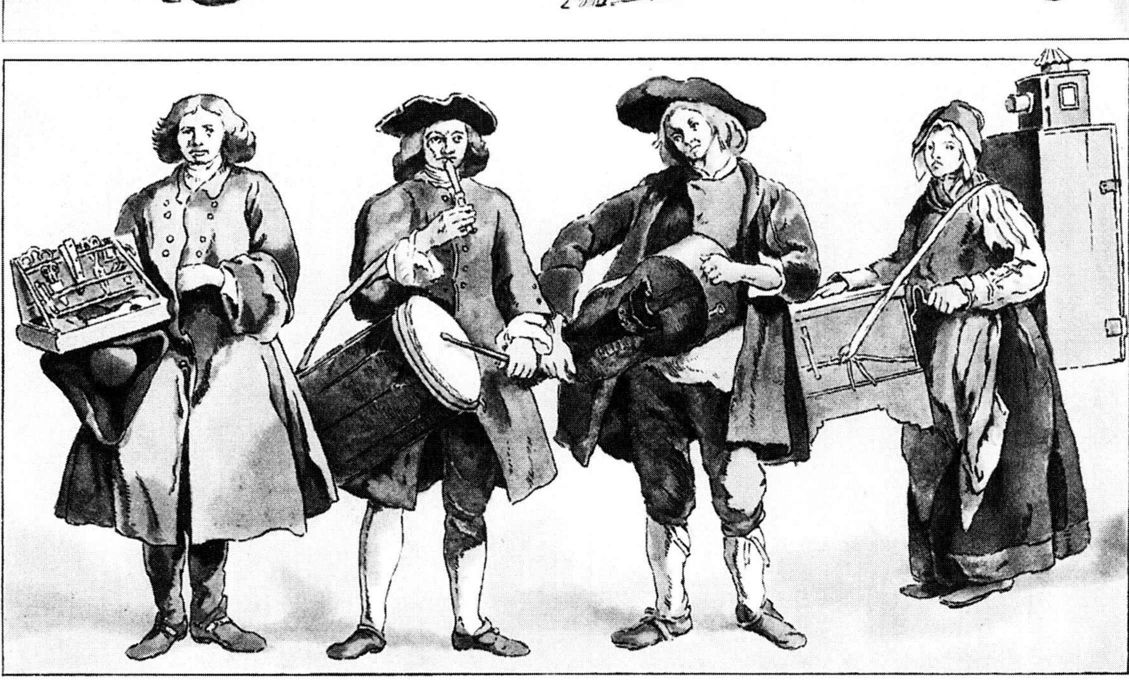

Itinerant Musicians
and Street-criers

11 12 13 14

VIENNA AND VENICE
Street Life 1770–1790

Viennese Street-criers 1775

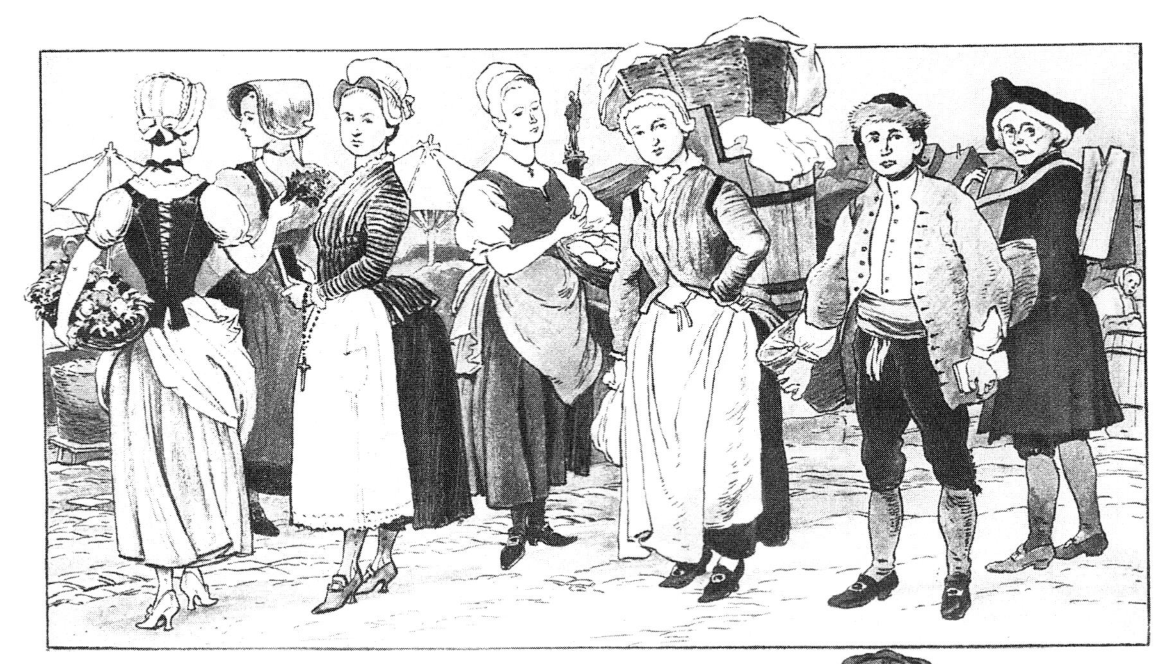

1 2 3 4 5 6 7

Viennese Street-criers 1775

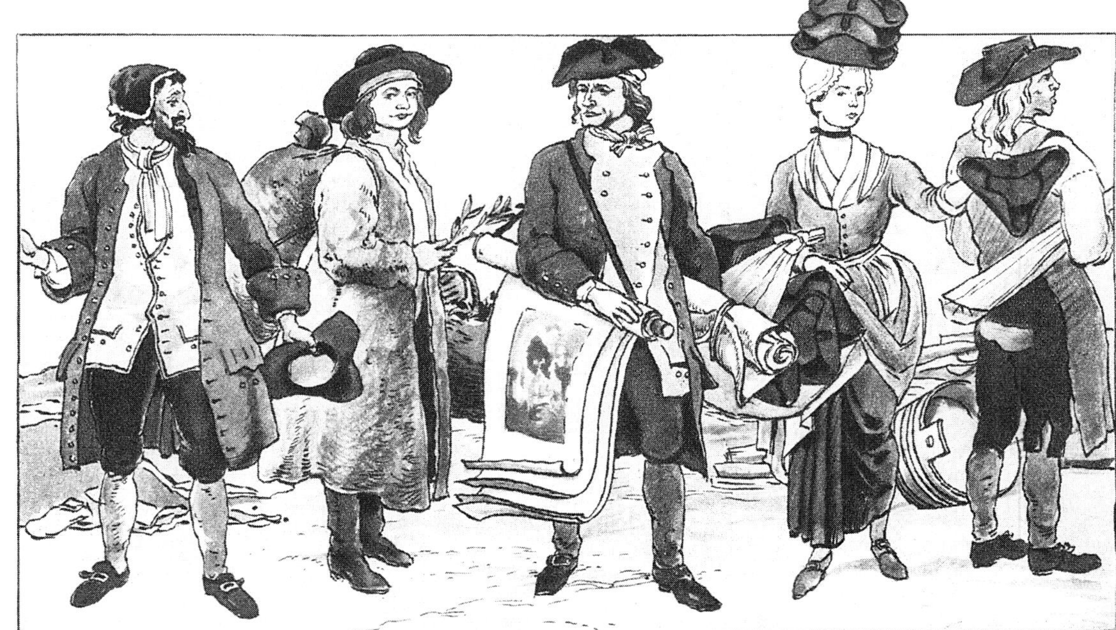

8 9 10 11 12

Venetian Street-criers 1785

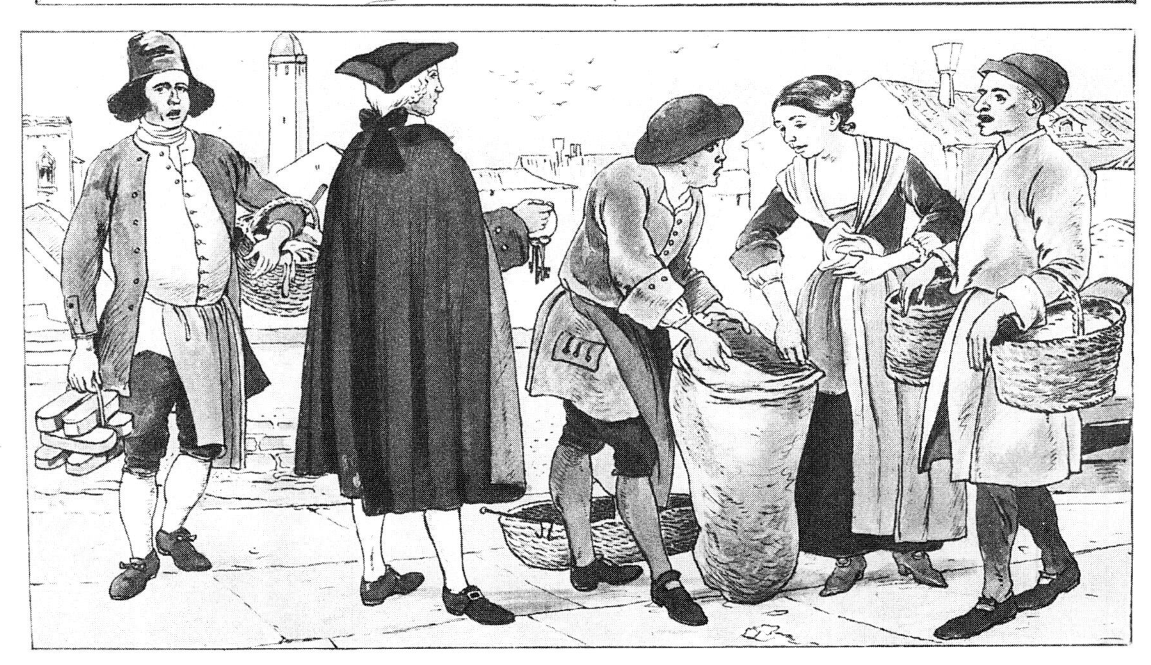

13 14 15 16 17

FRANCE 1770–1780

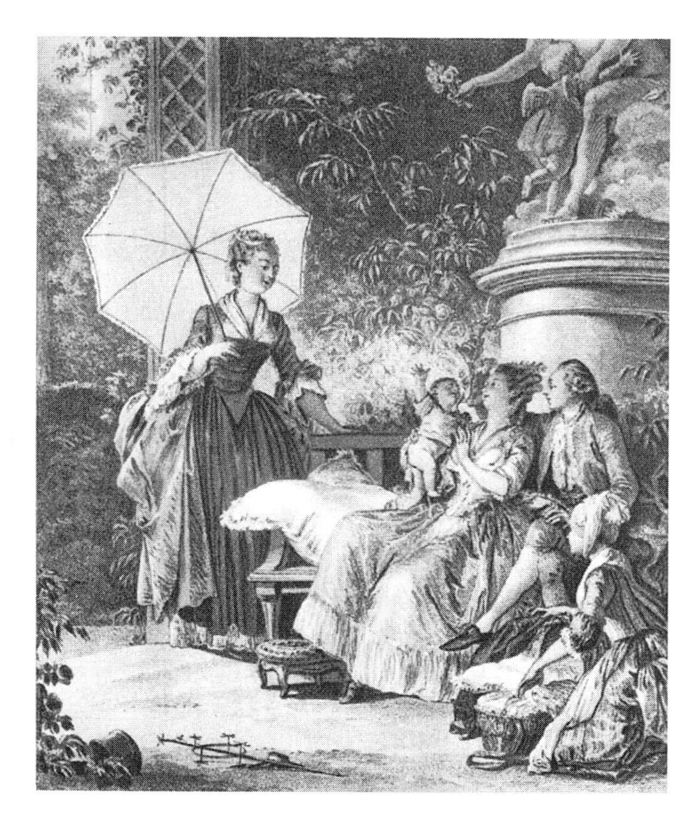

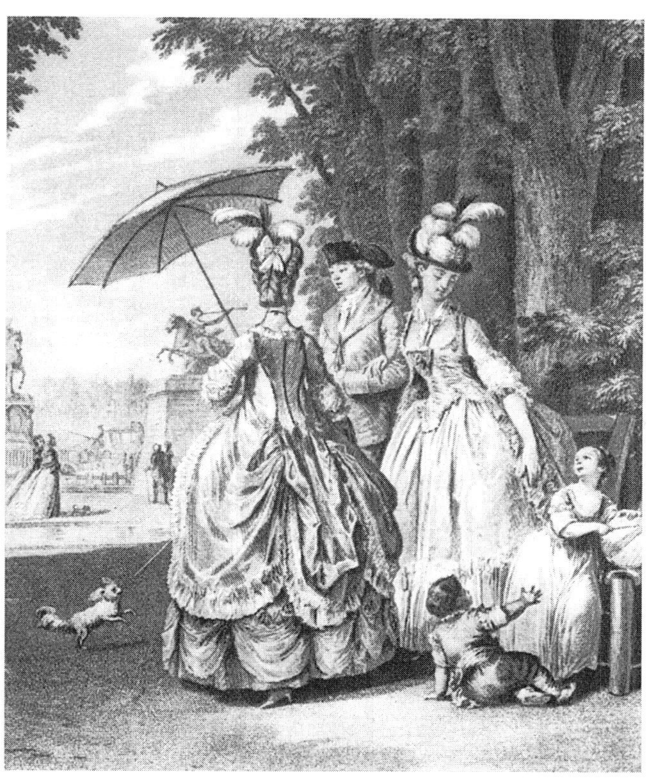

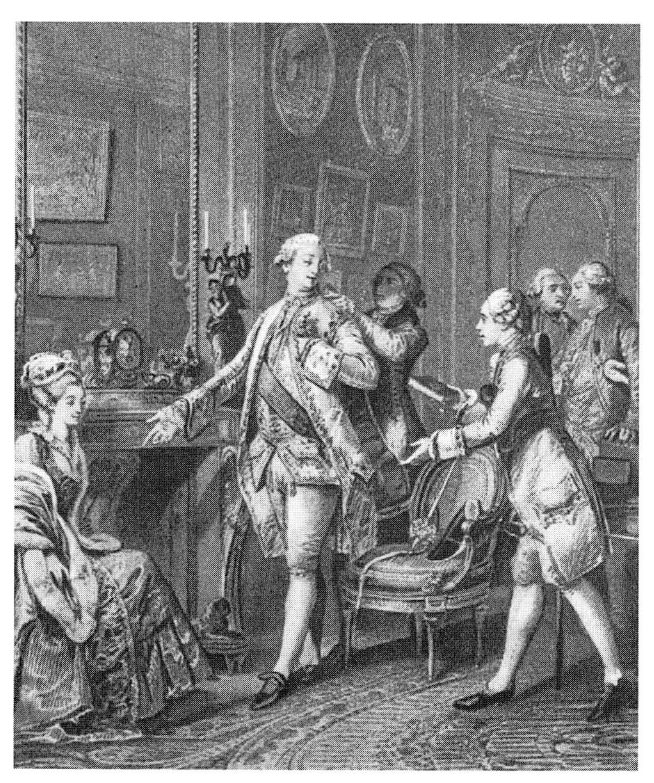

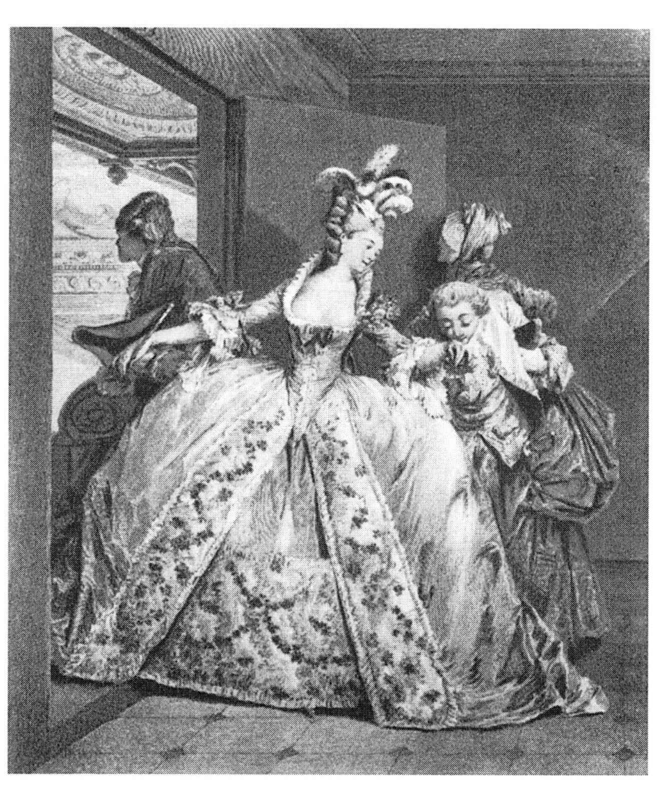

Parisian Society

ENGLAND
1770–1800

Noble Women

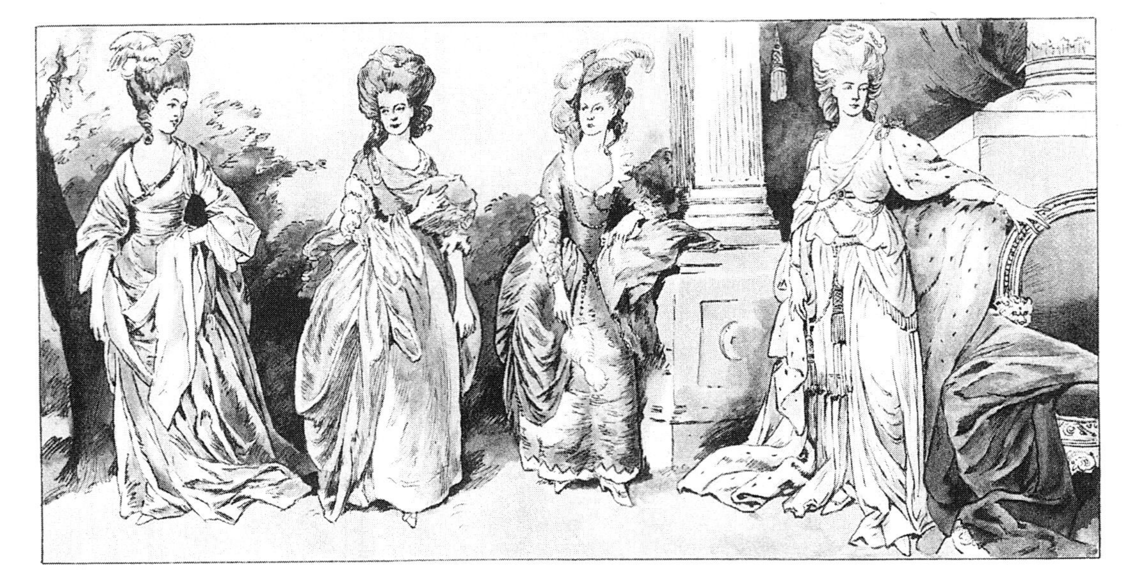

1 2 3 4

English Fashions 1770–1795

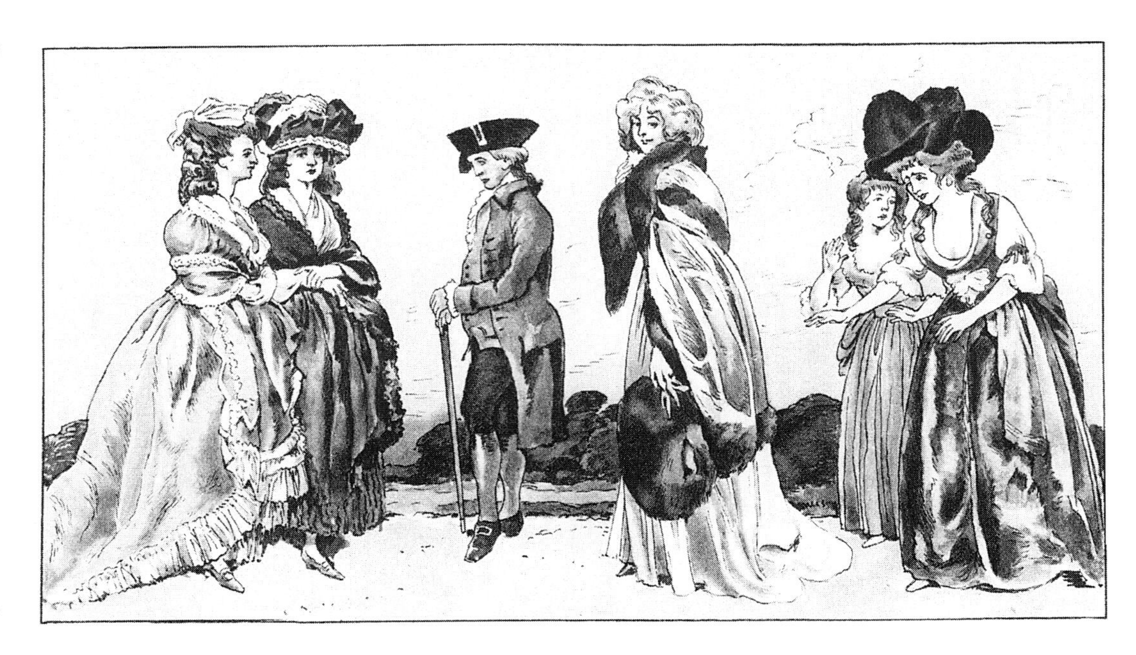

5 6 7 8 9 10

English Fashions 1795–1800

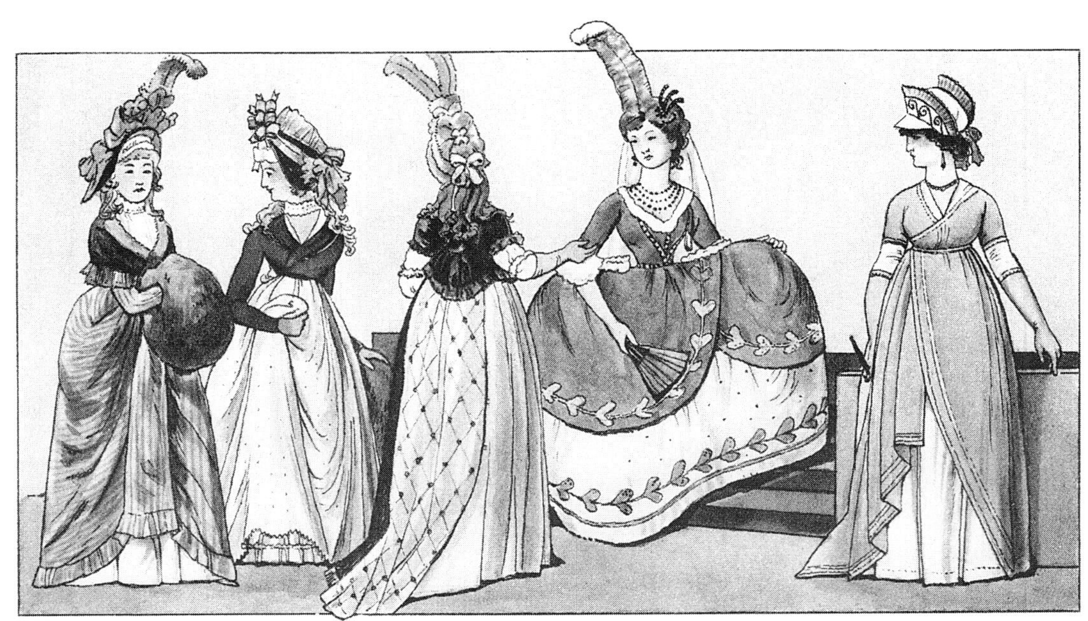

11 12 13 14 15

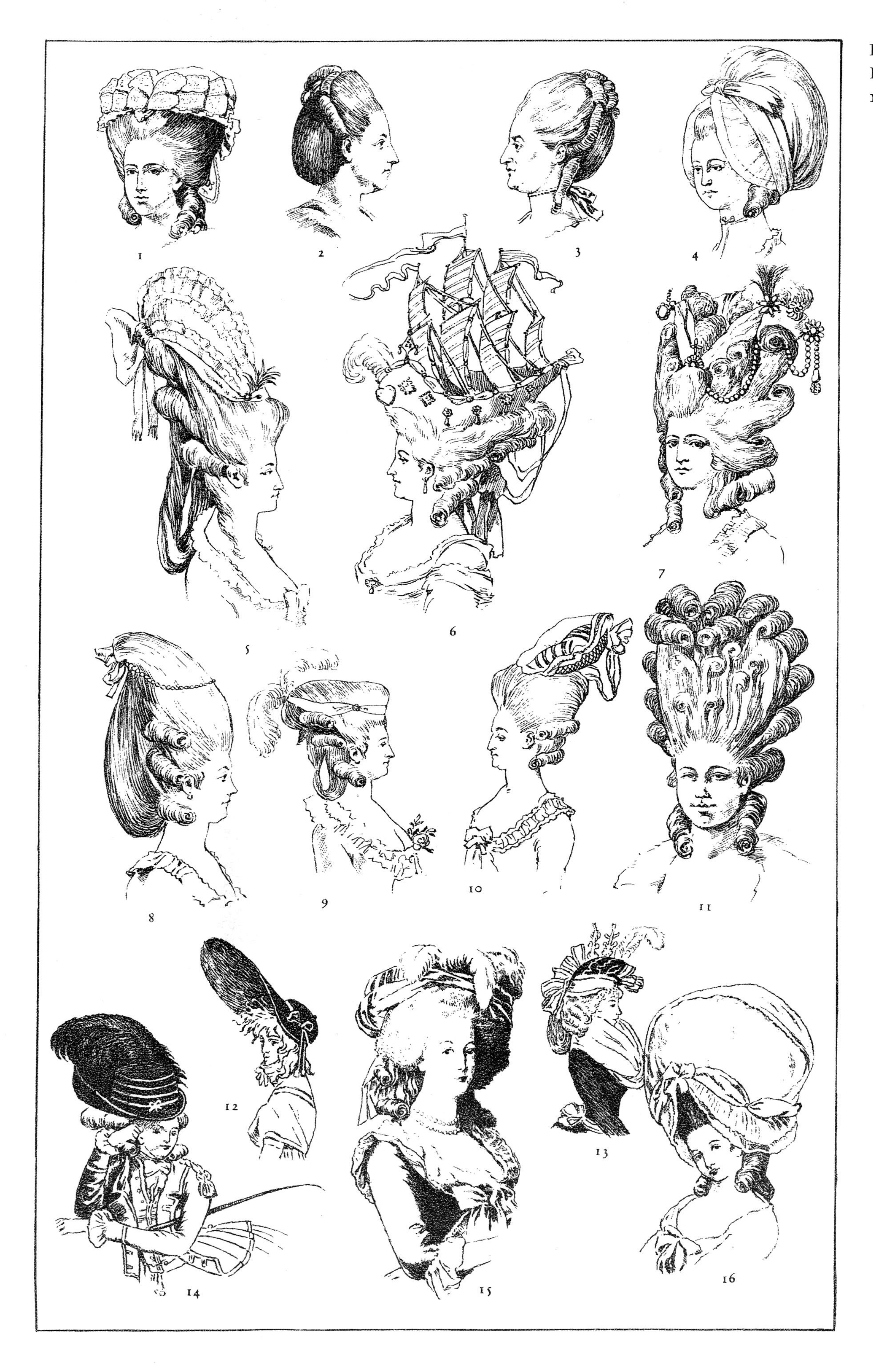

EUROPE
Rococo Hair Styles
1770–1790

GERMANY AND AUSTRIA
1750–1775
Costume in China Figures

Höchst and Frankenthal
1760

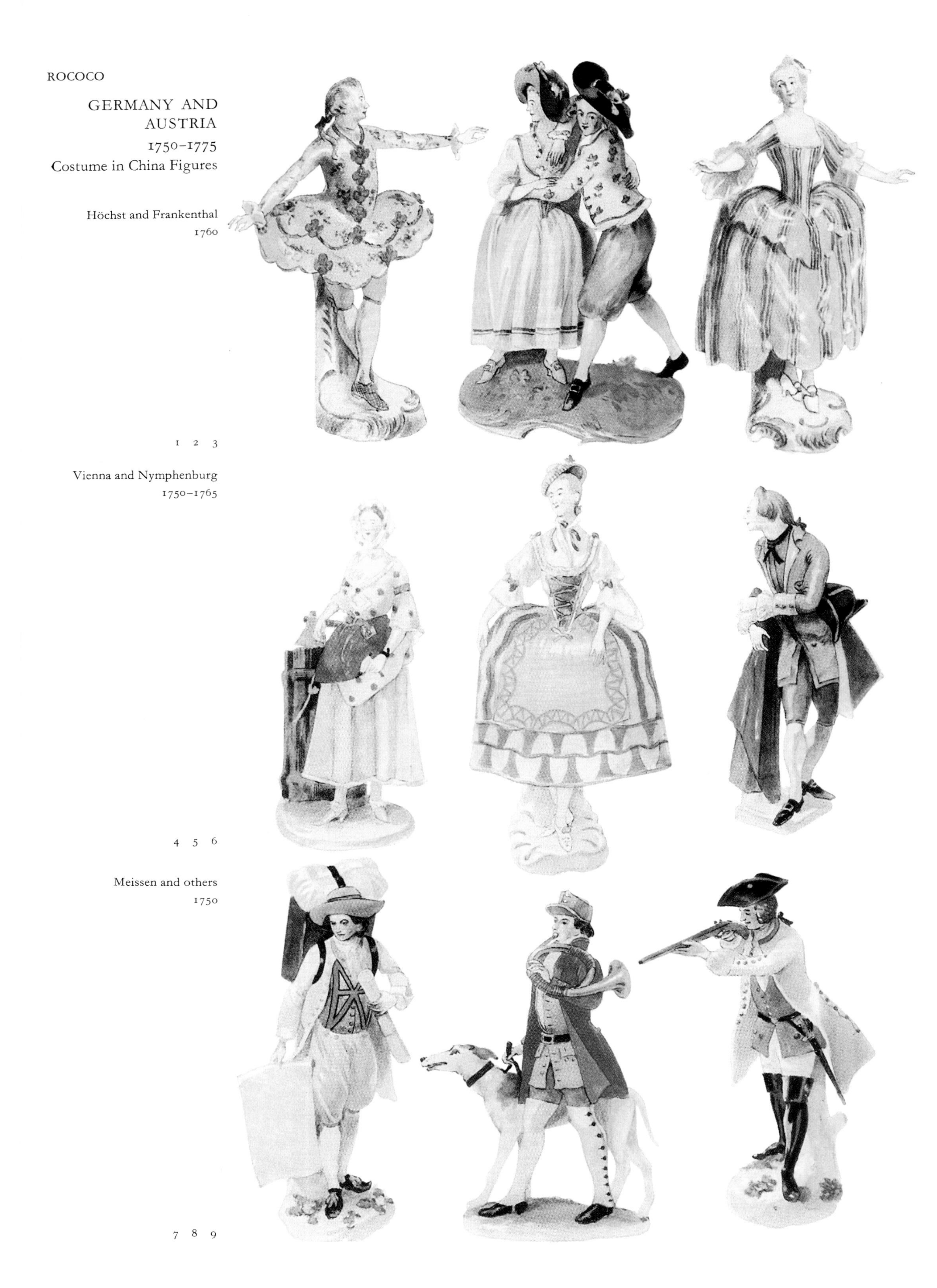

1 2 3

Vienna and Nymphenburg
1750–1765

4 5 6

Meissen and others
1750

7 8 9

FRANCE
1730–1770

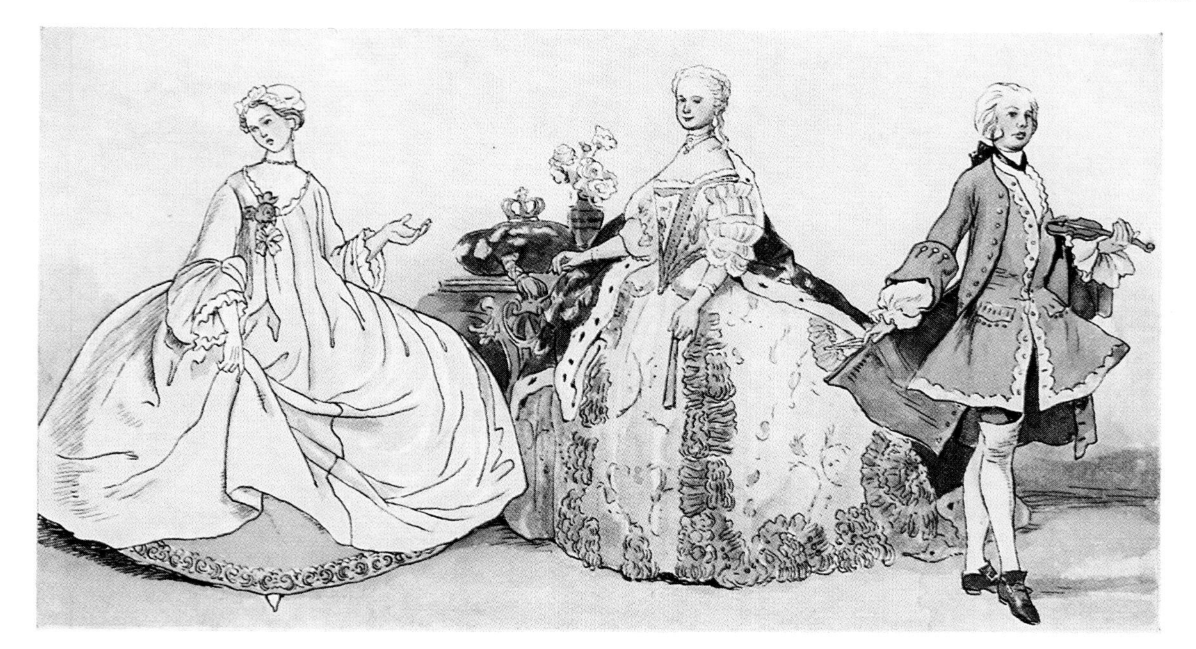

1730–1745

1 2 3

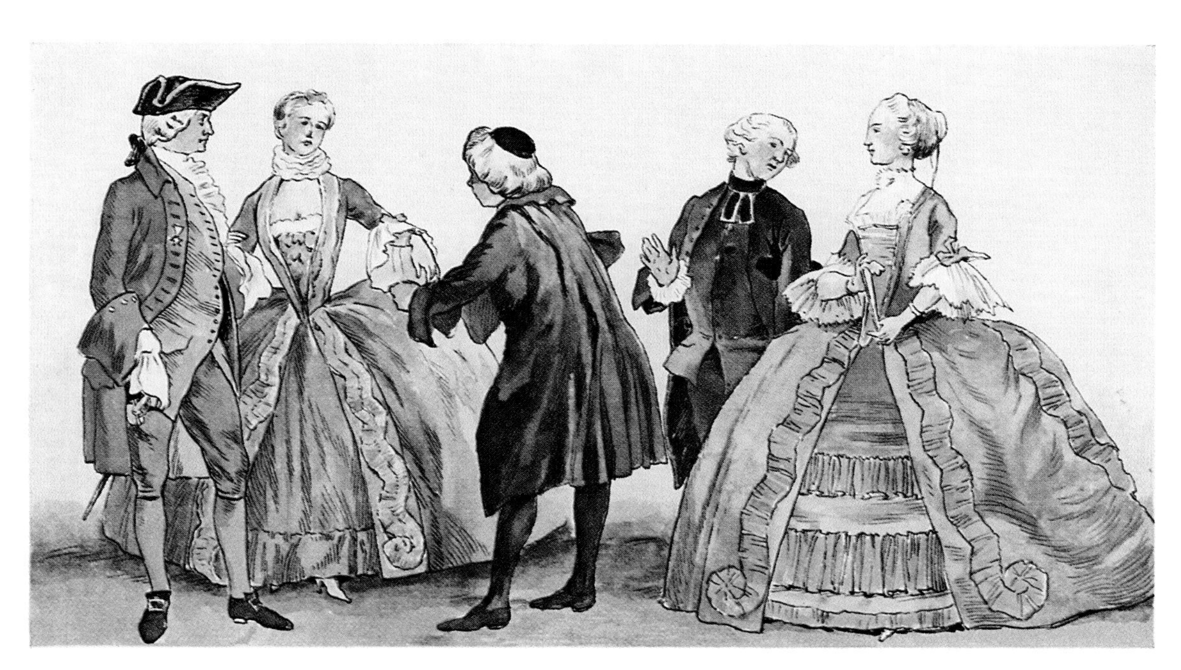

1755

4 5 6 7 8

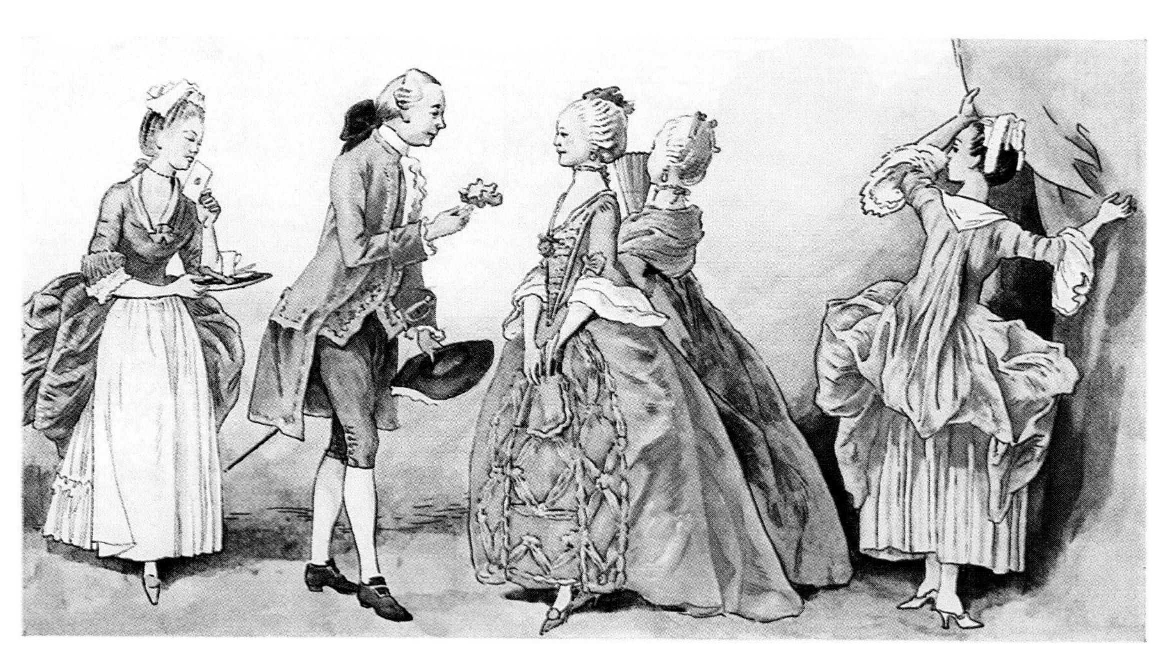

1760–1770

9 10 11 12 13

FRANCE
Louis XVI.
1775–1785

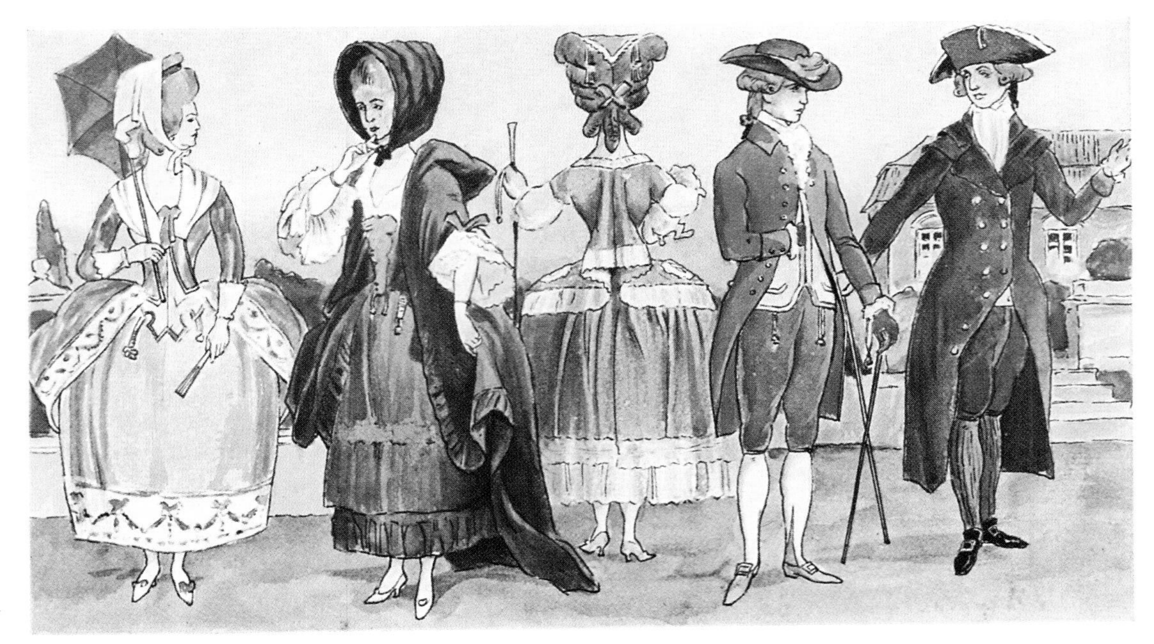

1 2 3 4 5

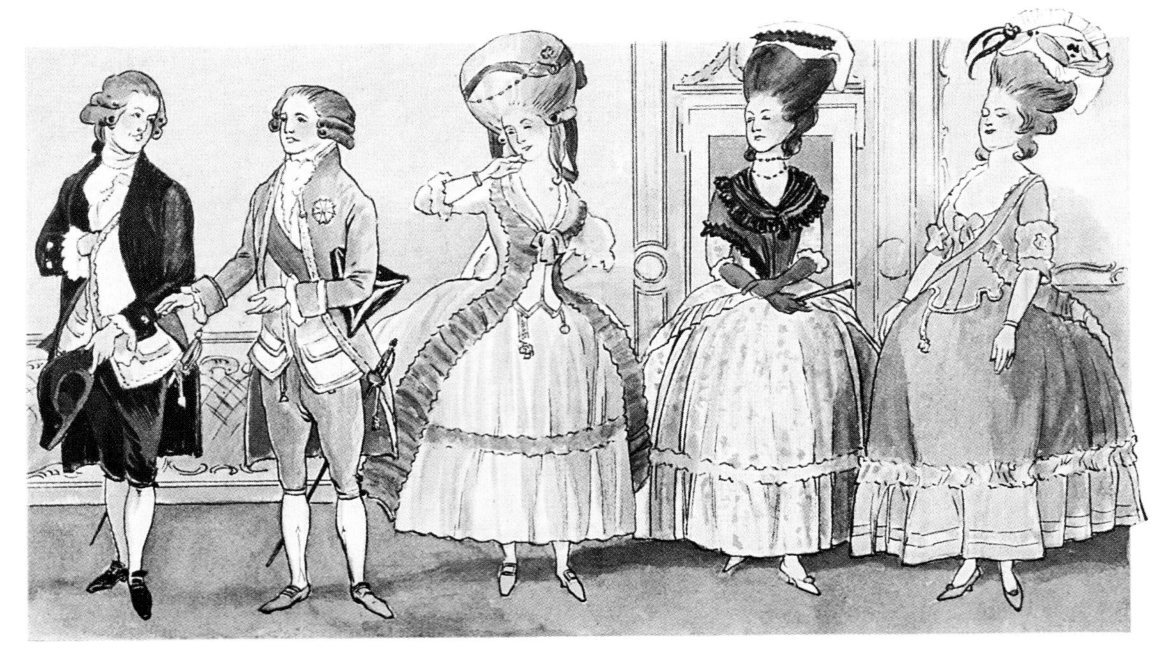

6 7 8 9 10

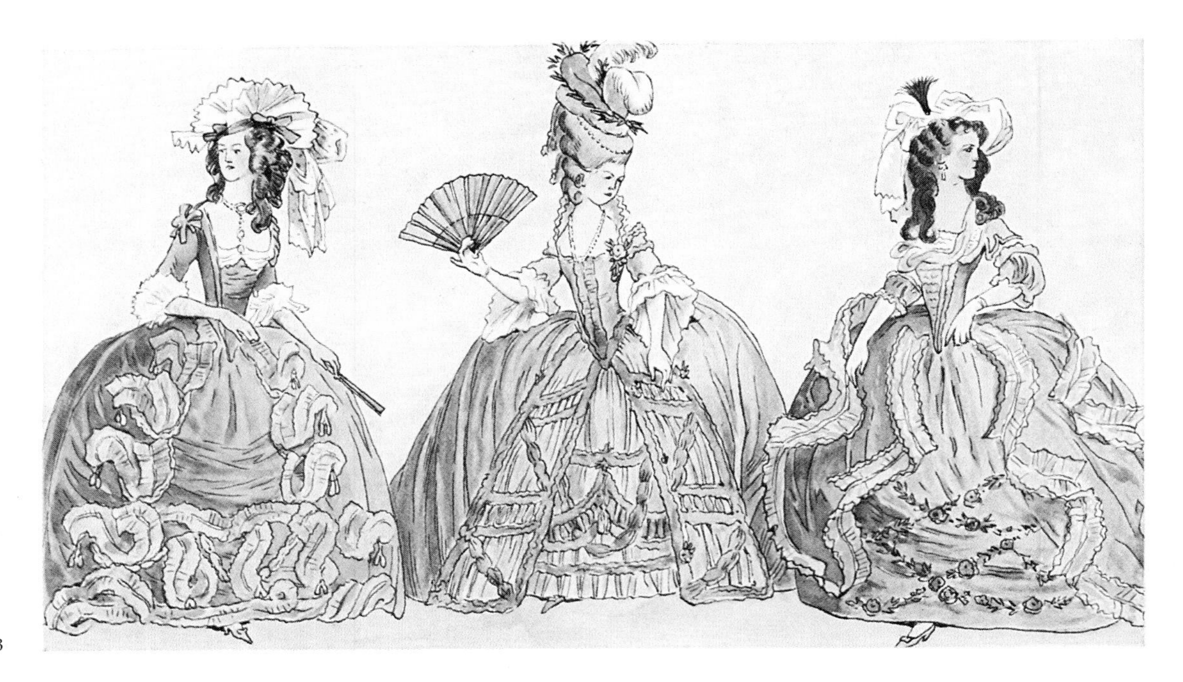

11 12 13

FRANCE
1780–1789

1780

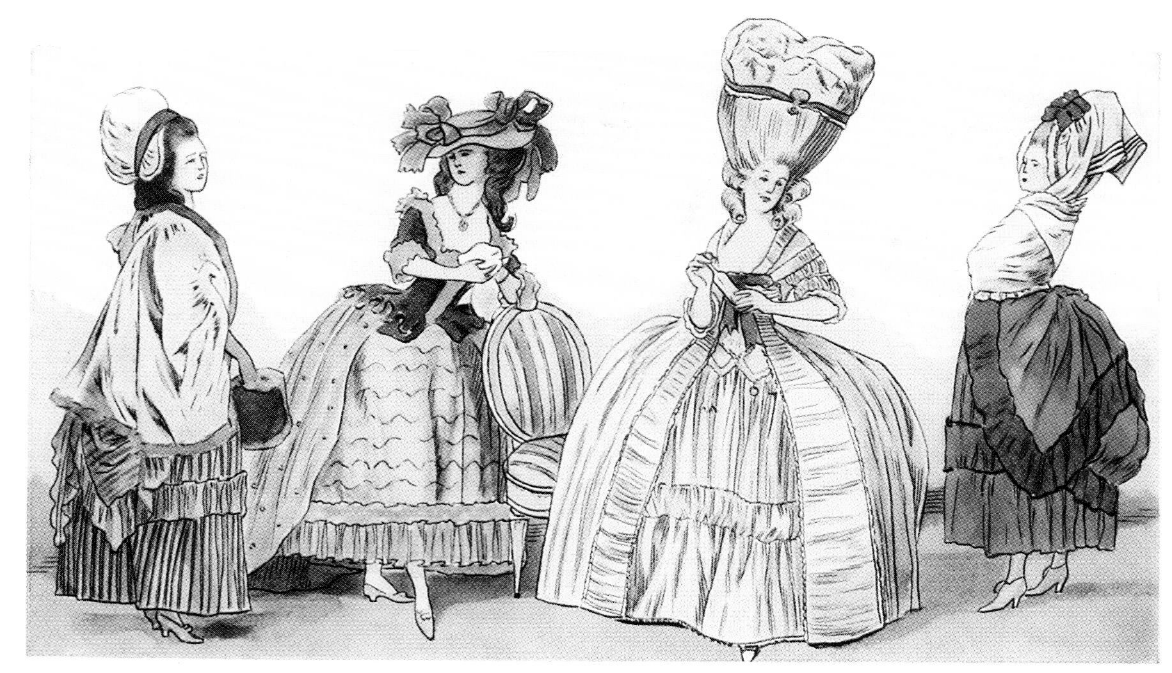

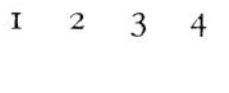
1 2 3 4

1780

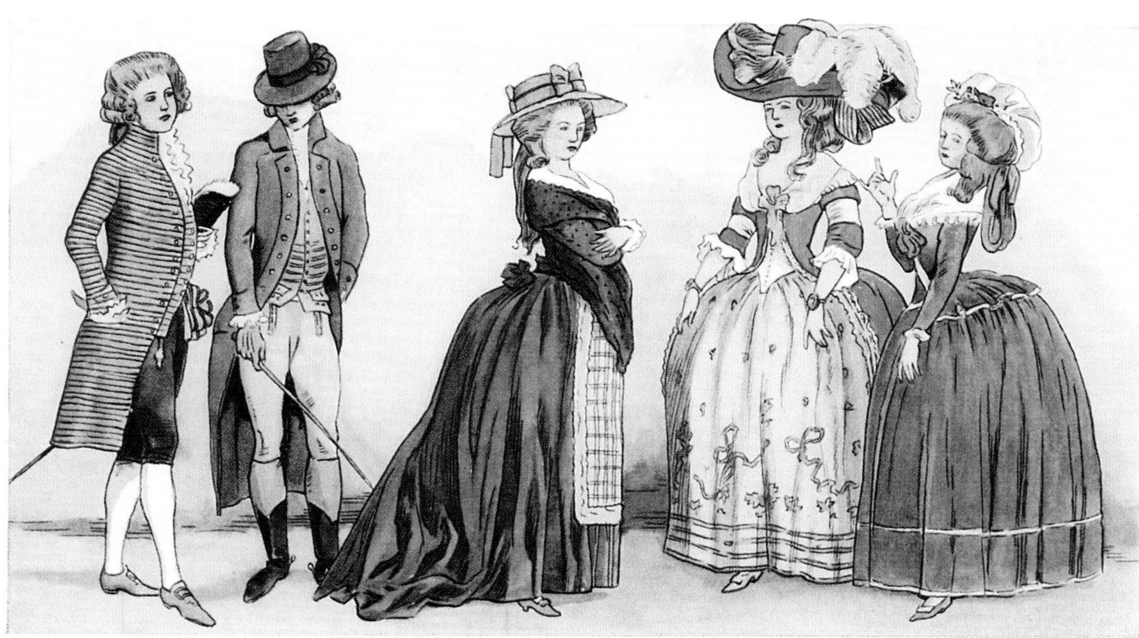

5 6 7 8 9

1789

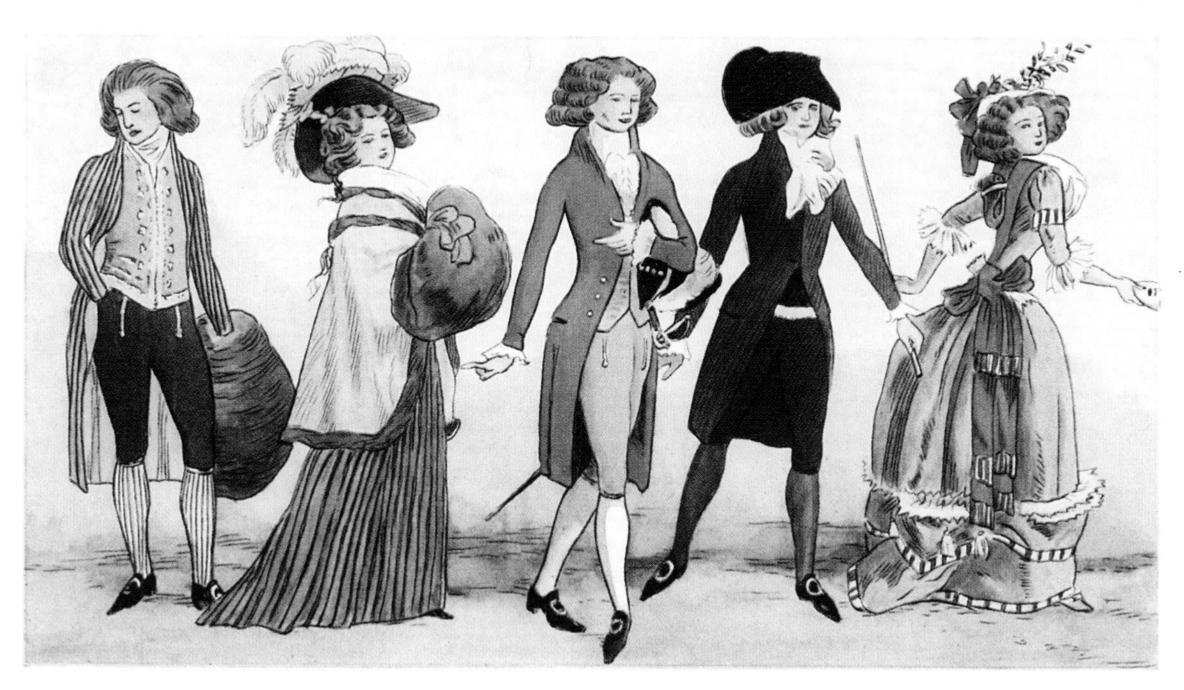

10 11 12 13 14

FRANCE
1790–1795

Revolution 1790

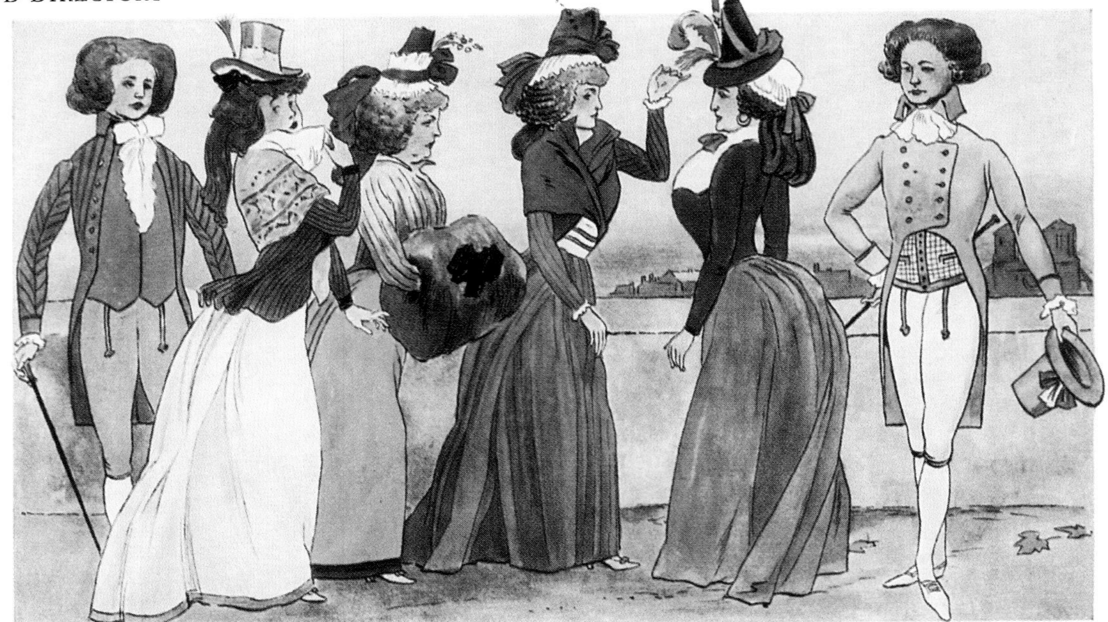

1 2 3 4 5 6

Revolution 1790

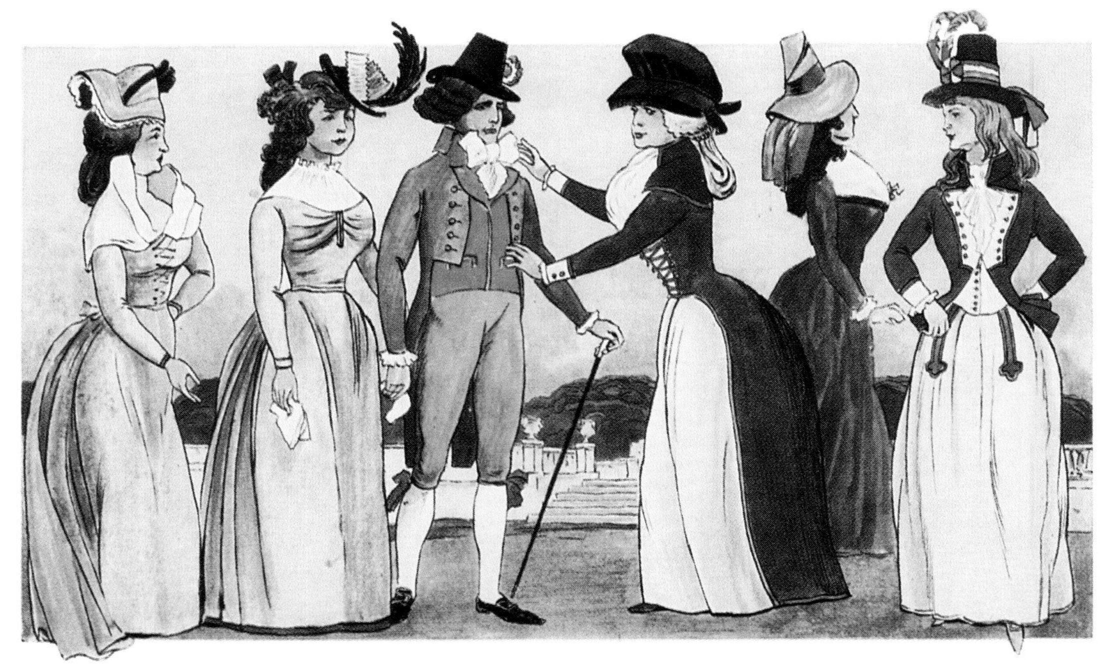

7 8 9 10 11 12

Directory 1795

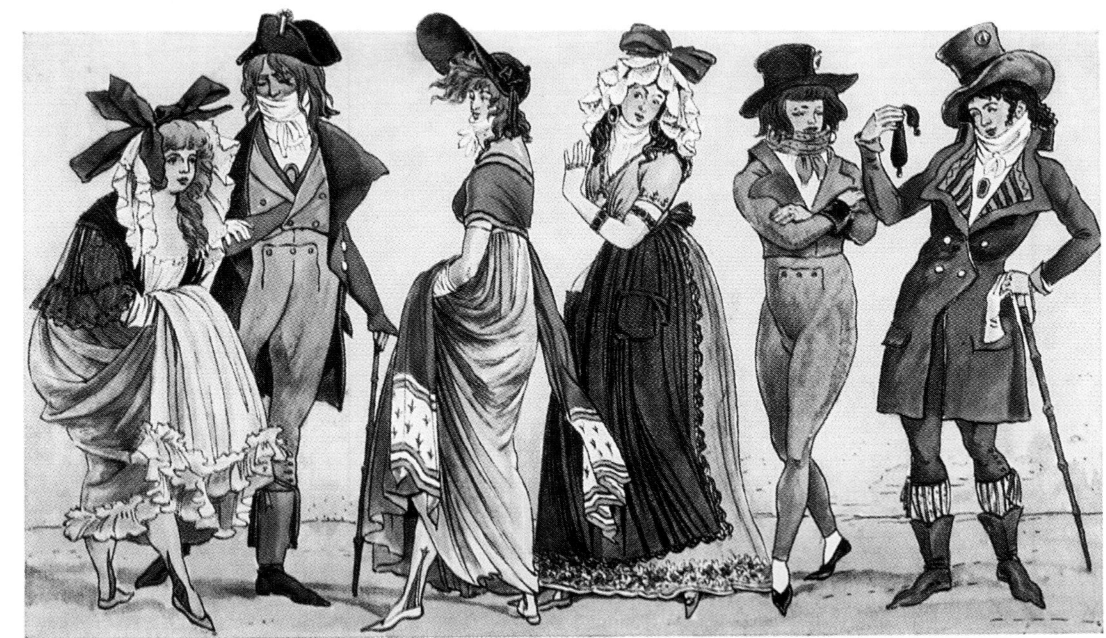

13 14 15 16 17 18

FRANCE
Revolution, Directory,
Consulate

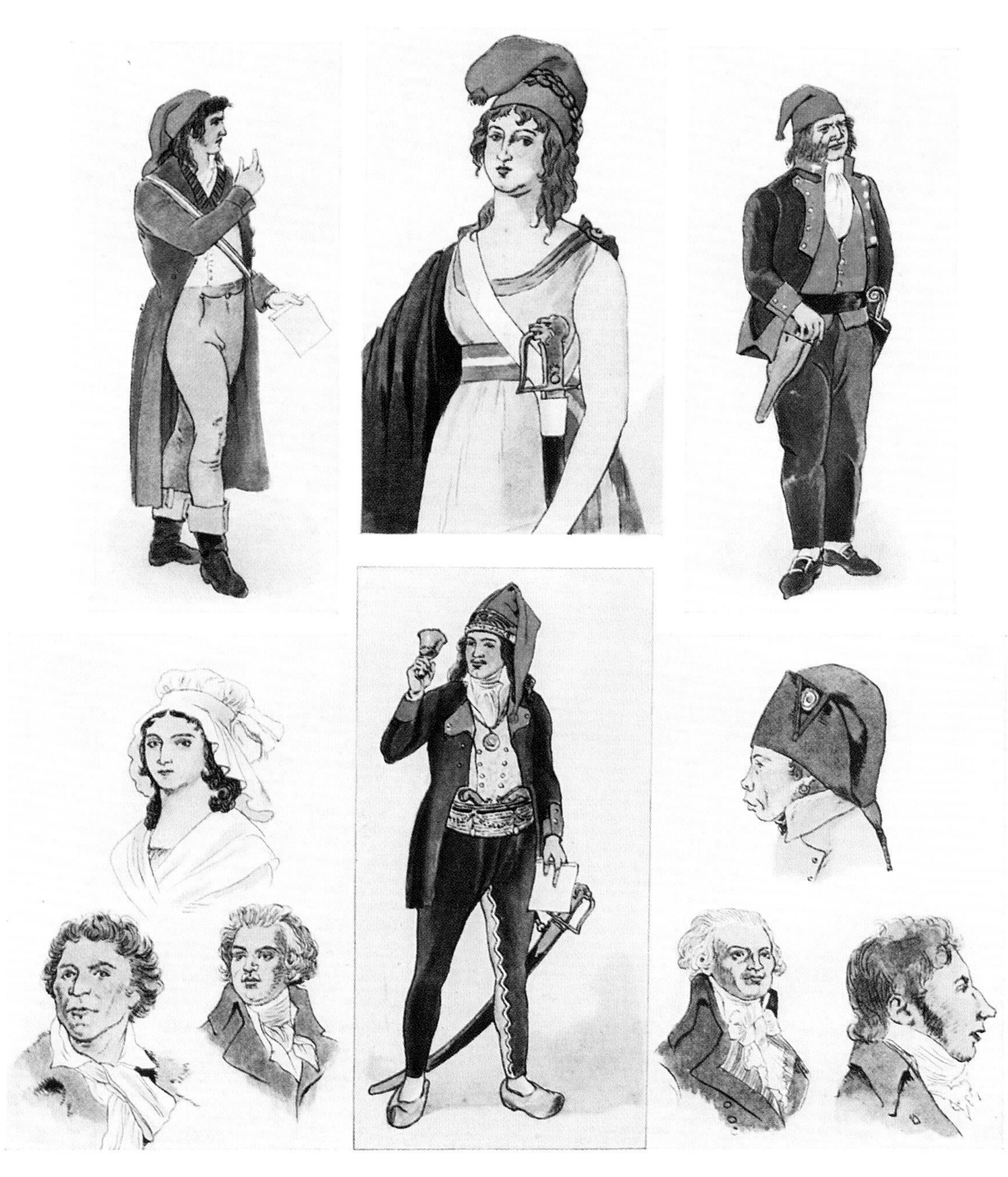

Costume of the Revolution 1792–1795

1 2 3

Head-dress, Collars and Neck-cloths 1790–1795

4 5 6 7 8 9 10

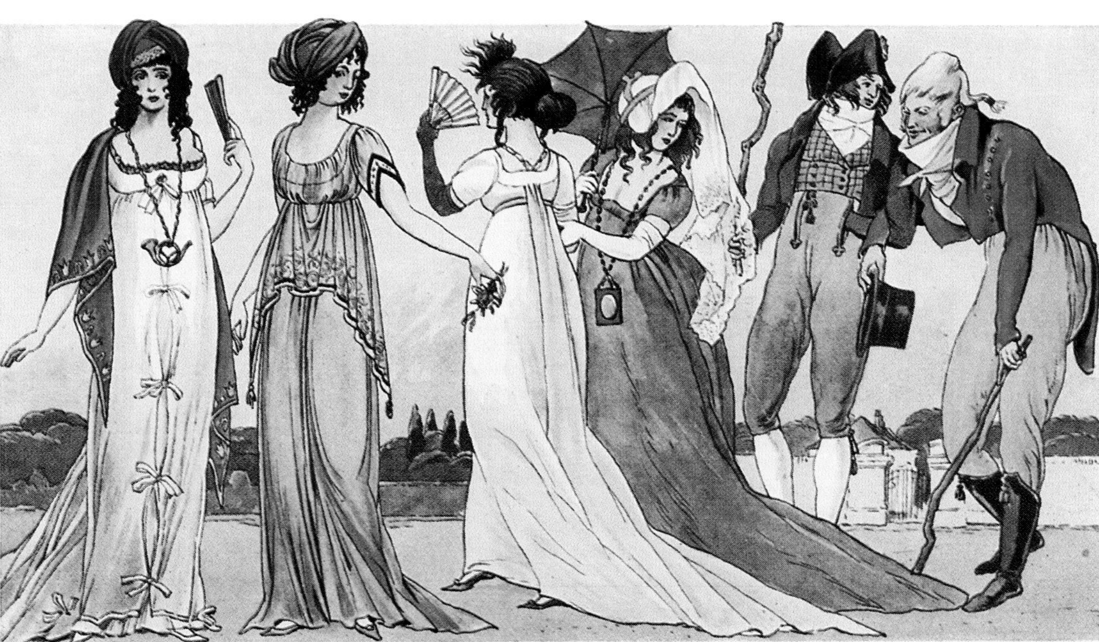

«Incroyables et Merveilleuses» 1795–1803

11 12 13 14 15 16

GERMANY AND FRANCE 1680–1790

German Uniforms
1680–1690

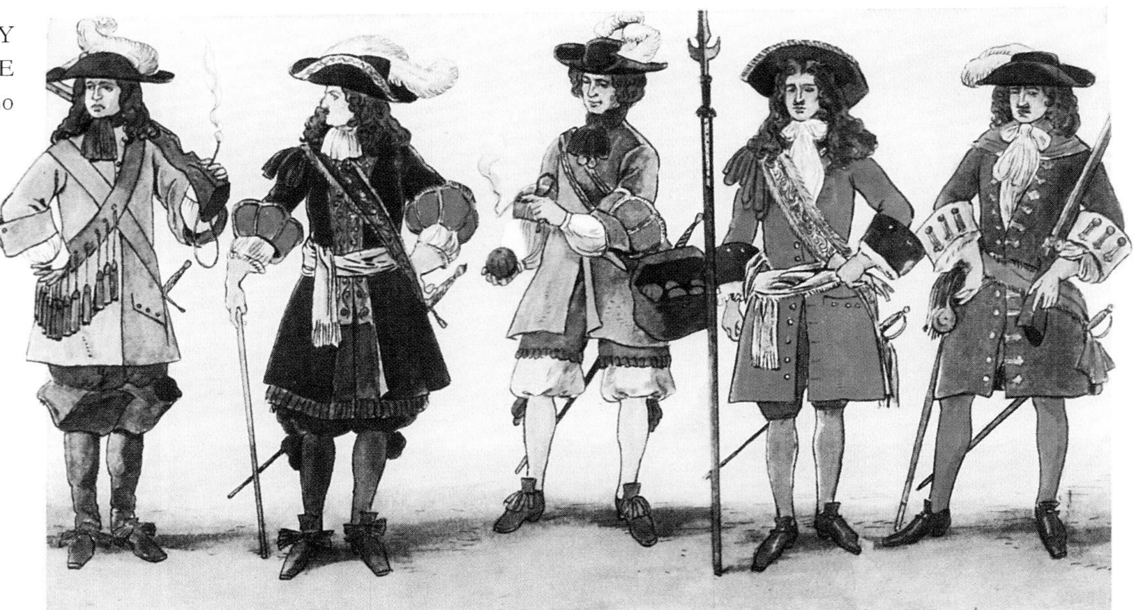

1 2 3 4 5

French Uniforms
1725–1757

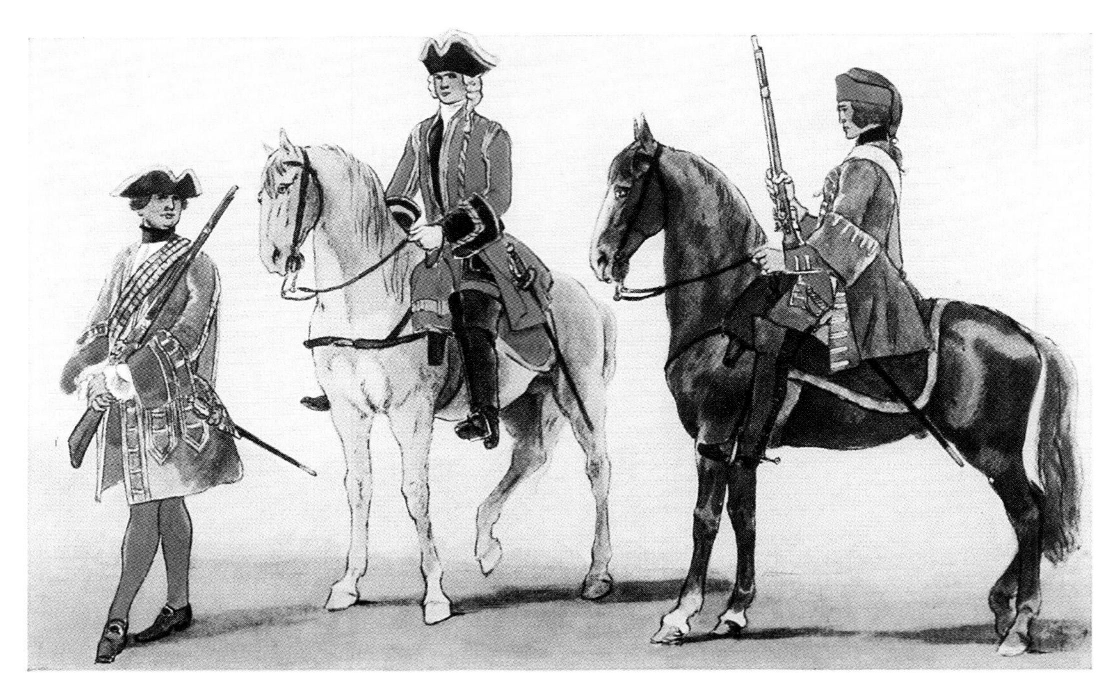

6 7 8

French Uniforms
1757–1790

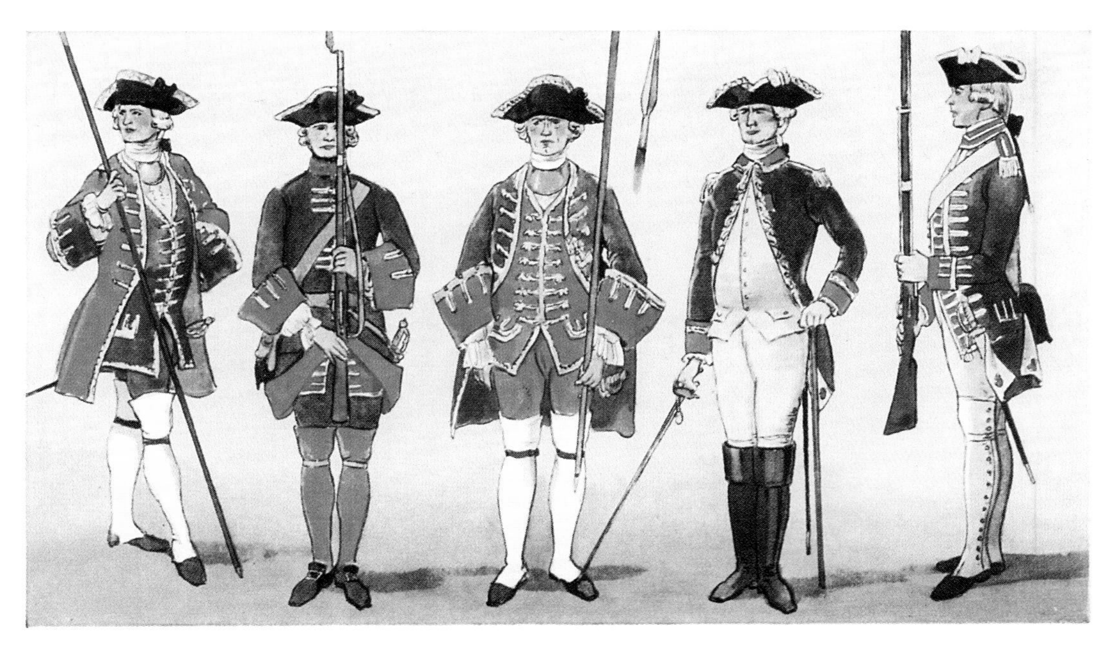

9 10 11 12 13

ENGLAND AND FRANCE 1800–1830

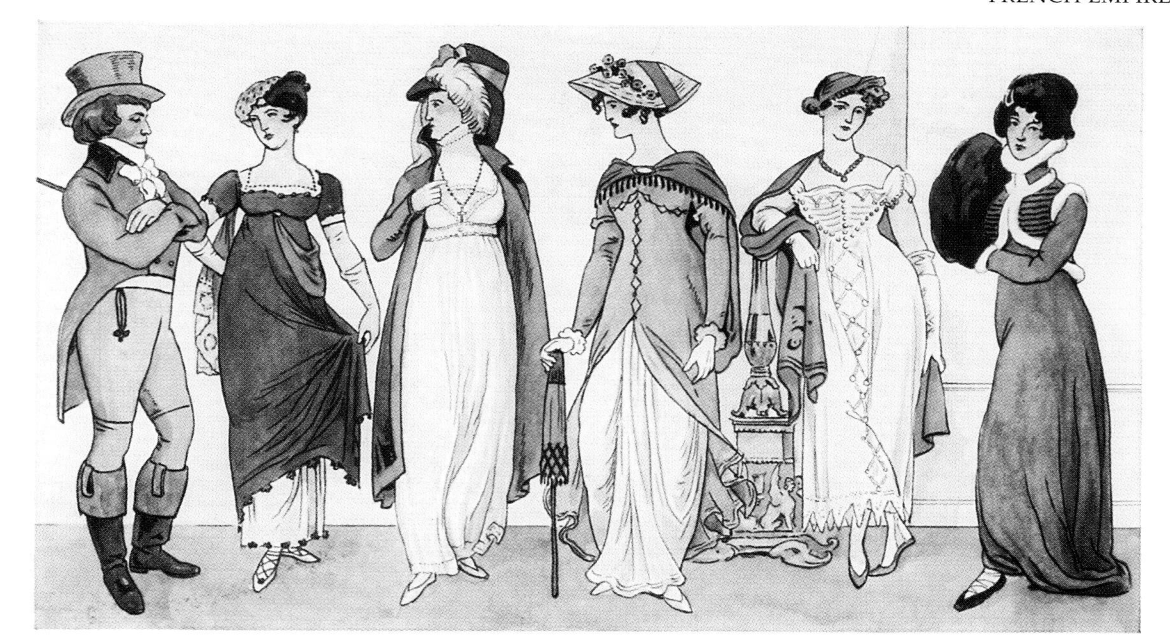

England about 1800

1 2 3 4 5 6

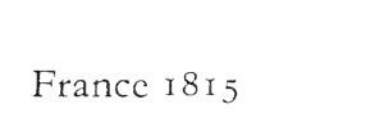

France 1815

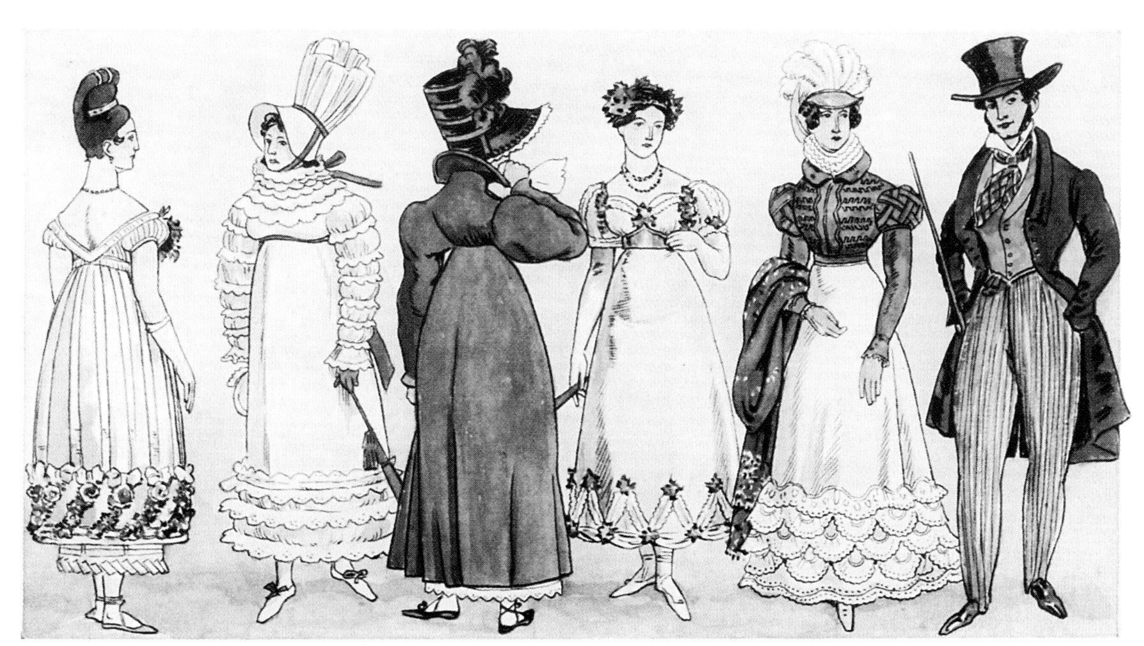

7 8 9 10 11 12

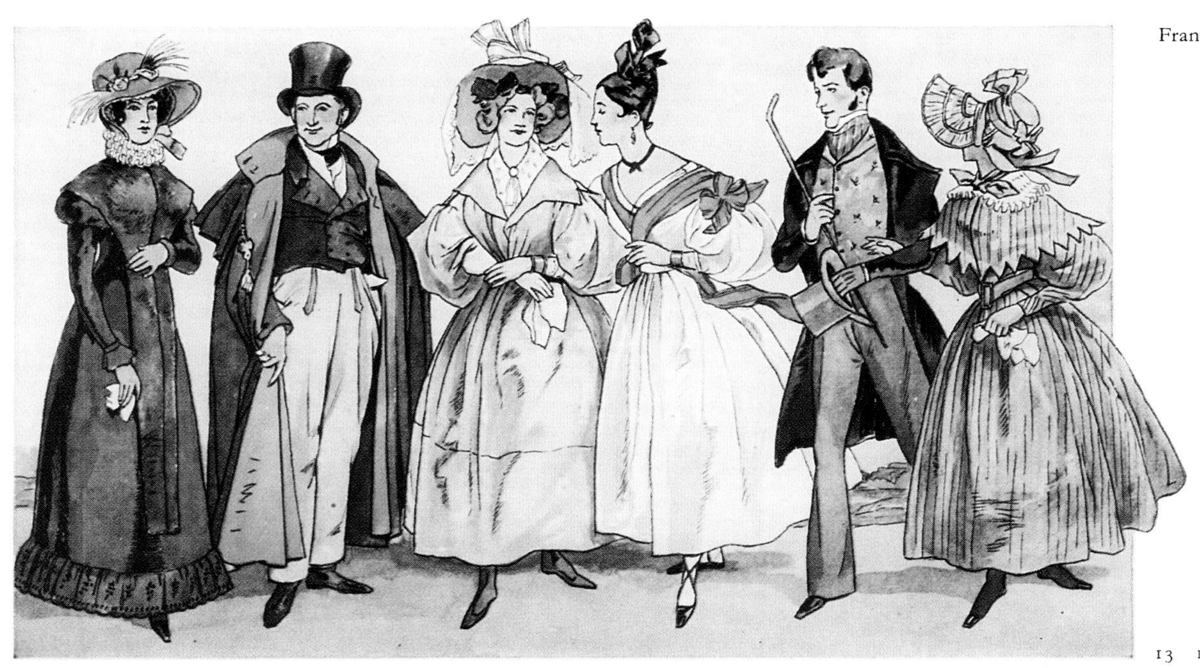

France about 1825–1830

13 14 15 16 17 18

GERMANY
1815–1835
"Biedermeier" Fashion

Fashion 1815–1819

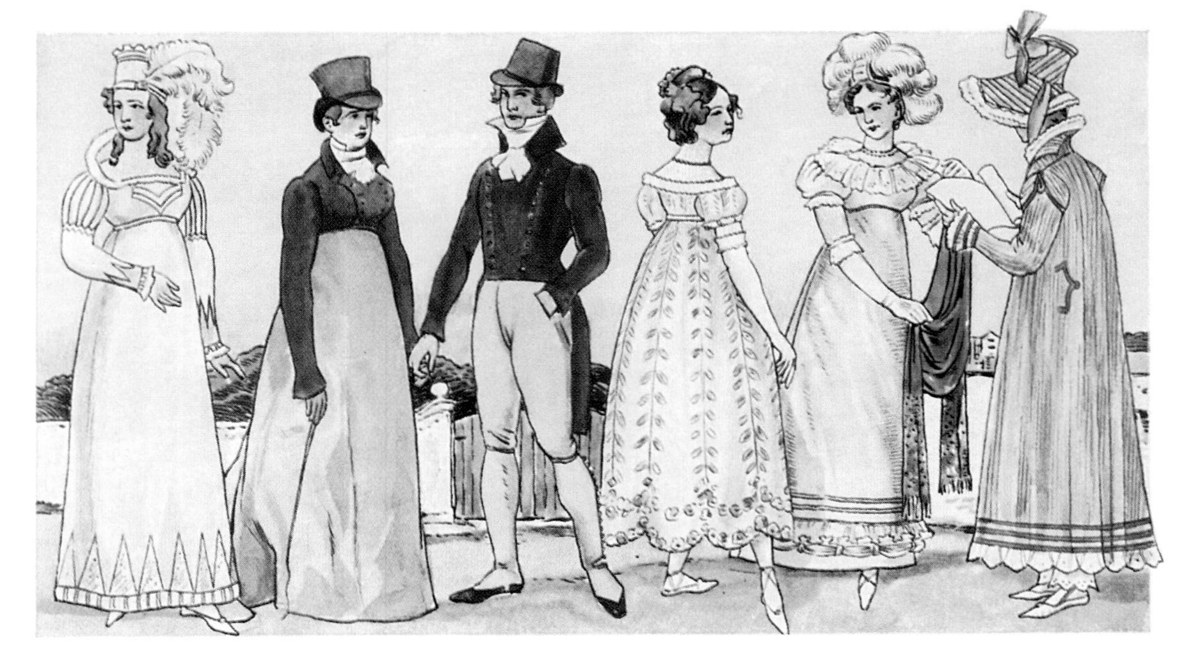

1 2 3 4 5 6

Fashion 1820-1832

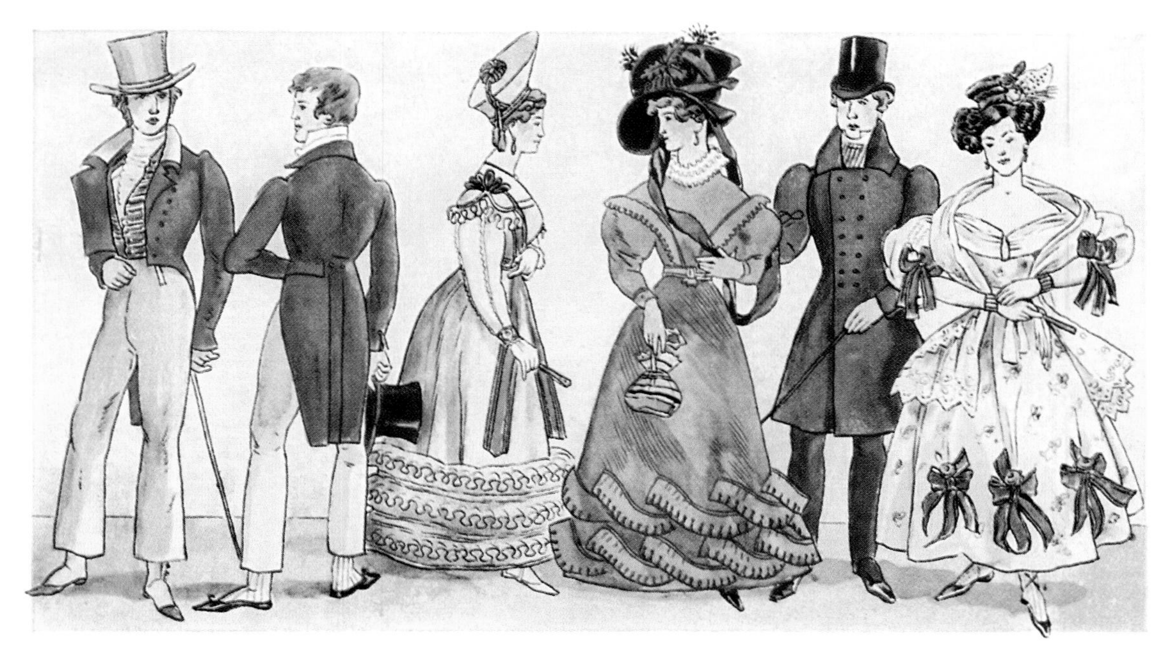

7 8 9 10 11 12

Fashion 1834–1835

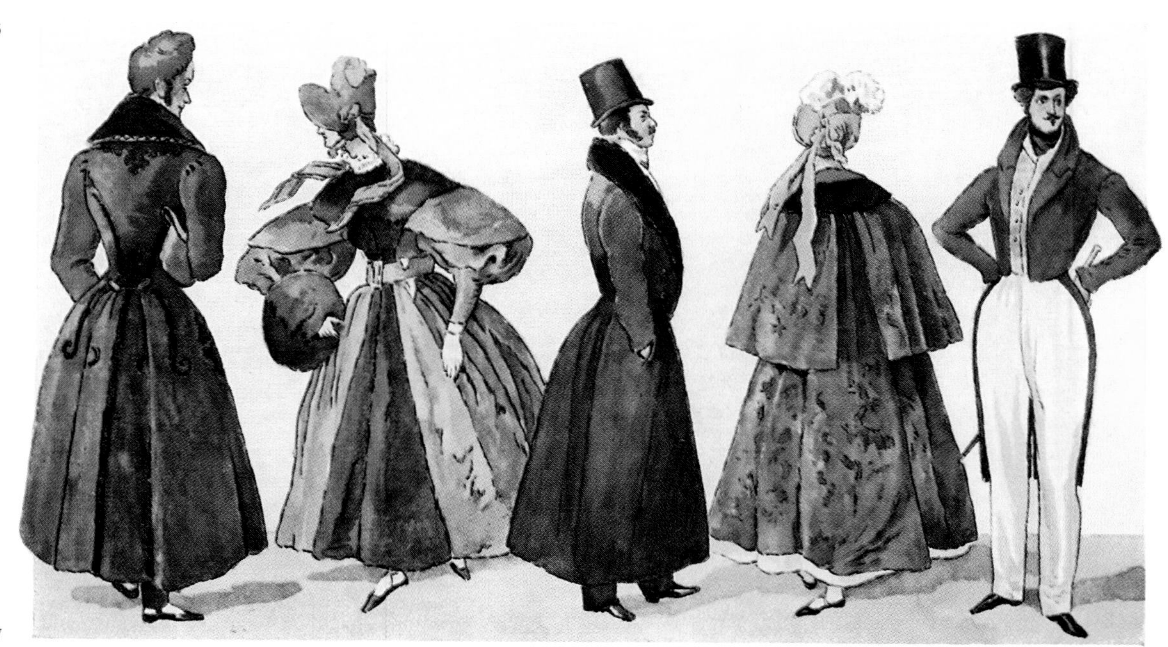

13 14 15 16 17

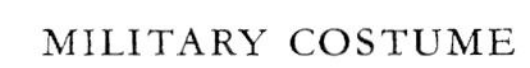

EUROPE,
Uniforms
1795–1813

Prussia 1806–1813

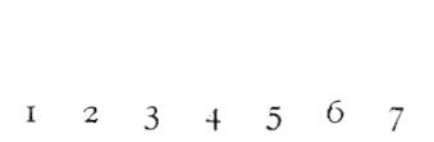

Russia and others
1800–1815

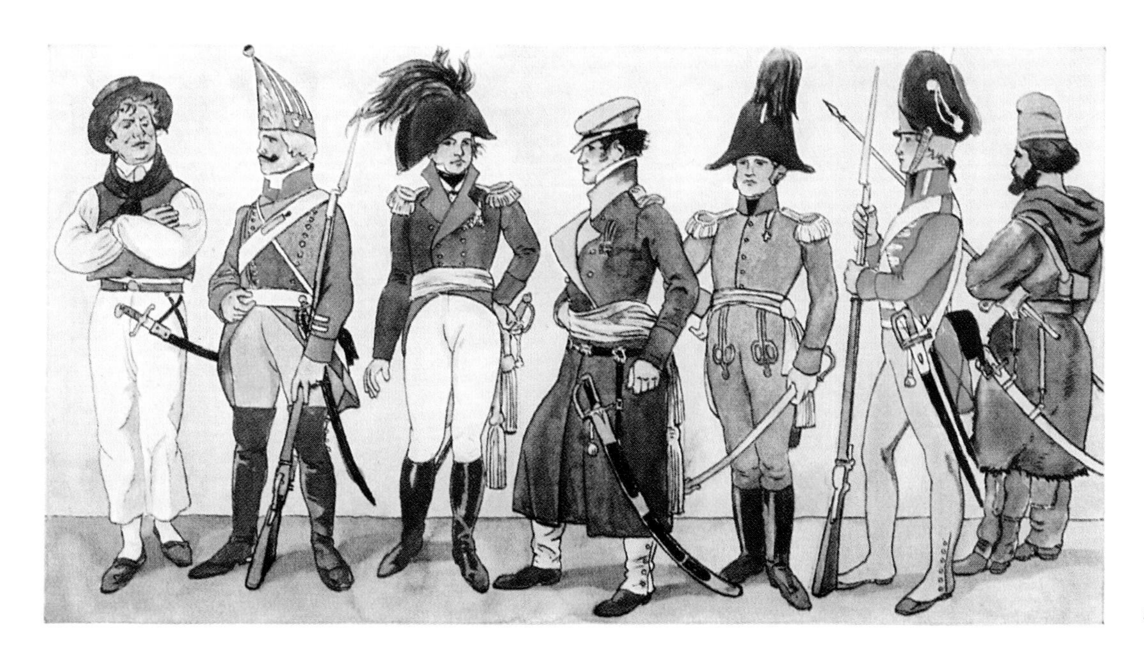

8 9 10 11 12 13 14

France
1795–1813

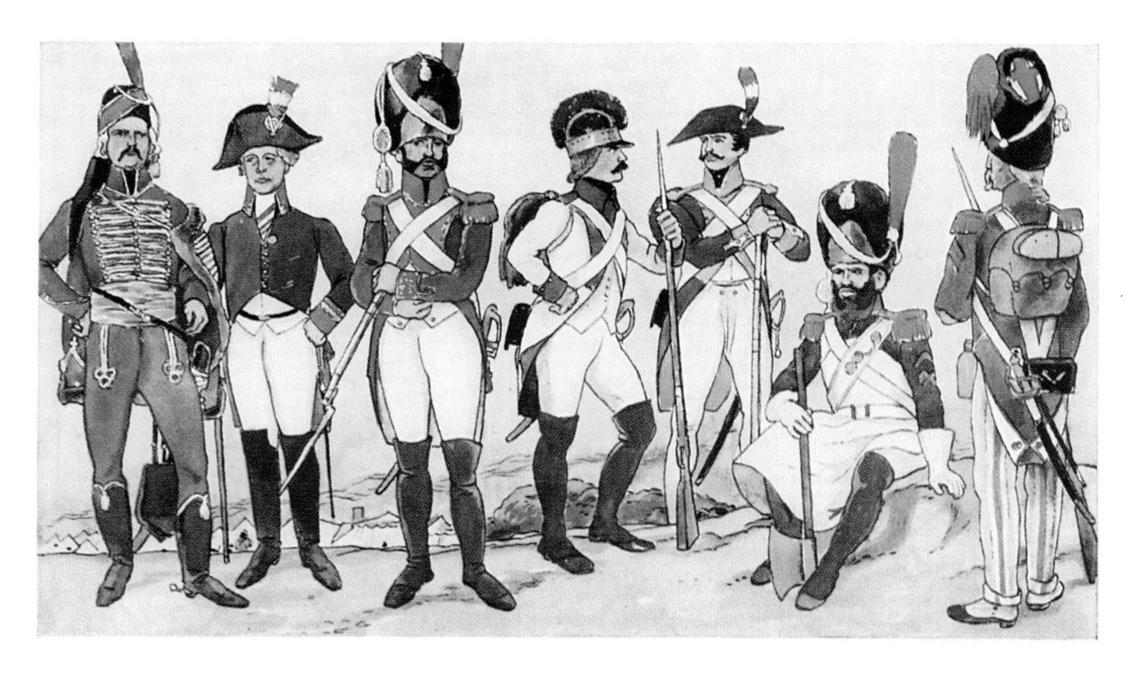

15 16 17 18 19 20 21

GERMANY
Uniforms
during the Reign of
Frederick the Great
1740–1786

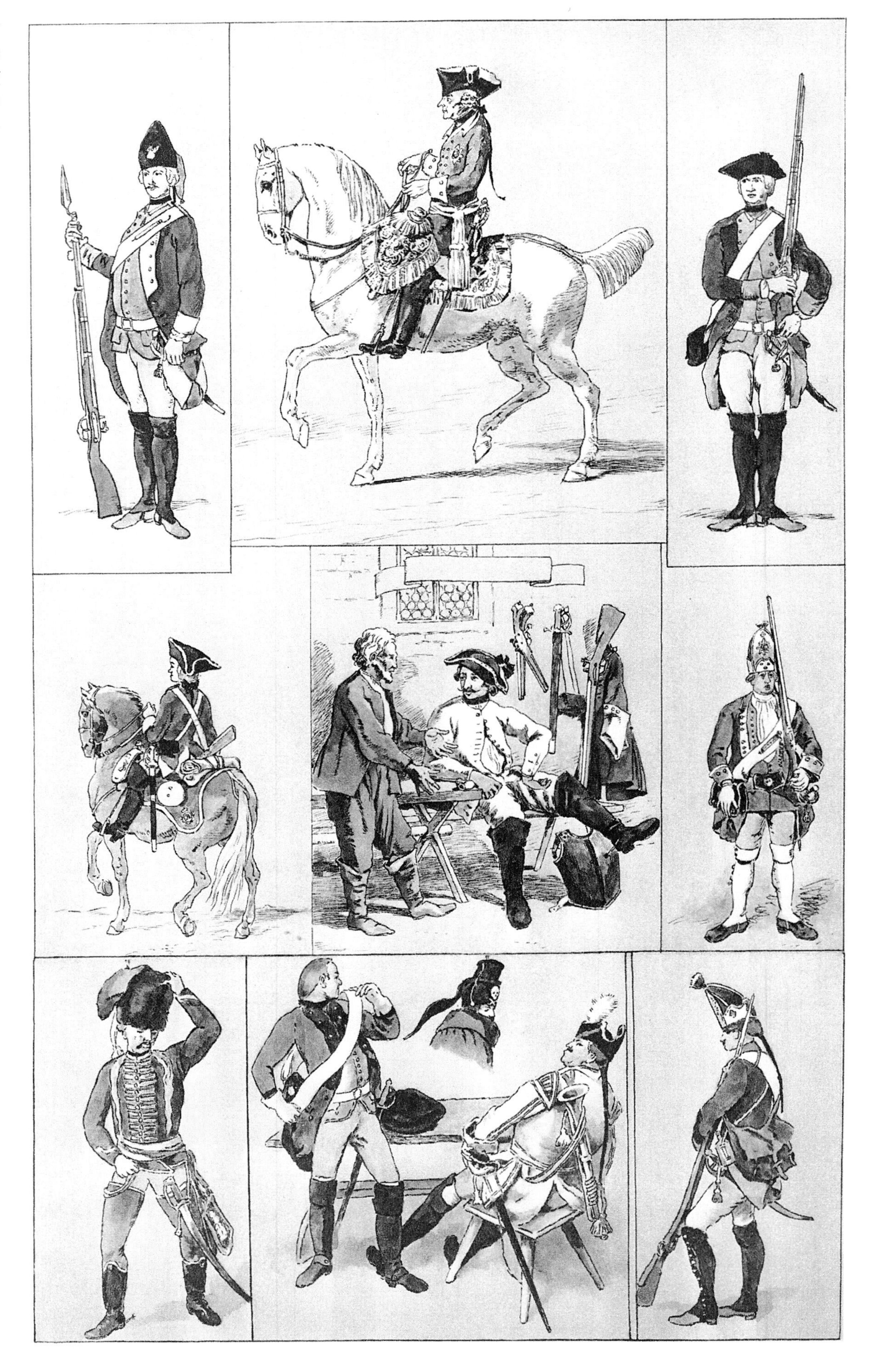

GERMANY

1786–1788

Fashion Almanacs

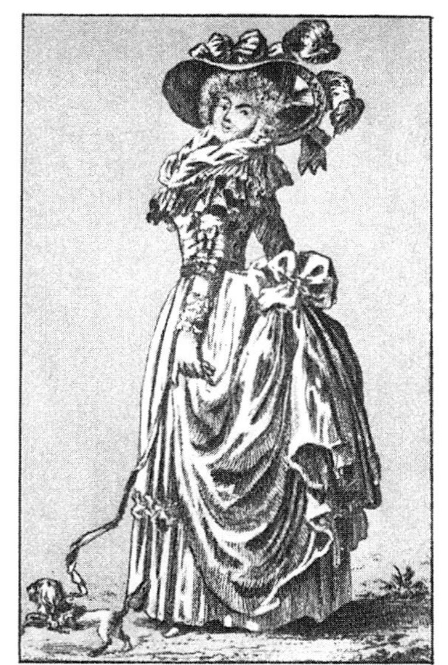

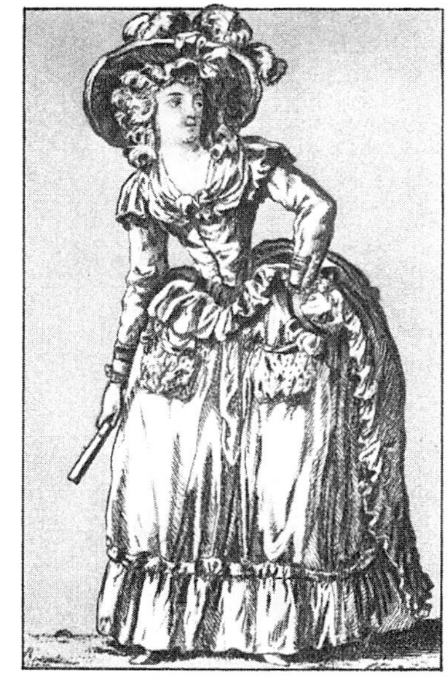

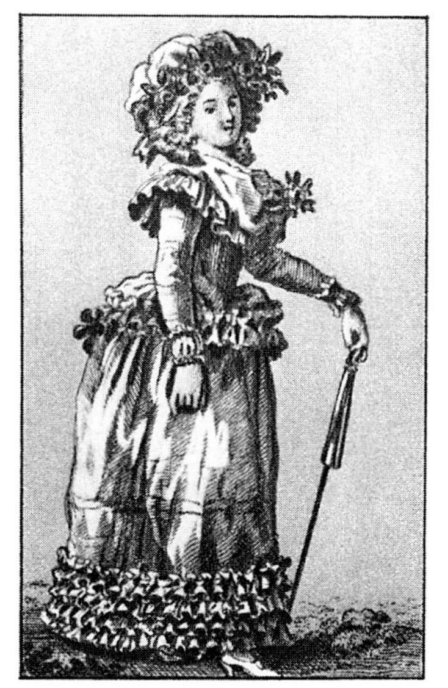

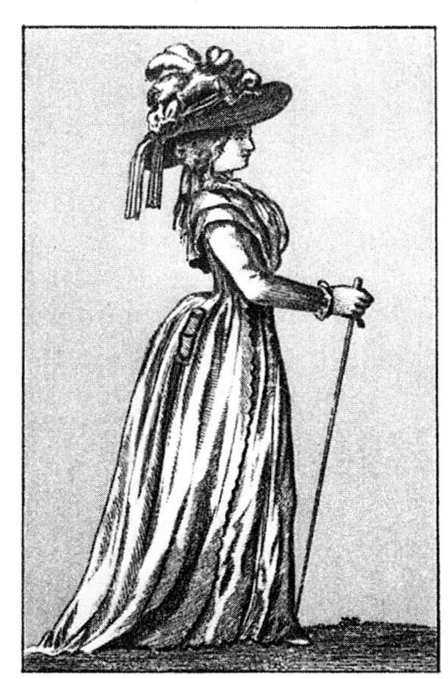

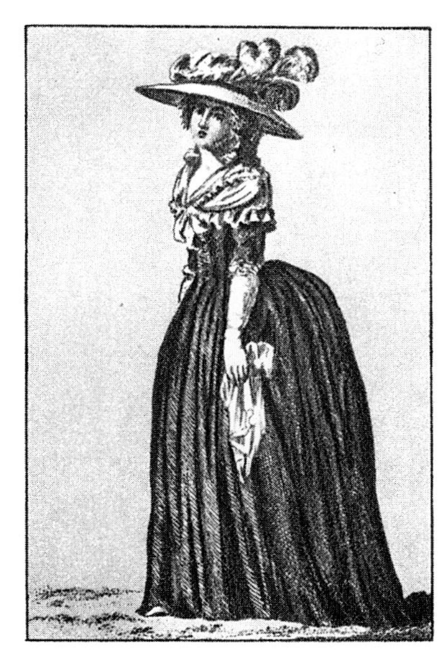

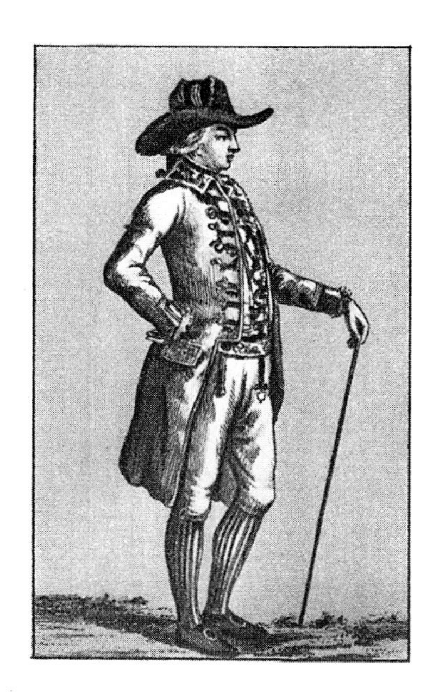

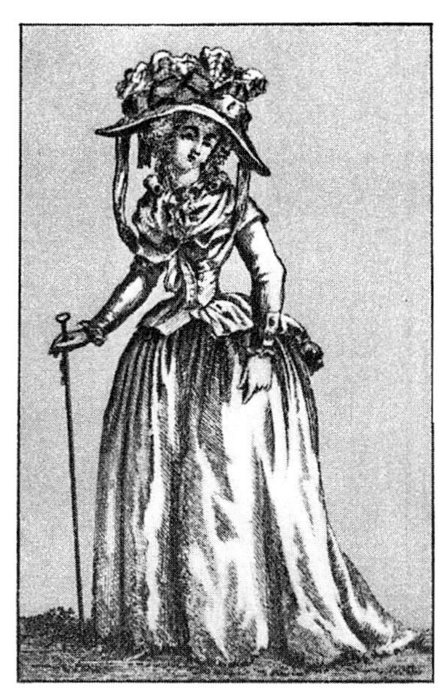

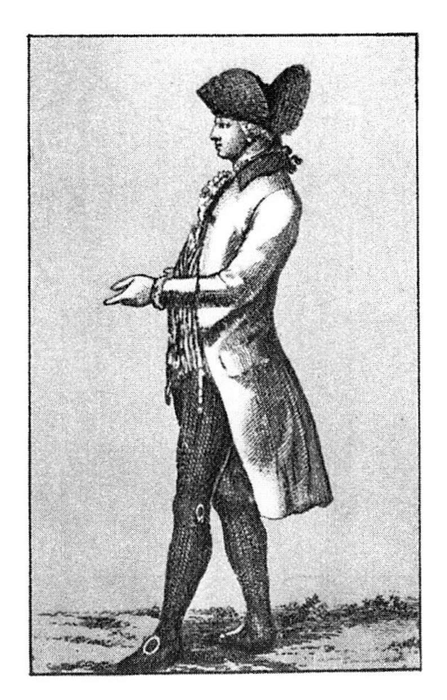

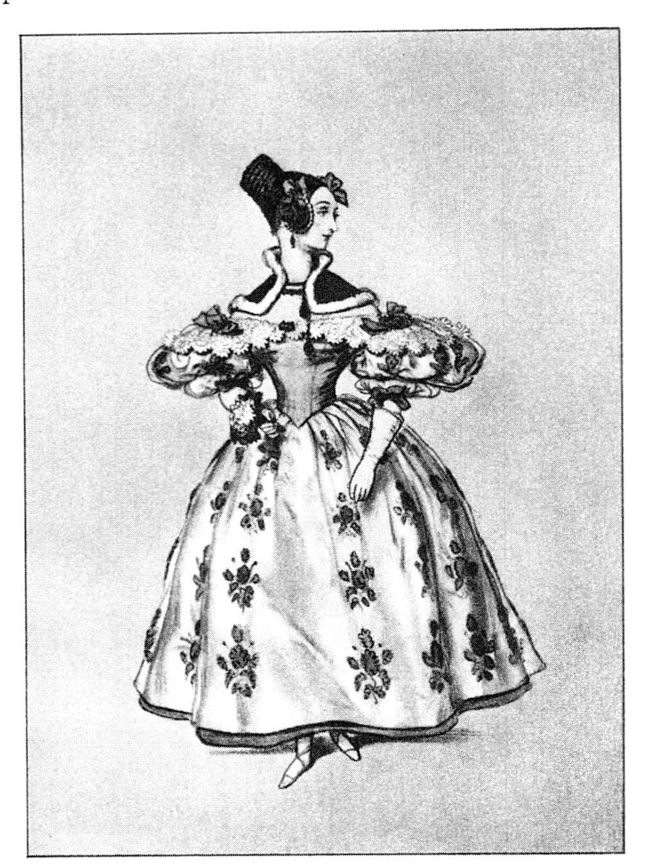

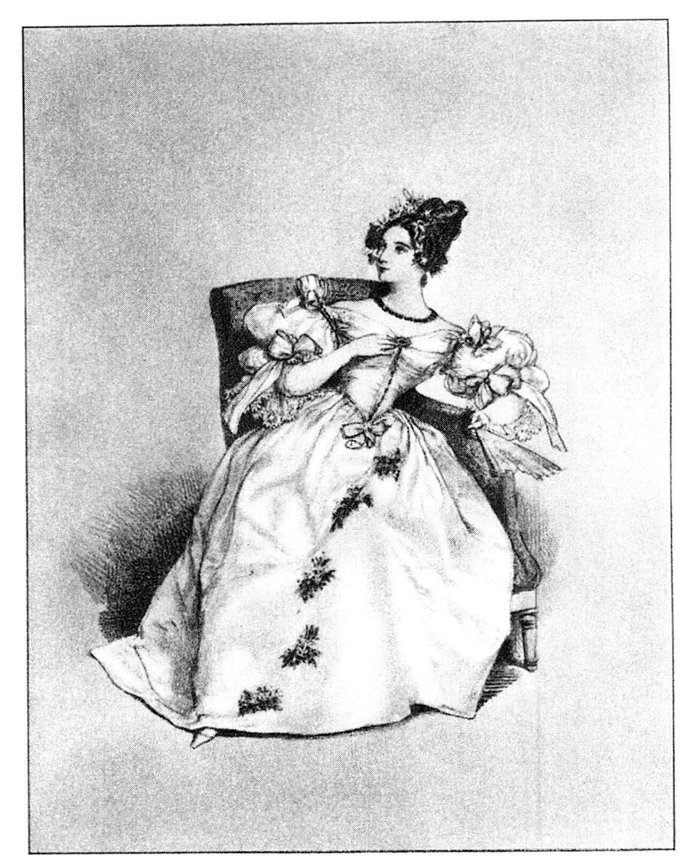

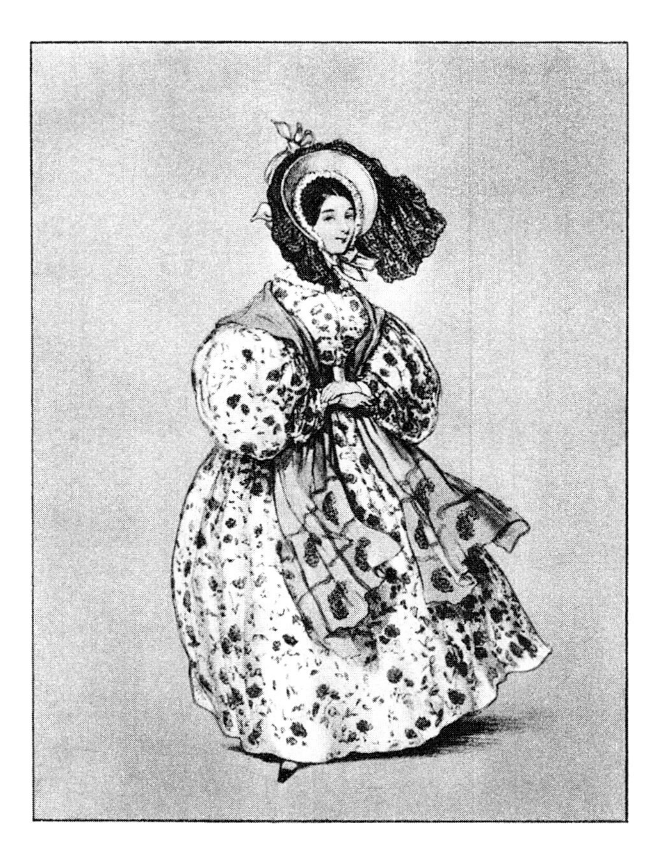

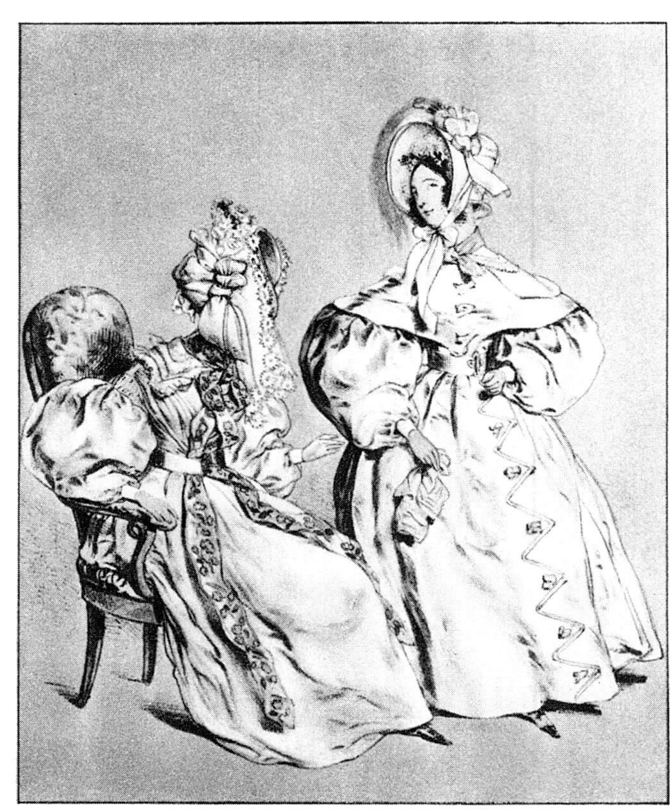

Paris Fashions 1830–1835

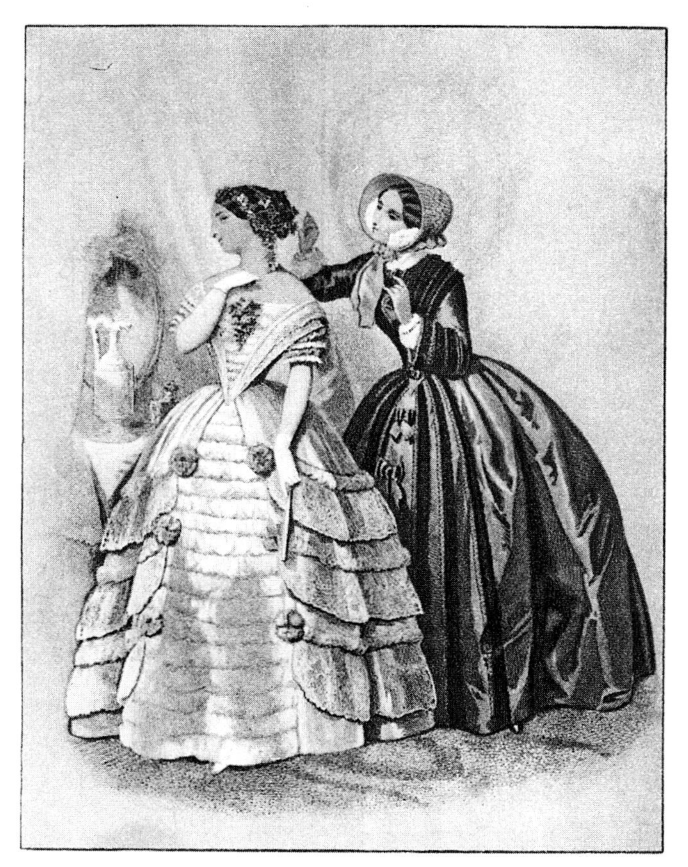

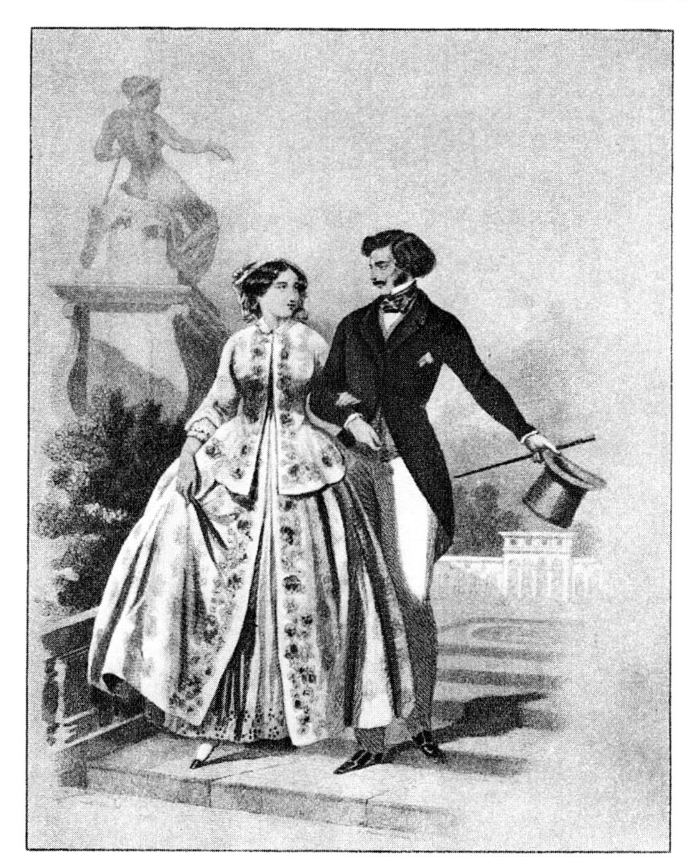

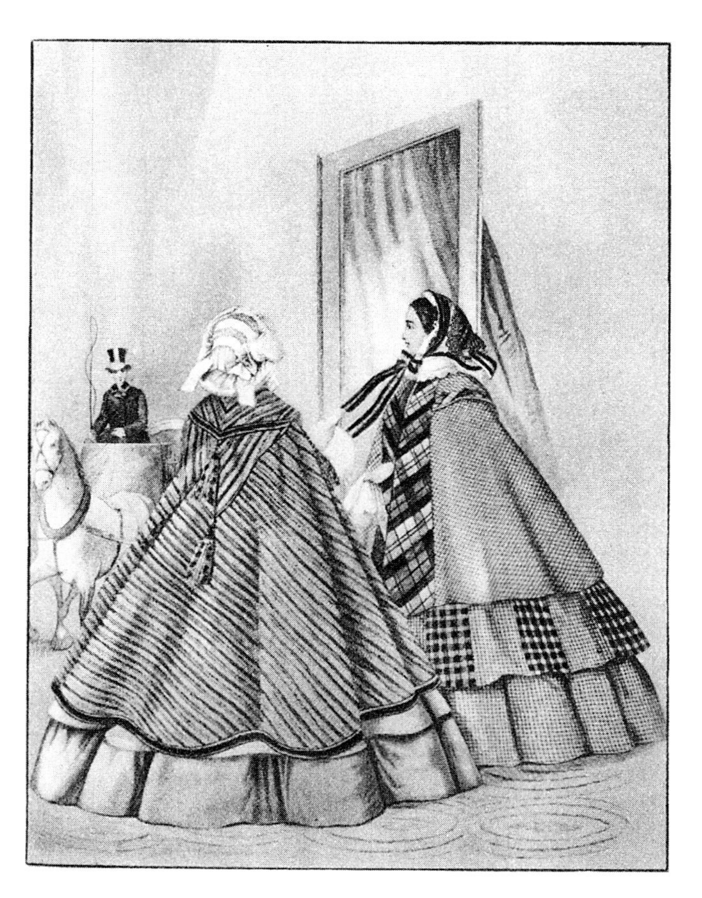

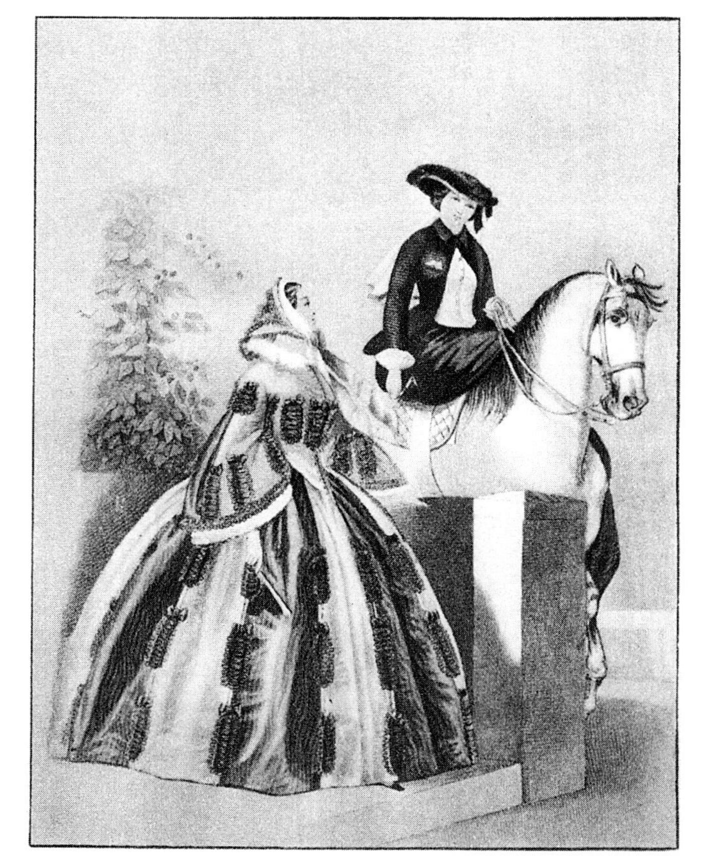

Paris and Berlin Fashions (Crinoline) 1850–1860

FRANCE AND GERMANY
(Cul de Paris)
1870–1875

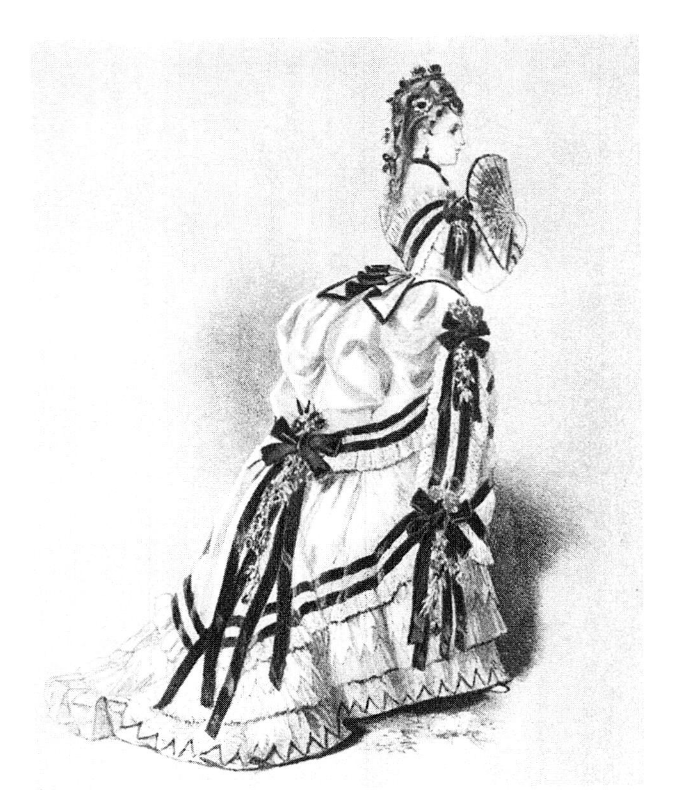

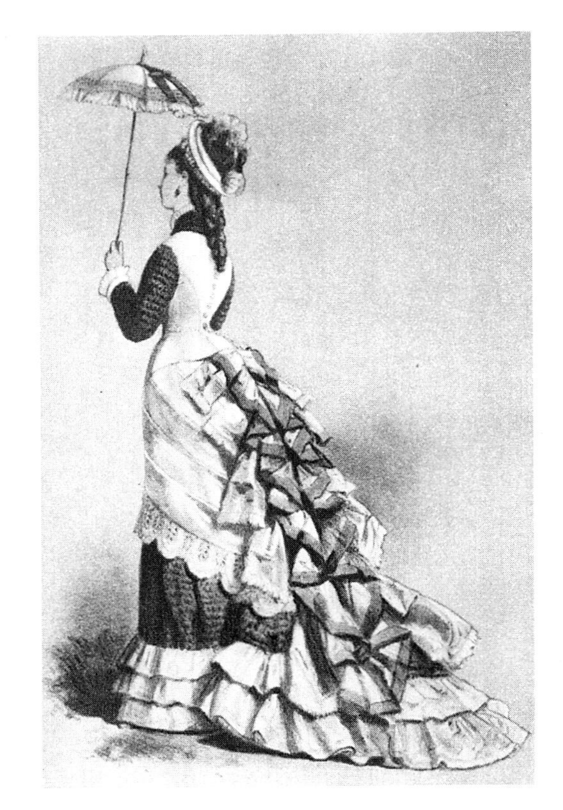

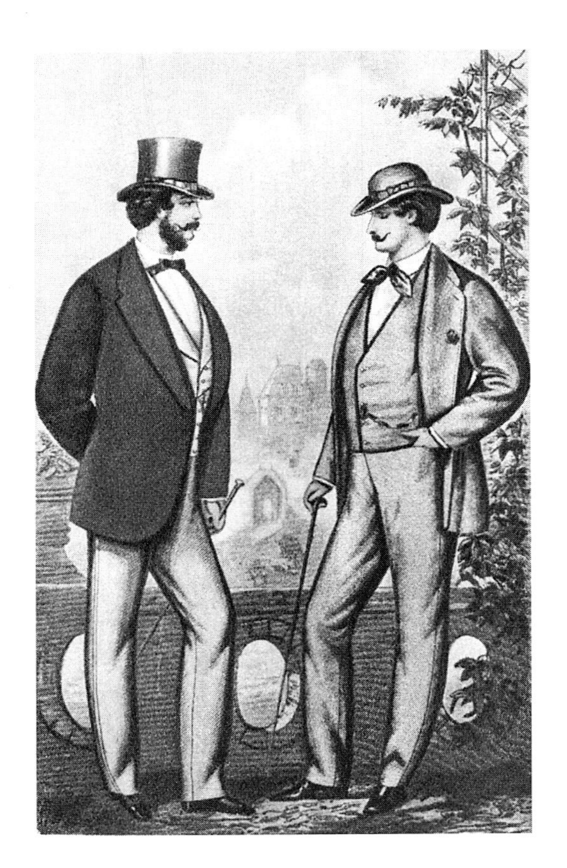

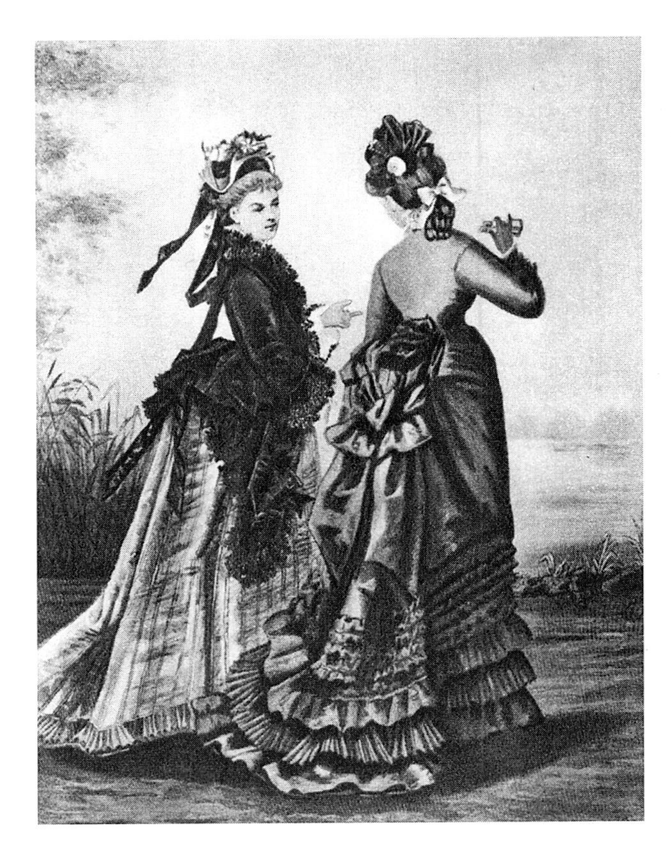